Clinical Addiction Psychiatry

Clinical Addiction Psychiatry

Edited by

David Brizer and Ricardo Castaneda

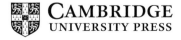
CAMBRIDGE
UNIVERSITY PRESS

CAMBRIDGE UNIVERSITY PRESS
Cambridge, New York, Melbourne, Madrid, Cape Town, Singapore, São
Paulo, Delhi, Dubai, Tokyo, Mexico City

Cambridge University Press
The Edinburgh Building, Cambridge CB2 8RU, UK

Published in the United States of America by
Cambridge University Press, New York

www.cambridge.org
Information on this title: www.cambridge.org/9780521899581
© Cambridge University Press 2010

First published 2010

Printed in the United Kingdom
at the University Press, Cambridge

A catalog record for this publication is available from the British Library

Library of Congress Cataloging in Publication data

Clinical addiction psychiatry / edited by David Brizer and Ricardo
Castaneda.
    p. ; cm.
Includes bibliographical references and index.
ISBN 978-0-521-89958-1 (hardback)
1. Substance abuse. 2. Compulsive behavior. I. Brizer, David A., 1953-
II. Castaneda, Ricardo, 1955- III. Title.
[DNLM: 1. Substance-Related Disorders–therapy. 2. Behavior,
Addictive–physiopathology. 3. Behavior, Addictive–therapy. WM 270
C6401 2010]

RC564.C546 2010
616.86–dc22
2010020572

ISBN 978-0-521-89958-1 Hardback

Contents

Contributors   vii
Preface   ix

Part 1 – Theory

1   **Death, drugs, and rock & roll**   3
David Brizer

2   **The disease concept – controversies and integration**   12
Mark Schenker

3   **Medical sequelae of addiction**   24
Michael Weaver

4   **Suicide and substance abuse**   37
Samoon Ahmad

5   **Abstinence as a goal**   45
Laurence M. Westreich

6   **Ibogaine therapy for substance abuse disorders**   50
Deborah C. Mash

7   **Therapeutic communities in the new millennium**   61
George De Leon

8   **Cosmetic psychopharmacology: drugs that enhance wellbeing, performance, and creativity**   72
Richard N. Rosenthal & Laurence M. Westreich

9   **Psychotherapeutic paradigms and the prescription pad: treating drug addiction with drugs**   88
Ed Paul

10   **Six key areas when working with addicts**   92
Kathleen Tracy

Part 2 – Real World

11   **The twelve-step approach**   97
Marc Galanter

12   **Alcoholism**   102
Jerome Levin

13   **Alcoholism in primary care**   125
Mack Lipkin, Andrea Truncali & Joshua D. Lee

14   **Nicotine addiction and smoking cessation**   133
Neil Hartman

15   **Clinical aspects of cocaine and methamphetamine dependence**   137
Arnold Washton

16   **Methadone treatment**   147
Robert Maslansky

17   **Psychoactive prescription drug abuse**   154
Bernard Salzman & Peter Micheels

Part 3 – Praxis

18   **Pain management and addiction treatment**   163
Robert Maslansky

19   **EEG neurofeedback therapy**   169
Siegfried Othmer & Mark Steinberg

20   **The new pharmacotherapies for alcohol dependence**   188
Barbara J. Mason & Marni Jacobs

21   **Dialectical behavior therapy adapted to the treatment of concurrent borderline personality disorder and substance use disorders**   207
Lisa Burckell & Shelley McMain

22   **Addiction and emergency psychiatry**   218
Richard Gallagher, Gregory Fernandez & Edward Lulo

23   **Ear acupuncture in addiction treatment**   230
Michael Smith

Index   251

Contributors

Samoon Ahmad, MD
Bellevue-NYU Medical Center, New York, NY, USA

David Brizer, MD
Mind-Meds.com, Nyack, NY, USA

Lisa Burkell
University of Toronto, Toronto, Ontario, Canada

Ricardo Castaneda, MD
New York University School of Medicine, New York, NY, USA

George De Leon, MD
National Development and Research Institutes, New York, NY, USA

Gregory Fernandez
Westchester Medical Center, Valhalla, NY, USA

Marc Galanter, MD
Professor of Psychiatry, New York University School of Medicine, New York, NY, USA; Research Scientist, Nathan Kline Institute for Psychiatric Research

Richard Gallagher, MD
Department of Psychiatry, Westchester Medical Center, Valhalla, NY, USA

Neil Hartman, MD
VA Medical Center, Los Angeles, CA, USA

Marni Jacobs, MPH
Scripps Institute, La Jolla, CA, USA

Joshua D. Lee, MD Msc
New York University School of Medicine, New York, NY, USA

Jerome Levin, PhD
The New School, New York, NY, USA

Mack Lipkin
New York University School of Medicine, New York, NY, USA

Edward Lulo, MD
Psychiatrist, Danbury, CT, USA

Shelley McMain, PhD
Centre for Addiction and Mental Health, Department of Psychiatry, University of Toronto, Toronto, Ontario, Canada

Deborah C. Mash, PhD
University of Miami Medical Center, Miami, FL, USA

Robert Maslansky, MD
Bellevue-NYU Medical Center, New York, NY, USA

Barbara J. Mason, PhD
Scripps Institute, La Jolla, CA, USA

Peter Micheels, MD
Bellevue-NYU Medical Center, New York, NY, USA

Siegfried Othmer, PhD
Mark Steinberg, PhD and Associates, Los Gatos, CA, USA

Ed Paul, MD
New York, NY, USA

Richard N. Rosenthal, MD
Bellevue-NYU Medical Center, New York, NY, USA

Bernard Salzman, MD
Bellevue-NYU Medical Center, New York, NY, USA

Mark Schenker, PhD
Caron Treatment Centers, New York, NY, USA

Michael Smith, MD
Lincoln Hospital Medical Center, Bronx, NY, USA

Mark Steinberg, PhD
Mark Steinberg, PhD and Associates, Los Gatos, CA, USA

Kathleen Tracy, MD
Bellevue-NYU Medical Center, New York, NY, USA

Andrea Truncali, MD MPH
New York University School of Medicine, New York, NY, USA

Arnold Washton, PhD
Recovery Options, New York, NY, USA

Michael Weaver, MD
Virginia Commonwealth University, Richmond, VA, USA

Lawrence M. Westreich, MD
Bellevue-NYU Medical Center, New York, NY, USA

Preface

We do not yet know whether our century will yield encyclopedists comparable in scope and stature to the historic champions of the genre such as Larousse and Diderot.

Clinical Addiction Psychiatry is not an encyclopedia. Thirty or forty years ago such a project would have been feasible: now, however, thanks to the convergent vectors of molecular biology, psychopharmacology, sound clinical research, and the demand for outcome measures, the addiction field has literally exploded.

The book's table of contents overflows like a Vesuvius, each chapter covering one or more of the dozens of provocative, fascinating, and essential subdomains of the field.

Granted, editorial decisions (such as what to include, what to exclude, what to emphasize, whom to subpoena to Grammarians' Court) can be arbitrary, whimsical, even random at times. We have attempted to avoid these kind of lapses by addressing three major topics in addiction.

Part 1, Theory, takes us to the 21st century – and beyond. It is fairly safe to assume that most, if not all, clinicians in the field have discussed the 'causes' of addiction with concerned patients and families. The 'addictive personality' discussion comes up perennially and reliably, appearing on talk show television, the cover of *Newsweek*, and in the minds of successive generations of students and teachers. The section emits both fire and ice.

For example, the first chapter – standing on the shoulders of giants long gone – temperately explores the "co-variance" of drug use, passion, and art. The succeeding chapter on the disease concept brings a (still) fairly new perspective into intelligent and contemporary focus. Like most diseases, the disease of chemical dependence often features numerous and at times deadly consequences. Readers – including those with an MD! – will find the chapter on medical sequelae of addiction to be fresh, informative, and very much up to date.

Some of the theoretical constructs described in Part 1 are very recent. Is drug addiction a crime, a disease, or both? (Or is it none of the above?) The chapter on dual diagnosis emphasizes current research and clinical approaches and perhaps just coincidentally proves that mentally ill chemical abusers cannot and should not be viewed from a dualistic point of view!

No doubt the book does leave some stones unturned, but ritual ibogaine use (and ibogaine's potential utility for addiction treatment) and 'cosmetic' psychopharmacology are not among them. Most clinicians would agree: DSM axis I disorders are just the tip of the epidemiological iceberg. For each patient with major depression, there are probably ten others with "subclinical" mood and/or anxiety disorders who never surface. As our field evolves, the overlap between "treating" illness and pharmacologically enhancing wellbeing and creativity will increase. The arrival of buprenorphine on the scene demands a new look at more traditional approaches to opiate/opioid addiction (such as therapeutic communities). Dr. Galanter's contribution is a most welcome gift.

Dr. Levin's chapter on alcoholism (which kicks off Part 2, Real World) is encyclopedic. Whoever said that understanding alcoholism was pretty much equivalent to understanding all of medicine happened to be right. But the story doesn't end there. Understanding alcoholism also requires righteous attention to psychology, genetics, family interactions, neurophysiology – and more.

The chapters on cocaine, nicotine, and methadone are sumptuous and are a pleasure to read. The respective contributors have brought together history, street culture, and medical science in their masterful discussions of these drugs.

The book's third and final section is about Praxis. Praxis makes perfect! Dr. Maslansky's chapter on the protean dimensions of pain (and painkillers) and methadone is a gift from a true expert in the field. Dr. Mason's chapter on the new anticraving drugs provides further proof that psychopharmacology can subdue demons (such as smoking) long written off as unshakeable.

Dr. Michael Smith's chapter on the use of acupuncture in treating addictions represents the robust and extremely promising outcome data of more than two decades of clinical experience.

Clinical Addiction Psychiatry is not a fashion victim. The book is not an anthem to pharmacology. Mind matters! Dr. McMain's chapter on dialectical behavior therapy (DBT) tells the tale of a new but very powerful kid on the block. Those who are unfamiliar with DBT will find the complex blend of spirituality and cognitive behavioral therapy absolutely fascinating. Dr. Gallagher brings extensive experience to his excellent chapter on emergency scenarios in addiction.

We hope that this collection of essays by *the* experts in the field inspires readers to always question more, know more, and do more (or less!)

David Brizer, MD and Ricardo Castaneda, MD
April, 2010

Part 1 Theory

Death, drugs, and rock & roll

David Brizer

Whether we like it or not, death is *the* universal concern.

The most cogent writing on the subject, aside from theological and spiritual tracts, is found in Ernst Becker's (1972) *The Denial of Death*. Becker, a philosopher gifted with a brilliant writing style, devotes each chapter in his book to a different human remedy for "the sickness unto death" (Kierkegaard, 2009) – mortality. Becker's conclusion, echoing that of his luetic predecessor, Friedrich Nietzsche, is quite simply, "Human, all too human." Devotion to work, family, love, sex, addiction…in the final analysis, each falls short of allaying the pandemic fear. The final chapter of the Becker book takes a surprising leap straight toward heaven: the only way out of this literal "suffering unto death" is to embrace a spiritual belief.

Becker's perspective is of course based on fear. His perspective is dualistic, since he subscribes to the universal belief that death is the opposite number of life – that death is something bad, something we constantly strive to contain, minimize, or deny.

The terror, the abject fascination inspired by death, finds expression in countless works of art, music, and science. From epoch to epoch, from one civilization to the next, death is the chief catalyst of some of mankind's greatest cultural achievements. Consider, for example, the Faust motif, which sprouts like poison mushrooms after rain, taking innumerable forms in art, music, and in literature. The idea of trading one's immortal soul for infinite wisdom and riches and power, right here and now, is inextricably bound with the fear of death.

Of course, if one actually *has* an immortal soul, then there is little to fear. Such a belief was no consolation to Mann's (1948) *Doktor Faustus*.

Becker's ominous maunderings aside, most of us somehow manage to sidestep the issue – by means of work, relationships, and creativity—until it is staring us straight in the face. The performance and appreciation of great music is for many the apex of their spiritual pyramid. The creative apogee, whether realized in music, writing, or any other form of artistic expression, is a secular variant of spiritual arrival.

How many have devoted – *sacrificed* – their lives in the pursuit of art? The lives of the composers, the painters, the actors and actresses, often read like Grand Guignol, like a soap opera dripping with blood, sweat, and tears. Alternately, their biographies read very much like *The Lives of the Saints* (Butler, 1788). The artist is a shaman, a kind of freak who suffers for the rest of us to keep our connection with "eternity" alive. The artist, struggling with his craft, shut away in his garret to wrestle with demons, is "Byronic." "You can't fool with Mother Nature." And, "You've got to suffer to play the blues." Anyone daring to loiter in Parnassus always pays, pays in unimaginable ways.

Beethoven's life – his interior life, in particular – is often considered a prime example of bartering "agony for art." Thomas Mann's novel, *Doktor Faustus*, depicts in shattering detail the legendary barter that this fictive Beethoven could have made. Mann's protagonist, Adrien Leverkuhn, is a nineteenth-century version of Ludwig B., in Mann's *roman à clef*. Leverkuhn, already an enormously accomplished pianist and composer, strives to reach his "personal best." His striving is so powerful – so persistent, so cosmically *loud* – that it is heard on the other (darker) side. A minion of Lucifer arranges the swap, and Leverkuhn gets his wish: he becomes the greatest composer in the world. The price? The composer must suffer the death by childbed fever of the only person he has ever loved, his adored and beautiful grandson. Would Leverkuhn have signed on had he known the real terms of the pact?

Would you?

No doubt there are many who would grab the opportunity. The "peak" experience, the incomparable sensation of being "in the pocket" (described as "oceanic bliss" or as "flow"), is without question supremely appealing and supremely addicting. Some clinicians actually advise their patients to accept life on a more even keel – to avoid moments of ecstasy or intense wellbeing intentionally, since the down side potential (craving for more!) is quite significant. This advice may sound puritanical, or repressive; on the other hand, the proffered wisdom is similar to some of the basic tenets of Buddhism, and, for that matter, of Alcoholics Anonymous.

Most of the suffering in life, it is held, is due to *attachment* and *desire.* "Desire" contains the potential (or promise!) for both fulfillment and often for devastating disappointment. If you can't take the heat – namely, the troughs that invariably follow peaks – well, then, stay out of the sun.

The dividing line between clinical issues and spiritual ones is ambiguous here. Bipolar disorder is more common among creative artists (Redfield Jamison, 1993), but the temptation to ascribe all artistic, mystical, and other intense states of mind to manic-depressive illness is a vast oversimplification that should be avoided. Oceanic bliss, whether experienced by musician, yoga master, or lover, should not be confused with psychiatric illness. William James' masterwork *The Varieties of Religious Experience* (originally 1902; then Dover Publications, 2002), is basically a 400-page travel guide to these perilous regions of oceanic bliss.

With all due respect (to Ernst Becker), who is to say which devotions are spiritual in nature, and which are "merely" secular? To confound the issue even further, death itself often takes on the allurement of erotic love.

The depiction of death – as final surrender to the vastness of the cosmos – is often highly erotic. The period of romanticism, especially in the culture of pre-Victorian Europe, is supercharged with depictions in art and literature of the allure of death. The works of Aubrey Beardsley, Charles Baudelaire, Lord Byron, Algernon Swinburne, Edgar Allan Poe, Joris-Karl Huysmans, to list but a few, are synonymous with the fetish of, and fascination with, death.

The artist's spiritual twin is the vampire. Once you have "touched the flame," there really is no turning back. The appetite for oceanic bliss only grows with time. Like Faust, like the vampire, the artist has sold his soul for an eternal life that seems abhorrent, inhuman, and freezing cold to the touch. Perhaps art conquers death by living on in the minds and hearts of those who follow.

Why has orgasm been described as "la petite morte" ("the little death")? The surrender of the forebrain (=ego), the letting go of the survival/vigilance/hunting and gathering functions, is common to artistic achievement – and is also a necessary ingredient of great sex, intense physical activity, and deep meditation.

Unlike our puritan clinician promoting bland living, good morals, right living, and squeaky clean fingernails, some consider the pursuit of oceanic bliss a core human drive. The fusion of protons releases thermonuclear energy. The single-minded pursuit of oceanic bliss, to the exclusion of all else, can also be monstrously destructive (when it takes, for example, the form of addiction, incessant exercise, or incessant *anything*).

Fusion? Hydrogen bombs? What do they have to do with rock music and catastrophe and death?

Rock & Roll

Rolling Stone magazine, reporting on the contemporary musical scene for more than four decades, has from time to time published roll calls of the "greatest" guitar players, blues players, and rock musicians of the century. A moment's glance at any of these makes it plain that this craft is, to put it mildly, *dangerous.* The life trajectories of the greats (such as Jimi Hendrix, Brian Jones, Duane Allman, Jim Morrison, Lowell George, and others) are absolutely rife with disaster. Most of the top blues players of the twentieth century (60% or more) died young and died tragically, victims of violence, fatal accidents, and of alcohol/drug overdose.

The conditions of death, dismemberment, disaster, and all out alcohol and drug dependence are present among these players more often than not. Many of the players' biographies read like eulogies, like body counts in an invisible and endless war.

For the sake of brevity – but also for shock value – I will describe the amazing parallels of mischance in the lives of four widely known musicians (three of whom are very much alive!). Each spent his formative years, creatively speaking, in electric blues bands. Each has been considered "the greatest" blues guitar player of his time. One – Eric Clapton (vide infra) – provoked hysterical fans to spray paint walls with the pronouncement, "Clapton is God." Each is British, each began their meteoric careers in John Mayall's Bluesbreakers, and to a man each went on to even greater celebrity with groups like Fleetwood Mac and the Rolling Stones.

Two of the three became (for a time) drug devotees; the other fell prey to psychosis. Even more extraordinary, each had the staying power and resilience of spirit to overcome his demons and to return to the world stage, where each always belonged.

Robert Johnson

No discussion of deals with the devil would be complete without mention of the original blues genius, Robert Johnson.

Johnson was a laborer in the cotton fields of the Mississippi delta during the second and third decades of the twentieth century. He was also (and certainly not by choice) a myth-maker. The tradition of "you've got to pay your dues to play the blues" began with Johnson.

Do you have to suffer to play the blues? What's up with that, anyway? It's a tragic tradition that goes way back. Johnson's lyrics are comic, tragic, and utterly transparent. Johnson was a womanizer, too.

Many people really believe that to make it big, you must sell your soul to the devil. The legend goes like this: Johnson met up with Satan at a country crossroads at midnight and made a deal. In exchange for his immortal soul, Johnson would (for a very short time, as it turned out) be the greatest blues player in the world. Listening to the scratchy primitive recordings that survived, the legend seems less far-fetched. Johnson worked the guitar strings like three virtuosi playing at once. Many Johnson tunes became hits (and then standards) for world famous rock bands like Cream and the Rolling Stones.

The man had hell to pay. When he wasn't working, he was playing, and much of the time he was living hard and fast and dangerous. Johnson was a handsome man, a drinking man, and his appetite for women didn't discriminate between those already spoken for and those who were not. Within 2 years of achieving local fame, Johnson was fatally poisoned by a very angry, very jealous husband.

The idea that extraordinary artistic talent and success come at a high price is not new. The medieval playwright Christopher Marlowe's character *Dr. Faustus* was the prototype of the artist in search of perfection – no matter the price. In more recent times, music (especially blues music) lovers still lower their voices whenever the name Robert Johnson comes up.

The songs were deadly serious – these are songs about love, loneliness, sadness, and pain – but that didn't stop Johnson from poking fun at himself and this doom-ridden world. Christopher Marlowe,

Thomas Mann, Robert Johnson: three men who at least on paper were galaxies apart.

Still, it is easy to imagine the three nefariously communing around song.

The curse didn't stop there. Art and doom have remained coevals right up to this day. The death or dissipation of *many* (former) key associates of the Stones is not the stuff of legend – it is a fact. Brian Jones (the first of several guitar players to "pass through" the band) died violently, mysteriously. Thirteen years ago, Eric Clapton's toddler tumbled out of an open window of a Manhattan high rise to his death. And the list goes on: Janis Joplin, Mike Bloomfield, Gram Parsons, Stevie Ray Vaughan, Kurt Cobain, Lowell George…

Eric Clapton

Most people old enough to remember have their own stories of joy, nostalgia, horror, and extremity about the late, great "sixties." The end of the seventh decade of the twentieth century was a kind of Rabelaisian tempest, or perhaps feast, an international transcultural carnival where everything exploded at once. Although no single event or personality was to blame, the rock and roll heroes of that time certainly took center stage. (Which was more compelling: the Stones' epochal album *Let It Bleed* [Rolling Stones, Decca Records, 1969] or the astronauts on the moon?)

EC was right up there. After deciding that his mentor – John Mayall – and Mayall's tyrannical adherence to the three-chord melodic structure of blues was too limiting (for him, that is), Clapton moved on. His next venue, a three-man band called The Cream, created an international stir and a taste for a very new kind of music. The tunes were recognizable, very basic: Cream's melodic structures were often even simpler than the blues. At the heart of these performances were the virtuoso's (very) extended solos. On stage, Clapton and cadre used the recorded material as launch pads for other-worldly, often brilliant, improvizations that dipped up, over, sideways, and down. At the heart of these performances were the extended solos, sometimes lasting an hour or more, that each player took. During these, the band – their hearts and spirits "in the pocket," their souls at peak flow – weaved complex tapestries of super-amplified freefall through fantasy realms of minor and major and most everything else in between scales. (During one interview, Clapton described these forays as musical highwire acts often fueled by LSD. Specifically, he noted that he felt "evil" when lapsing into a minor chord pattern or scale; he felt at peace when returning to the land of the major scale.) This kind of experience, for him and other musical champions of the era, was nothing out of the ordinary.

Spiritually, Clapton's experience in Cream was compelling. How does a human brain create cogent and complex and brilliant art, while traversing a landscape of melting forms and unbidden synaesthesiae? The explanation is not readily forthcoming. Historical parallels certainly exist: da Vinci noted in his journals that he often hallucinated complex figures and beings by continuous staring at highly grained pieces of wood. Perhaps unhinging the doors of perception is the preamble to a dance with "Mr. D.," Old Nick himself.

This is where the mysteries, allusions and scandal come full circle. Recall the terrain of the still unexplained miracle of Robert Johnson's delta blues: a dark and desolate crossroads, always at spiritual nadir in the middle of the night. This is where the deal-making, the signing of blood pacts, takes place. Johnson's tunes all gave witness to dark, grave proceedings.

Throughout his musical career, playing in different bands at different points in time, EC paid homage to these tunes. Many fans consider Clapton's rendition (on Cream, *Wheels of Fire,* Polydor Records, 1968) of Johnson's *Cross Road Blues* (Robert Johnson, Vocalion Records, 1937) to be one of the supreme examples of guitar virtuosity.

How long can a brilliant flame burn? During Clapton's decades'-long reign (an arbitrary designation, since he continues to play to adoring audiences around the globe), parties and drugs and many thousands of altered "states" danced in tandem with EC's guitar. He took most every drug around yet had a very long and productive run. Eventually, however, he seemed to tire of occupying that center panel of the Brueghel triptych and he literally slowed down. Musically, after 4 or 5 years with Cream, his taste and artistic requirements changed again. Cream disbanded, but Clapton played on, his records still selling by the millions. His work took on a distinctly more traditional sound. He was tired of the pandemonium and he wanted to play songs, wanted to play ballads, wanted to turn down the heat.

Rather than disinter and rehash biographical information that has been covered in great detail elsewhere, this monograph will explore and emphasize the musicological ("pyrotechnical") and consequent artistic and spiritual dimensions of this "holy trinity" (Eric Clapton, Peter Green, and Mick Taylor).

Eric Clapton was born and educated in England. Clapton did not meet his biological father until he was 30 years old. Like the other British musicians discussed here, EC was socioculturally poised for the life of a skilled laborer, or, failing that, for a working class life. Instead, in the years that followed, Clapton became one of the greatest if not *the* greatest electric blues player of all time.

It is tempting but perhaps specious to speculate how Clapton's life turned out the way it did. No doubt part of the explanation was Clapton's seething ambition to succeed at his art.

Clapton's earliest visible years, as he moved from one band to the next – usually as the showcased player – were already rife with hints of the success and virtuosity that lay ahead. The mysterious quantum leap from the Ripley teenager who went on to achieve world musical fame remains a puzzle. What is perfectly clear, however, is that this young man practised his music steadily, doggedly, honing his musical ear and tormenting his bleeding fingers mercilessly during many thousands of intensely driven hours of practice. While most of us recall our youth as a time of exploration, a phase of quick nervous forays from one new thing to the next, it seems that Clapton singlemindedly devoted his formative years to learning the blues. His study of music was extensive; he describes listening to endless collections of discs, recordings of Mississippi delta players, Chicago blues masters, folk guitarists, jazz players – absorbing the spirit and technique of any genre or player who touched his creative core.

The early 1960s, particularly in England , were an exciting time for emerging young musicians. First, the sentimental and often spiritually banal artists and songs of the previous decade were on their way out, replaced by a new generation of players and bands who believed in their hearts that their mission – to capture and convey the essence of a largely overlooked musical tradition (American blues) – was for all intents and purposes a *holy* one. Mayall, for example, titled the second Bluesbreakers album "Crusade" (John Mayall & the Bluesbreakers, *Crusade,* London Records, 1967).

Further, the instruments themselves had greatly changed. While acoustic guitar remained prominent in pop music, the newfangled thing – a guitar of solid wood, equipped with two or more microphones ("pickups") that amplified the strings – opened up new worlds of sound for players. These were sounds that had never been heard before. Thanks to the efforts of guitar makers like Leo Fender and Stanky Gibson, players like Clapton could turn a gently weeping note into a wall-shaking thunderclap at the turn of a dial or the slash of a guitar pick.

Early on, EC played "riffs" that were recognizably *his*. His playing, while touted for its seemingly inhuman speed and accuracy, was most notable for its gorgeous and passionate "feel." EC, as the saying goes, "had the touch." He often put his personal stamp on a solo by somehow intuiting the exact moment in a passage when extra volume or muting or a moment of electronic feedback would be absolutely "right."

Clapton chronologies are widely available. His first internationally known band was the YardByrds, a five-man "combo" that interpreted and put rocket fuel into the music of their heroes – Muddy Waters, B. B. King, Elmore James, among others. The YardByrds, like the Mayall outfit, also became a graduate school of sorts for artisan-grade guitar players. Clapton was ultimately replaced by other brilliant players, guitar gods like Jimmy Page and Jeff Beck (each of whom went on to world-rocking careers; their recordings and concerts still ignite the hearts and gonads (!) of fans the world over).

Another intense personality of the time – John Mayall – made musical history by recruiting EC into his squad of dedicated British bluesmen, John Mayall & The Bluesbreakers. Mayall, like Clapton and the other artists under review, was a devoted if not fanatical student of American-based blues. Mayall's record collection was a bluesman's Library of Congress; to his further credit, Mayall loaned discs from his priceless collection to players he considered dedicated, like himself, to the artistic and spiritual challenge of the blues. If you worked for Mayall, you didn't do much else. Mayall was obsessed with his work, and he insisted that his players work and always do better according to his empyrean standards. The Bluesbreakers, featuring Clapton, flourished between 1965 and 1966. The band toured widely, and sleeplessly, to the growing acclaim of hundreds of thousands of fans – fans who had never heard this kind of music before. The best known recording, *The Bluesbreakers with Eric Clapton* (Decca, 1966) is a sacred relic among fans. Collectors and Clapton cultists have been able to salvage a number of archival tracks, including out-takes,

rare sessions with other players, and the like. But the total collaborative musical output was, many feel, never enough.

What was so special about EC and his playing? His intensity, in both appearance and musical sensibility, and in the way he handled the guitar – all these were very special. Much of the rock music of the time was easy to listen to – and just as easy to forget. But very few players crafted a twelve-bar blues solo in the same life or death manner that Clapton did. Armed with his Gibson Les Paul (a guitar that soon became the "hammer of the gods" among players and enthusiasts), Clapton attacked his solos with a vengeance, with a heartfelt ferocity that was at once primal *and* technically flawless. For EC, bending a note was never a casual thing; every note, every bend, every inflection, had its deadly serious purpose. A personal favorite is the soul-piercing solo EC takes on Mayall's version of "Have You Heard" – a slow and majestic slow blues that unflinchingly builds from the first opening note to the orgasmic burst of notes at the very height of the solo.

Afficionados of other musical genres (such as opera or jazz) can relate to the superlatives and apostrophes that are enlisted in any serious attempt to describe this music in words. Lovers of opera, of symphonic orchestra, use similar language when attempting to describe peak moments of their treasured music. Although electric blues seems at quite an aesthetic distance from the work of Verdi, Mozart, and Puccini, both forms capture the spirit and express the passions of the human heart with equal intensity, fervor, and majesty.

Clapton's time with Mayall was a tiny blip – a flea on an elephant – compared with what was to come. Clapton told reporters that he felt hemmed in, limited, by Mayall's tyrannical devotion to the blues – blues, more blues, and nothing but the blues! Deviations from the genre? In Mayall's band, there was no such thing. Either you loved the blues or you left.

Clapton chose to leave.

EC rising

Signing a pact with the devil is not light opera. Even the saddest and sorriest "bottoms" that seasoned clinicians encounter over the course of a busy career pale in comparison to the life-changing horror that could have swept Clapton completely away. Recent biographies, including those of Clapton (2007), Marianne

Faithfull (2000), and Patti Boyd (2007) document the gory detail of EC's drug abuse years.

The absolute nadir, however, must have been his 4-year-old son Conor's fatal fall from the 53rd floor of a midtown Manhattan high rise in 1991. The closest we can get to that experience is the horrifying narrative of Adrien Leverkuhn, the fictive Beethoven in Thomas Mann's *Doktor Faustus.*

That's when EC turned his life around. His soul and his music softened, became humble, and many of the songs from this period are filled with an almost intolerable freight of sorrow.

Clapton's story, a model of human endurance and courage, continues to this day. Perhaps the absence of a father steeled him for what was to come.

EC began to prefer playing unamplified ("unplugged") guitar. He also founded a toney rehab program in the Caribbean. Clapton's most recent work – his acoustic interpretations of Robert Johnson – will easily rise to the top of the canon and resist erosion by the mournful friction of time.

As Clapton sweetened his music – and frustrated countless fans by holding back the banshee attacks and fighter jet solos – he became more thoughtful, more open, and generally more remorseful about his drinking, drugging, and womanizing ways. His recent autobiography (Clapton, 2007) reads like a puritan's travel guide to the bars, clubs, and concert halls of his past: there is minimal mention of the chemical extremes, of the drug-primed bacchanals of his earlier days. Clapton went in and out of collaborations with various musicians whose sensibilities – and talent – diverged, sometimes greatly from his.

Then everything came to a halt. "Mr. D." came to collect his due. Clapton's 4-year-old son fell to his death from a Manhattan high rise.

EC had already embraced sobriety. Now he was really done. Too many things had gone out of control. Clapton toned down his look and he toned down the music. He began recording ballads – many from the Robert Johnson songbook – on an acoustic guitar, sans band. Now he produced very mournful, very elegant lieder, songs about his absent father and his lost son. These songs are painful: they are sweet, lugubrious, and overwhelmingly sad.

Those with grit and intestinal fortitude can handle the jeroboams of sorrow packed into these songs. In one song, Clapton mourns the father that, as a child, he never knew.

In real life, EC didn't get to look into his father's eyes until he was 30 years old. Yet the song succeeds brilliantly at evoking both the joy and the sorrow of having no one to show you the way. The death of Clapton's 4-year-old son Conor may have been EC's final payment to the Great Deceiver. Perhaps Satan and his minions have stopped knocking on Clapton's door, evermore.

The supernatural

Similarities, strange coincidences, parallel universes, doppelgangers, synchronicity…Peter Green, another young working class Englishman, signed on with John Mayall's Bluesbreakers the moment Clapton left.

Born Peter Greenbaum, son of an English butcherman, PG – like his predecessor in Mayall's "college of electric blues" – was an autodidact who devoted his adolescence and young adulthood to a steady diet of study, practice, and playing the blues. Rarely was he seen without guitar in hand.

His ascension to the very "top of the pops" ran the usual (usual for emerging superstars, that is) obstacle course of short-lived engagements and gigs in the highly incestuous world of English blues players, pubs, and clubs.

During his pre-Bluesbreakers period, Green (with great trepidation) watched Clapton perform; not only was the Les Paul guitar on fire – but Clapton's singing was awesome, too!

Undaunted, Green played on – and his success took him down a hard and rocky road.

A Hard Road (John Mayall & the Bluesbreakers, Decca, 1967) was the second Bluesbreakers album, Peter Green at the helm. The recording features the identical twelve-bar blues structure, scales and fingerings that Clapton used. None the less, Green's sound was totally unique.

Green and Clapton even used the same equipment, early model Gibson Les Pauls. But the sounds each achieved were worlds apart. On guitar, Green could twist a note, bend it and turn it, and then sustain it for what sounded like forever.

Green's sound: that of a high voltage shaman, an oracle, launching fire and brimstone portents from the Dark Side. Green's preference for minor seventh chords explains some of the uncanny sounds he achieved. The technical aspects of his playing, such as his use of reverb and extreme sustain effects, do not fully account for the music's power. Green's instrumental and vocal magic bore witness to his personal crucifixion in strange and unearthly realms.

All told, Green did one album with the Bluesbreakers; this album, *A Hard Road,* is a masterwork of the genre. The guitar sound is unmistakable. Each passage – the solos in particular – rises and then falls from astonishing heights of passion and brio. Further, Green's signature "attack" sounds faster and more technically perfect each time you hear it.

One of the best examples of Green's guitar is his instrumental, *The Supernatural* (on *A Hard Road,* op cit.). Even those sworn to scientism – card-carrying atheists, too – will hear shadow and séance and tenebrous possibility in the unforgettable two and a half minutes of this very strange song.

Mayall's Schoolmen each went on to international recognition and fame. After Mayall, PG founded what was arguably *the* band of the era, Fleetwood Mac. Many "Mac" devotees are unaware of the band's solid foundation (thanks to Green) in the blues. Again, the Peter Green tunes are crepuscular, other-worldy, and they begin to point toward his imminent collapse into apocalyptic and gnostic-type beliefs.

Green quit Mac at the height of its success. Pumping out one chartbuster after another, the young men of Mac were practically millionaires.

Green, already a mendicant in his mind (he wore long flowing garments, a long beard and a halo of unshorn locks, very much the latter-day Christ), then gave all his money away. Green the anchorite disavowed all commercial attachments and inducements and ignored the desperate pleas that he remain with Mac. He continued to write and play, recording a number of songs that became increasingly eccentric, almost messianic in tone.

Green had found God.

Then he disappeared. According to rumor, PG had joined a cult called The Children of God and had moved to Israel. The last album-length recording was a record aptly entitled *The End of the Game* (Peter A. Green, *The End of the Game,* Reprise Records, 1970). The album art (featuring a tight head shot of a ferocious tiger) very much matched the music within. The album tracks – instrumental forays into odd sound effects and melodic blind alleys – were disturbing and very different from anything PG had ever done before.

Decades later PG re-emerged, this time with a bona fide band (The Splinter Group), international concert dates, and a more recognizable and more traditional sound. Green had wandered into stygian precincts, with LSD as his guide. Psychosis soon followed. His second coming, likely facilitated by psychiatric treatment, was a triumph and an inspiration.

Before his extended sojourn into mysticism and madness, he (yes, he too!) recorded an archival Robert Johnson tune (Robert Johnson, *Hellhound On My Trail,* Vocalion Records, 1937).

Michael Taylor

Michael ("Mick") Taylor, the third panel of the metaphorical triptych, was the last superstar graduate of the Mayall/Bluesbreakers school.

Taylor's profile will sound familiar: English, working class, intensely dedicated, afficionado of blues. In many photos Taylor is seen wielding a Les Paul. Unlike Clapton and Green, he stayed with the Bluesbreakers long enough to record at least three world-class LPs.

Taylor was 16 years old when he was recruited by Mayall. His sound – again, within the same melodic and rhythmic structure, the twelve-bar blues – was totally unique. Descriptions of his work capture elements but never the entirety of the sound. He perfected a finger vibrato style that took the instrument and its electronics to the peak of their potential. Further, he has been an acknowledged master of electric slide guitar. His sense of timing is simultaneously brilliant, surprising, and filled with passion. Taylor's listeners continually react to his solos, almost by reflex: "*Of course, how could it be any other note but that?*"

It is unclear exactly how or why Taylor left the blues band.

We do know that he was drafted by The Rolling Stones following the drug death of their guitar player, Brian Jones. Taylor was with the Stones from 1969 until the mid-1970s. During this period the band astounded the world with one creative triumph after another. The recorded material was brilliant; the concerts are still talked about in hushed, devotional tones. On stage, Taylor took the Stones' overplayed trademark tunes to new and exotic places. Taylor's extended solos on stage were comparable in both majesty and invention to the sumptuous musical excursions of Ravi Shankar. In fact, Taylor often surprised and amazed listeners with forays into exotic "Far Eastern"-sounding intervals and scales. These extended passages were usually improvised; their spontaneity added to the musical power. Taylor's guitar solo on *Sway* (Jagger/Richards and Mick

Taylor, from the album *Sticky Fingers* (Rolling Stones/ Atlantic Records, 1971) – 16 bars from start to finish – is one of the supreme guitar passages in rock and roll.

Are drugs bad? The challenge here is to consider the question from a non-dualistic point of view. The Stones' best album, *Exile on Main Street* (a double album, containing 18 original songs; Rolling Stones/ Atlantic Records) was recorded in 1972 at a rented chateau in the south of France. During their months'-long stay, the band's unabashed drug consumption took on almost heroic proportions. None the less the Stones and their precocious virtuoso managed to craft music that was rapidly (and appropriately!) canonized. Some argue that creative triumphs sometimes occur *despite* the drugs.

Taylor did pay the devil his due.

His life and career took an extended nose dive, no doubt related to some of the appetites he had cultivated as a Stone. Taylor spoke of his drug use publicly and actually continued to perform and record during those difficult times. Taylor, like Clapton and Green, overcame his demons. The best part of the happy ending is that he is still out there, at the top of his spiritual form, playing out music miracles just like before.

CODA: how to treat VIPs

Everyone is a VIP, especially when they come to you for help. Individuals with damaged self-esteem (along with everyone else) should always be treated as VIPs.

Life and doctors and treatment programs, however, often fail to rise to this level of compassion.

VIP patients (celebrities, artists, musicians, actors, politicians, plutocrats) often have the following in common:

1. They expect (boundless) individual attention, unconditional love, and immediate gratification of expressed (or even covert) needs.
2. Substance use history is often marked by intake of massive and costly amounts of drugs and/or alcohol.
3. Substance use is not only condoned but actually encouraged by fans and those trying to gain entry to the Olympian social circle.
4. They are often irritable, and have intense feelings of both entitlement and self-loathing.
5. Self-regard roller coasters between heavenly aeries and self-created dungeons of despair.
6. They have been courted many times by healers and would-be miracle workers, so they are suspicious of any new Buddhas on the block.

7. They expect shallow superficial relationships; they often expect very little of others – "*everyone wants something from me.*"
8. Attempts at honest, direct communication may be perceived as more efforts to manipulate and to connive.
9. "The show must go on:" they *must* have their drugs because of a critically important rehearsal, performance, recording session, etc.
10. Often dismissive or suspicious of attempts to gather background information on family of origin, childhood, personal issues: "*Hey Doc, been there, done that…how many milligrams can you write me?*"
11. Beneath the bravado and the tough as nails exterior there is often an extremely fragile and sensitive soul, who over-personalizes events and behaviors, and reacts to even neutral content conversations as though being criticized or rejected.

On the other side of the smoking gun sits the therapist, who needs to monitor both the client–therapist interaction and his/her own feelings, which are also to some extent predictable:

- Why me? What makes him think I can possibly help him?
- He's got serious money, inconceivably more than I do. Which of us really needs help?
- With all that money, all that power at his beck and call, how can he possibly be so depressed/ messed up/self-destructive?
- He has no idea what real pain is about.
- How come he can get away with all this? Anyone else would be in prison by now!
- This person loves drugs. There's no way he's going to be interested in any meaningful change.
- I must have listened to his second album 400 times. Here he sits, in my office, asking for help. I used to worship this person!

And so it goes. Usually the second meeting is far more comfortable and informal than the first. It's probably helpful to back off on systematic information gathering during the first meeting, unless issues related to acute withdrawal or other potential medical crises are imminent. It's best when VIP and doctor can establish a relationship where each recognizes the humanity and (to some extent) the limitations of the other. More often than not the VIP is from New Jersey or Brooklyn, not Mount Olympus; although the clinician is rife with diplomas, certifications, and academic honors, he too is a human being, a human being who will try to do his best by his patient but who is certainly not infallible, certainly not equipped with all the answers and quick fixes that his high roller patient wants. It's also helpful to spend some time trading life stories, so each gets to see the other as real, as capable – yet fallible, too.

So if and when the shade of Robert Johnson comes knocking on your office door, parchment and blood ink and wax seal in hand, find the nearest exit and head for the hills!

References

Becker, E. (1972). *The Denial of Death*. New York: Free Press.

Boyd, P. (2007). *Wonderful Tonight: An Autobiography*. New York: Random House.

Butler, A. (1788). *The Lives of the Saints*, recent publication, New York: HarperCollins, 1991.

Clapton, E. (2007). *The Autobiography*. New York: Broadway Books.

Faithfull, M. with Dalton, D. (2000). *Marianne Faithfull: An Autobiography*. Princeton, NJ: Princeton University Press.

Kierkegaard, S. (2009). *The Sickness Unto Death, first published 1843*. New York: Feather Trail Press.

Mann, T. (1948). *Doktor Faustus*. New York: Knopf.

Redfield Jamison, K. (1993). *Touched with Fire: Manic-Depressive Illness and the Artistic Temperament*. New York: Free Press.

2

The disease concept – controversies and integration

Mark Schenker

In no other area of research and social or medical endeavor have slogans so extensively replaced theoretical insight, as a basis for therapeutic action, as in alcoholism. The emotional impact of the statement, "Alcoholism is a sickness," is such that very few people care to stop to think what it actually means.

> Wexberg (1951), quoted in Jellinek, The Disease Concept of Alcoholism (1960)

There are few more controversial topics within the area of addiction treatment than the disease concept of addiction. This construct, or set of constructs, has been debated in the scientific literature for over a hundred years, and it remains a bone of contention between those oriented toward biological conceptions of addiction, and those preferring more behavioral or social explanations. The question of whether addiction is a disease or some other sort of entity has both theoretical and practical implications.

That alcoholism is a disease is an article of faith for those in Alcoholics Anonymous (AA); it is only secondarily that it is noted that this term is not used in the major works of AA (Alcoholics Anonymous, 2001). Bill Wilson, one of the founders of AA (and the primary writer of most of the early AA literature), consciously avoided using the word "disease" for fear of arousing controversy and a negative reaction from the medical profession; Bill used words like "malady" and "affliction," less incendiary terms, instead. Interestingly, Bill did not spend a great deal of time in describing the nature or etiology of alcoholism, but was more concerned with the person of the alcoholic, and with the pragmatic task of recovery.

The closest the "Big Book" of AA (Alcoholics Anonymous, 2001) comes to defining alcoholism is in the preface, "The Doctor's Opinion," in which Dr. William Silkworth describes alcoholism as an allergy combined with a craving. For the majority of AA members this is all the explanation that is needed. For the more scientific-minded among us, this formulation is just the beginning.

For better or for worse, our common notion of the disease concept of alcoholism, and, by extension, other addictions, derives from the AA depiction. However, there are other sources for this formulation, and the history of the disease concept goes back much further than Bill Wilson or E. M. Jellinek. Benjamin Rush, a signer of the Declaration of Independence and a Philadelphia physician, is often cited as providing an influential early formulation of the disease concept. He published a pamphlet in 1784 which had an enormous impact on subsequent generations of physicians and thinkers in the field (White, 1998). While he concluded that alcoholism was a disease, he vacillated between describing its origins as psychological or biological in nature. In either case, he advocated abstinence as the only resolution of alcoholism, once it had developed.

Models of addiction

To fully understand the radical departure of construing addiction as disease, it is useful to place this view in the context of other perspectives on addiction (Rogers & McMillin, 1988). The "moral models" are the early alternatives to the disease concept. The moral model views addiction as primarily a moral issue. The abuse of alcohol in general, much less the habitual abuse of it, is seen as emerging from personal preferences and poor moral choices. In one variant, sometimes termed the "wet moral model," alcohol itself is seen as the culprit – alcohol is inherently evil and will corrupt, sooner or later, anyone who uses it. Any use of alcohol is bound to result in a bad outcome for the user, and for those around him. The logical alternative, from this perspective, is the total prohibition of alcohol; the grand experiment of the 18th Amendment to the US Constitution is the clear result of this kind of thinking. The "dry moral model" sees the problem as the inappropriate and unmoderated use of alcohol; the fault lies in the moral failing of the person who uses alcohol recklessly and intemperately. For these adherents, alcohol must be used moderately or not at all; abuse represents poor moral fiber.

Before we dismiss these models as whimsical echoes of the past, it is important to note that these views underlie some of our current approach to our drug problem. The criminalization of drug users, the logical outcome of the "war on drugs" which we've been waging since the 1980s, represents the categorization of the problem as a legal and moral issue, not a medical one (Humphreys & Rappaport, 1993).

The mid 20th century saw the advent of psychological models of addiction, spurred by both Freudian and behavioral psychology. The most common formulation of this model centers on the idea of the "addictive personality." This construct presumes that underlying personality dynamics form the core of addiction. Such characteristics as immaturity, impulsivity, inability to delay gratification, selfishness, and lack of conscience are part of this presumed personality formation. The analytic formulation of addiction as a regression to a more primitive state, whether to an oral fixation or further back, is a clear example of such thinking. It is notable that as recently as DSM-II, alcoholism was classified as a personality disorder (American Psychiatric Association, 1968).

However, empirical support for an addictive personality has been sparse (Vaillant, 1995). This theory has eroded not only because the support for the construct has not been forthcoming, but because the treatments based on it have not been fruitful. It has long been accepted that psychoanalysis and psychodynamic therapy have fared poorly in studies of effectiveness with this population. However, this has not stopped many members of the public, many addicts, and many professionals (e.g. Melzack, 1990) from invoking it regularly as an explanatory vehicle. Dodes (2002) provides an example of a "new" approach to a psychological interpretation of the issues underlying addiction.

A second stream of psychological models flows from behavioral psychology. Whether through strict operant principles or social learning theories, addiction is depicted as primarily a phenomenon of learning and conditioning. Studies of "expectancies" as well take a cognitive behavioral view of alcoholism and addiction.

In the 1970s, "family systems models" appeared to be a more progressive approach to understanding and treating addiction (Stanton *et al.*, 1982). Rather than locate the addiction within an individual, the addiction was placed in an interpersonal context, one with powerful resonance. "Addiction is a family disease" became a popular phrase in addictions treatment centers, and renewed efforts were made to engage families in treatment. There were several variations on this theme. For some, "family disease" simply meant that all members of the addict's family were affected and merited therapeutic attention. For others, behaviors of family members were assessed to detect causative factors, or reinforcing variables. The "new" model of family therapy was also available as a novel approach to treating addiction, and several different schools of family therapy were applied to deal with drug and alcohol addictions.

Like the fable of the blind men and the elephant (each one giving a different description based on the part he happens to be touching), each of these theories yields valuable perspectives, yet none is fully explanatory of the complex behavior of the addict or alcoholic. Despite debate about which of these perspectives is the most valid for understanding the self-destructive compulsions of the alcoholic or drug addict, it is clear to me that the only way to explain this phenomenon is by pulling each of these theories into a comprehensive integrative framework.

The disease concept

A fundamental assumption of the classic disease concept is that addiction is a clearly delineated illness, defined by specific symptoms, and following an identifiable course. The idea of alcoholism as a disease centers on these primary symptoms (Milam & Ketcham, 1981):

- Loss of control over one's consumption of alcohol
- Physical dependence
- Elevated tolerance
- Organ damage.

These symptoms form the core of the criteria for substance dependence found in the DSM-IV (American Psychiatric Association, 2005). The identifiable progression of the disease has been portrayed in the famous "Jellinek Chart" presented in Figure 2.1 (which was not actually developed by Jellinek, but was named in his honor).

A modern refinement of the disease concept sees this illness as founded on physiologic dysfunction, primarily dysregulation of neurotransmitter systems (Erickson, 2007). Although several different systems

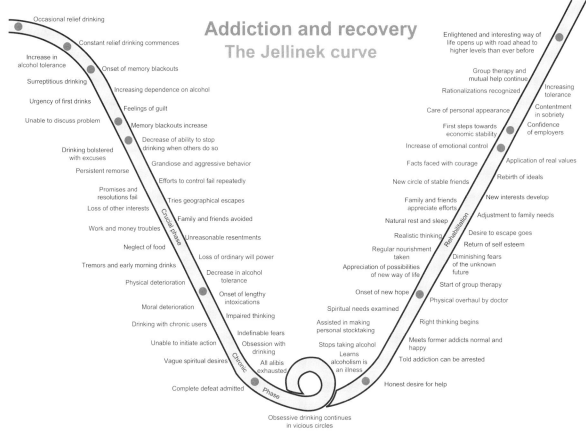

Figure 2.1 The Jellinek Chart.

have been proposed, there remains a lack of consensus about which system (endorphins, serotonin, GABA) is the primary culprit, and it is assumed that further research will clarify this picture. It may be that there are several variant "diseases" each with somewhat different characteristics. However, overall, this position is best expressed in NIDA's catch phrase, "Addiction is Brain Disease."

Addiction as brain disease, however, carries several limitations as a full explanatory system of addiction. For one thing, it is quite weak in explaining the persistence of addictive behaviors and craving beyond the period of detoxification. For example, why would someone return to drug use after detox, knowing that it results in misery? Even more puzzling, how are we to explain the relapse to full-blown substance abuse of an addict whose 15 years of sobriety have yielded a satisfying drug-free lifestyle? For another, many of the behaviors and attitudes which underline and maintain

addiction are difficult to explain merely on the basis of a sensitivity to substances of abuse.

Furthermore, the articulation of the disease concept has been marred by a kind of imprecise thinking that allows a wide variety of viewpoints, and has yielded a lack of consensus in the field. This has resulted in dissection of the word "disease" (at one extreme, an interpretation of alcoholism based on the "dis-ease" or discomfort of the sufferer) and the word "concept" (if this is merely a heuristic device, or a metaphor, the need to validate it becomes less pressing).

In keeping with the spirit of the twelve-step fellowship, many writers have simply treated the disease concept as a given, as a postulate which needs little defining. Many writers in this area appear more concerned with describing the characteristics of the addict or alcoholic, and have bypassed defining or explicating the exact nature of the disorder. As a result, the concept remains vague and undefined.

Major contributions to the disease concept

Two seminal sources in defining the disease concept are the work of E. M. Jellinek and George Vaillant.

Jellinek is famous for writing the first fully developed review of this topic, *The Disease Concept of Alcoholism*, in 1960. William White (1998) has written that this book "remains one of the most frequently cited and least read books in the alcoholism field" (p. 215). Much of the subtlety of Jellinek's work has been lost in subsequent generations, who have adopted the phrase "disease concept" from the title without noting the important distinctions that Jellinek draws in the pages of the book.

Jellinek provides a comprehensive review of a variety of theories of alcoholism, including psychological, metabolic, economic, cultural, and public health perspectives. He emerges with the view that none of these points of view are sufficient to explain the phenomena of alcoholism completely. Psychological explanations, for example, can explain the initiation of alcohol intake, but not the subsequent progression of the disease. Biological theories (whether posited on endocrine, metabolic or nutritional mechanisms) are weak in explaining the etiology of the disorder. His own integration suggests that the initiation of heavy drinking is determined by psychological factors, but "later a physiological X factor accounts for a disease condition outwardly manifested through loss of control" (p. 84). The nature of this "X factor" remains controversial, but more is known now than in Jellinek's day.

One of the more robust findings drawn from Jellinek's work is his identification of several subtypes, or "species" of alcoholism. Primary among these are his distinctions between alpha alcoholism, gamma alcoholism, and delta alcoholism. Alpha alcoholism is defined as a psychological dependence on alcohol, possibly to relieve psychological symptoms. Gamma alcoholism is characterized by the phenomenon of loss of control – the patient may maintain sobriety between drinking bouts, but cannot control his intake once he starts. Delta alcoholism is sometimes referred to as "maintenance drinking" (Milam & Ketcham, 1981) – the patient exhibits physical dependence and elevated tolerance, but no loss of control. His pattern consists of an inability to abstain, but he remains within limits defined by inebriation and withdrawal. Two other types, beta and epsilon alcoholism, are encountered less frequently and are not often discussed.

Two significant implications emerge from Jellinek's conceptualization. First is the idea that alcoholism may not be one unitary entity, but may consist of separate subtypes, which follow different patterns. (It may be possible, in the future, to identify different subtypes of alcoholism based not on behavioral criteria, as Jellinek did, but based on the neurotransmitter systems involved.) The second is Jellinek's contention that only two of these subtypes (gamma and delta) met his criteria to be categorized as diseases, in that the physiological aspects of addiction were clearly present in these two species. In this perspective, not all problem drinkers are alcoholic; this term is limited to the two varieties that provide evidence of physiological adaptation.

George Vaillant (1995) has a unique vantage point from which to assess alcoholism. He inherited several large datasets, begun in the 1940s, including a set of Harvard undergraduates and a set of Boston inner city youths, all white males. By following these subjects prospectively, he has been able to infer premorbid characteristics of those who developed alcoholism rather than suffer the limits of retrospective study. Subsequently, he has been able to follow some of these men for a period of 60 years (Vaillant, 2003), truly a unique situation in virtually any area of psychological research.

Vaillant (1995) reaches conclusions that agree with Jellinek in some aspects, but differ in some significant ways. Vaillant concludes that alcoholism "can simultaneously reflect both a conditioned habit and a disease" (p. 376), and that, rather than viewing it as consisting of subspecies, construes it as existing along a continuum. For Vaillant, alcoholism is defined by the number of problems it creates, not necessarily by a set of specific symptoms. Vaillant views alcoholism as occurring when the patient crosses a vague, but real, line. Once it has developed a life of its own, it becomes a chronic disorder, functionally autonomous from the conditions that may have created it. Vaillant's conclusion is that much of the behavioral and psychological problems that we generally associate with alcoholism are caused by this disorder; he does not find any significant evidence of premorbid psychological factors distinguishing between alcoholics and non-alcoholics.

Vaillant (1995; 2003) provides insight on several other areas of alcoholism, not directly related to the topic at hand. One relevant conclusion is that the disease of alcoholism may not be as progressive as

Jellinek (1960) or Alcoholics Anonymous (2001) has assumed; many of the men he studied (Vaillant, 2003) were able to sustain problem drinking for extended periods of time without progressing into more severe addiction. Furthermore, he concludes (1995) that the chances of a return to asymptomatic drinking decrease the further along the continuum the patient is.

Critiques and limitations of the disease concept

Of course, there have been significant critiques of the disease concept. Fingarette (1988) has provided one of the more coherent and significant challenges. A primary target for Fingarette is the phenomenon of loss of control, an essential element of the disease concept. He views this as a flawed assumption, and one that some research appears to invalidate (e.g. Marlatt *et al.*, 1973). Methodological limitations of the Marlatt study are not discussed, and the more nuanced disease model proposed by others is dismissed.

Another significant critique of the disease model by Fingarette, one shared by Stanton Peele (1989), is a moral one. These writers feel that the categorization of alcoholism as a disease allows patients to avoid responsibility for their disorder. Rather than face their disorders constructively, this label allows them to assume a passive "victim" stance.

This critique appears to have a strong emotional resonance, but it is a clear misunderstanding of the actual practices of those working in an active recovery program. The assumption of responsibility for one's own recovery is an inherent part of the program of AA, and is reflected in several of the Steps and Traditions of AA. Fingarette argues that AA's insistence that alcoholics are "powerless" encourages them to avoid responsibility. Vaillant (1995), in response, argues that "alcoholics who label themselves ill – and not bad – will be less helpless;…they, like diabetics, and in contrast to pickpockets, will try harder to change and to let others help them to change" (p. 378).

Peele (1989), a prominent critic of the disease model, views addiction as a matter of values. In his view, people suffering from addiction are lacking in more rewarding and meaningful life activities. As I have pointed out elsewhere (Schenker, 2009), it does not take a great deal of clinical experience to encounter patients whose lives would be entirely fulfilling and productive, if not for the destructive effect of addiction in their lives.

Both Peele (1989) and Fingarette (1988) point to strong economic incentives to endorse the disease concept. In Fingarette's case, the alcohol beverage industry has an interest in ensuring that the locus of the problem is to be found in the individual and not in the product. For Peele, the addiction treatment business is apt to label all sorts of aberrant behaviors as diseases worthy of treatment, which he characterizes as a lucrative industry. These criticisms may have more merit than the attacks on the disease concept themselves.

An integrative model

Given these concerns and viewpoints, I'd like to present an integrative model of addiction that serves several purposes. First, it helps to reconcile the various schools of thought that have struggled with the nature of addiction. Second, it works through some of the semantic difficulties that plague this field. Third, it provides a level of understanding of the phenomenon that can help inform and direct treatment efforts.

In some recent literature, addiction has been described as a "biopsychosocial" phenomenon. This model begins with that assumption, while teasing out more subtleties and specifics and adding other dimensions.

To present this model, I refer the reader to Figure 2.2. This model construes the disease of addiction as comprised of several layers of concentric, cumulatively reinforcing, variables. The outer layers serve to reinforce the conditions set up by the inner layers, although there is considerable reciprocal interaction between levels of the model. We will begin by describing the model from the innermost level, biological factors, moving on to the outer levels, involving cultural and existential dimensions. I will use alcohol as my primary focus, given the relative abundance of research in this area, but will highlight other relevant issues as well.

Biological factors

The model begins with processes of biological adaptation and with physiological reactions to alcohol. Examining this level is instructive, and basic to understanding the role of the subsequent levels of reinforcement. Studies of adopted-out twins provide evidence that the phenomenon of alcoholism is significantly mediated by genetic factors (Goodwin, 1988). However, they do not identify the mechanisms of such intergenerational transmission.

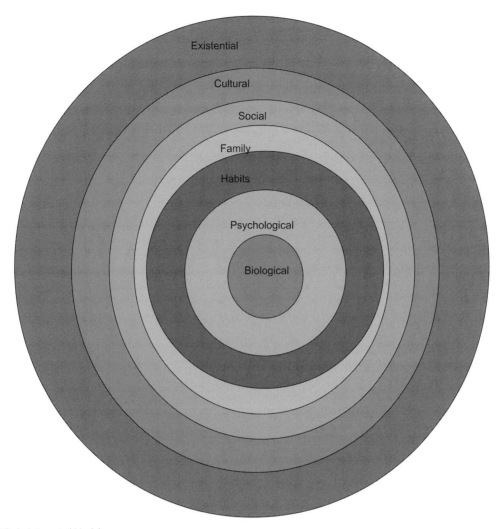

Figure 2.2 An Integrated Model.

The biological factors involved appear to be the same three criteria cited in the DSM: physical dependence, elevated tolerance, and loss of control.

Tolerance

Physiological and psychological markers of adaptation to alcohol are present in the sons of alcoholic fathers even prior to the onset of alcohol problems (Schuckit, 1988). Furthermore, these signs, particularly early evidence of alcohol tolerance, appear to predict the subsequent onset of alcoholism (Schuckit, 1994).

The phenomenon of elevated tolerance appears to be an early warning sign of the presence of alcoholism. The experience of rapid development of tolerance is also clinically observed in many alcoholics. This may be one of the key signs in adolescent substance abuse that allows us to distinguish between alcohol dependence and more typical adolescent misuse.

Dependence

One's vulnerability to alcohol dependence, one factor in the *diagnosis* of alcohol dependence, also appears to have physiological and genetic roots. Studies of other mammals suggest that this vulnerability is both heritable and selective – not everyone who is exposed to alcohol, even over extended periods of time, will become dependent on it. It is interesting to note that of the many American soldiers who became addicted to heroin during the Vietnam War, the vast majority gave it up upon their return to the United States and to more normal living (Stanton, 1976).

Loss of control

This appears to be the defining characteristic of addiction, which may even occur in the absence of the other two primary symptoms. This has been compared to the behavioral phenomenon of eating potato chips – once you start, it becomes difficult to stop. The AA saying, "One drink is too much and a thousand isn't enough" seems to capture this experience.

Perhaps the essence of the disease concept can be found in this one factor. Loss of control over substance use has been recently shown to be regulated by specific brain circuits involving pleasure centers in the brain (Baler & Volkow, 2006; Erickson, 2007). Increased sophistication in brain imaging techniques and similar diagnostic procedures have given us more evidence that, at least at this level, addiction is, indeed, a brain disease.

The limitations of utilizing dependence as the primary factor in diagnosing alcoholism or substance dependence is revealed in reviewing data of those who are prescribed painkillers or benzodiazepines, both readily addictive to certain people. Only a small proportion of those prescribed benzodiazepines become dependent on them. Many people become dependent on opiates for pain control, may even develop some degree of tolerance, yet never lose control of their use, and we do not think of them as addicted. The centrality of loss of control in determining the nature of addiction becomes clearer in this context.

It is also clear that these three factors underlie all behavior that will meet the criteria for substance dependence, and that all three are physiological in essence. However, as indicated earlier, this level of understanding does not fully explain the fullness of the phenomenon of addiction, nor does it explain addiction's resiliency in the face of extended abstinence. Vaillant's (1995) notion of addiction as both a disease and a behavioral problem points the way to a more complete understanding of this disorder.

Psychological factors

While I do not view addiction as a primarily psychological disorder, I do believe that psychological factors play a significant role in the etiology and maintenance of the disorder. While a full DSM diagnosis may not be necessary for this factor to come into play, certain psychological traits do appear to be related to the development of alcoholism and addiction. A clinical vignette will illustrate this:

A woman in her early 20s sought help because her alcohol use was becoming increasingly problematic. In college she could out-drink her peers, but this was not viewed as a significant issue, as heavy drinking was the norm among her friends. However, in the years since her graduation, her friends had curtailed their use considerably, whereas she had continued to drink at similar or greater levels. An evaluation revealed some classic symptoms of alcohol dependence: she had an elevated tolerance for alcohol, she clearly demonstrated loss of control, and she was beginning to experience withdrawal symptoms. Furthermore, she had a family history of alcoholism, including her father, who was a recovering alcoholic. However, this woman did not present with a significant level of denial or defensiveness around her drinking. She sought help relatively early in her awareness of this becoming a problematic issue in her life. It was relatively easy in this case to provide some educational counseling about the nature of alcoholism, the signs and symptoms of the disorder, and the likely outcome if she continued to consume alcohol. This woman was able to terminate her use of alcohol successfully at that time, given the information presented and her own openness around her problems.

The primary psychological dimension construed as relevant for the development of alcoholism at this level is the presence of a kind of defensiveness and/or denial, specifically around the issues of alcohol consumption. This denial may be a more pervasive style, active in other areas of life, or it may be confined to this one issue. However, the presence of a factor that allows the biological factors to develop unchecked appears to be instrumental for the progression of the disease.

The existence of defensive structures is hardly unique to alcoholics and addicts. The avoidance of dealing with the full force of reality appears to be present in a wide variety of both pathological and normal psychological processes. However, the combination of this factor and the underlying biological factors constitute the necessary and sufficient conditions for the development of addictive disease.

Other psychological factors come into play at this level as well. Actual psychopathology, including distortions in the perception of reality based on thought or mood disorders, may act to render the person more vulnerable to indulging in their substance of choice. Depression may play a role both in lowering the energy level necessary to "fight" the urges to use, as well as increase the desire to escape. Mania may increase the urge to feel better than good.

However, what is common to psychological variables at this level is their dynamic nature. The degree of defensiveness present is seen as contingent on the degree of threat posed. There is a motivated quality to this kind of defensive operation. To some degree, the actual defensiveness which emerges is related to the presence of the addiction itself, in the sense that we tend to protect ourselves from an awareness of vulnerability (Adler, 1929).

The role of expectancies may be best seen as operating at this level of the disease. A person's set of beliefs about drinking and about alcohol appear to be significant factors in the desire to drink, and in their perceptions of effect of alcohol (Brown *et al.*, 1980).

Habits and learned behavior

Beyond the dynamic forces of denial and defensiveness described above, the role of conditioning is highly relevant in maintaining addiction. While a purely behavioral model of addiction falls short of being a fully explanatory vehicle, many of the basic principles of learning theory are relevant in understanding some of the phenomena of addiction.

Simple classical conditioning is invoked in understanding the role of cues involved in perpetuating addictive behavior. The presence of a certain person in one's life when getting high becomes paired with the feelings associated with getting high, and that person eventually becomes a conditioned stimulus for that behavior. In recovery language, it is important to avoid the "people, places, and things" associated with one's addiction. These are considered "triggers," or cues that can stimulate cravings and/or addictive behaviors.

Operant conditioning is invoked, given the powerful reinforcement that the drugs themselves provide. The entire sequence of behaviors leading to drinking or to getting high form a chain of associations that become reinforced when the person begins to feel the effects of the drugs themselves.

A few simple examples can illustrate the behavioral principles involved. Imagine a man who comes home, hangs his coat in the closet, walks through the living room to the kitchen, opens the refrigerator door, and cracks open a cold beer. This entire ritual is reinforced by the high he experiences as he drinks. This sequence forms a habit, anchored by the end point of drinking. Returning home from an inpatient rehab experience of 30, 60 or 90 days, he will find that this set of behaviors continues to exert an influence on him. A patient who smokes cocaine with his brother will experience urges to use when he meets

with him, even if both are committed to sobriety; the brother's intent is irrelevant to the power of his simple presence in triggering an urge to use in the subject.

In the first case, the patient may derive benefit from breaking up the sequence of events, perhaps by beginning to hang his coat elsewhere, moving the furniture in the living room or the refrigerator. (Of course, removing the alcohol from the refrigerator itself is essential to anyone committed to sobriety!) The latter example may find little satisfaction except through avoiding the other person until one's sobriety is more established, or by only meeting in highly controlled circumstances.

The important aspect to remember at this level is that dynamic interpretations are not always relevant to some addictive behaviors. Examining these behaviors as "self-destructive" or "self-sabotaging" may miss the point entirely. These behaviors may not be highly motivated at all – they may simply be deeply ingrained habits. Insight will only be useful in helping to devise alternative behavioral strategies.

Cognitive factors may also be seen as relevant under this heading. Expectancies about the role of alcohol in social functioning can be powerful in determining both the decision to drink and the behaviors that occur when drinking. This issue will also come into play in the social context.

Family dynamics

The notion of addiction as a family disease has become almost a cliché in many treatment programs, resulting in a wide variety of interventions to involve the family in treatment of addicted individuals. However, there is a real lack of consensus about the presumed nature of family factors in addiction and recovery, ranging from theories that family dynamics are responsible for "causing" addiction to a simpler (and less controversial) idea that addiction in a family affects all members.

In this model, family dynamics are seen as reinforcers of addictive behavior, regardless of whether they are initially causal or not. Family dynamics can come to revolve around a member's addiction, just as they adapt to any other serious illness in a family. Family members learn to avoid dealing with dad when he is drunk and this avoidance prevents dad from experiencing some of the natural consequences of his behavior. By accommodating the addiction, the family serves to support it.

In its extreme form, "enabling" behaviors serve to keep the addicted person from experiencing negative consequences, and may serve a reciprocal purpose in the involved family members. A parallel process, "scapegoating," identifies the patient as the source of all family woes; the family members may seek to preserve this homeostatic balance, and avoid dealing with other disturbing facets of their family life.

Enabling is a more complex behavior than may initially be apparent. It is easy to view enabling as a negative set of behaviors that merely serve to reinforce the addiction. However, there are usually other factors at play, making the motivations and implications of the enabling (and the termination of such behavior) problematic on other levels. To use a familiar example, a wife may be persuaded to call her husband's employer to say he has the flu, when he is, in fact, hungover or on a binge. However, this call may be what saves the husband's job, and therefore preserves the health insurance and income of the family.

The important issue from the perspective of this model is that family factors may play a significant role in the development and maintenance of addictive behaviors, as well as in the recovery from the addiction.

Social factors

Social factors operate at two levels. The first level concerns actual social interactions. The role of peer pressure in the initiation and maintenance of substance abuse and dependence is profound. For certain people, this issue is one of the chief obstacles to recovery, and is a key relapse factor, as noted in the advice to recovering people to avoid "people, places, and things" associated with their addiction.

Rarely, peers will deliberately sabotage a recovering person's attempt to stay sober, either by spiking a drink, by encouraging drug use, or by direct interpersonal pressure. It is far more common, however, for the peer group to just "not get it," not understand the need for abstinence. Newly recovering people may also "not get it" and seek to re-establish regular contact with drug-using friends or drinking buddies, but hope to abstain in their company; however, most find that this is notoriously difficult to do, whether through their own cravings while in their company, actual inducements to use from the friends, or simply the social expectations of the situation.

Newly recovering people are often reminded that their sobriety may be seen as a threat by other addicted individuals, and that these friends may not be as supportive as hoped for. Addictions counselors will often advise patients that these drinking buddies are not really friends. However, this misses the point in that these friendships may have been experienced as real and sustaining, and may have been as good as it gets to the addicted person. We all need social contact, and, for many, the superficial camaraderie of a bar or a crack house may be a reasonable substitute for true interpersonal relationships.

At another level, addiction is supported by one's social self-definition. For many people, a primary marker of adulthood is the ability to drink legally. This translates into a self-image that relies significantly on one's substance abuse, whether that conveys sophistication, coolness, or alienation. For those whose substance abuse began in their adolescence, a quality of rebellion may be fused with the substance use, and may form a key part of their sense of self.

Cultural factors

It is an inescapable fact that we live in a culture that promotes substance abuse. There are reminders of substance use, particularly drinking, shouting at us from billboards, magazines, television, and all other forms of media. Our culture, deliberately and not so deliberately, cultivates the image of substance use as something tolerable, acceptable, even glamorous or exciting.

Although there have been some attempts to change this cultural message in recent years, this has made small inroads against the advertising budgets of the alcohol and tobacco industries. Musical messages also serve to promote partying and even some antidrug messages may subtly promote substance use.

More subtle than the actual drinking and drugging cues is the underlying cultural message that the solution to discomfort lies in chemical cure, and that discomfort itself is undesirable. One of the more difficult tasks for newly recovering people is in learning to tolerate some of the "normal" aches and pains of living, both physical and psychological.

In my office I have a cartoon posted. A psychoanalyst is addressing a patient lying on a couch. The analyst says, "I've concluded that you have an addictive personality." The patient exclaims, "That's awful! What can I take for that?"

A person seeking to recover in such an environment must face such cues and messages on an ongoing basis, and must find a way to have the message of sobriety reinforced in an equally powerful manner. The role of AA or similar support groups is invaluable in providing a strong message that abstinence is possible and is healthy, and that the message provided by the culture at large is dangerous and misleading.

Another problem is a prevailing underlying cultural belief in the moral model or the psychological model of addiction. Addicts and alcoholics are seen in an extremely negative light, as deficient creatures. The Reagan-era message of "Just Say No" continues to reverberate in the public consciousness, and those who find it difficult or impossible to do so are frequently seen as degenerates. Unfortunately, this message has also been internalized by many addicts and alcoholics, and the resultant shame has often discouraged them from seeking help or acknowledging their own problems. (As will be discussed below, this feeds into the level of psychological defensiveness and denial.)

Existential factors

The difficulty of accepting one's addiction is one of the first hurdles to be experienced in the process of recovery. It is often difficult in our "Do-it-yourself" society (Slater, 1970) to accept that one cannot do everything alone. Acceptance of our limitations can be the beginning of a calmer mindset, one of acceptance and surrender (Kurtz, 1982).

Writers on recovery topics describe the act and process of surrender as a turning point in the addict's acceptance of his or her disease state (Tiebout, 1949; 1953). This insight may lead to a larger shift in world view from a competitive to a complementary mode (Bateson, 1972). While this is one of the benefits of recovery, it is also one of the more significant obstacles, and one of the factors that keeps the addiction in place.

The messages of self-sufficiency and individuality that are so prevalent in our culture resonate at a more profound personal level as well. Acceptance of one's addiction brings an end to any lingering infantile notions of omnipotence (Kurtz, 1982). The need to accept help and support from others resurrects our earlier, preverbal, struggles with feelings of inferiority (Adler, 1929). This sense of incompleteness, which binds us to others, also violates our sense of personal autonomy.

However, these insights may also form the nucleus of a new sense of self, and a new relationship to others. This insight of incompleteness and limitation can lead

to a "spirituality of imperfection" (Kurtz & Ketcham, 1992) based on mutual interest and affiliation. This is closely related to the spirituality central to the fellowship of AA and other such twelve-step groups.

Implications of the integrative model

I believe that some of the confusion in this area of discourse arises from confusion around levels of interpretation. For some, the "disease" of addiction resides purely in the biological aspects of the disorder. For these theorists (e.g. Milam & Ketcham, 1981) the physiological aspects of the disorder define it – there is little need to search further to explain the phenomenon. These theorists have been described as "unidimensional" (White, 1998) in their reliance on biological factors, even if there are differences about the precise mechanisms involved.

Recent advances on brain imaging and related technological breakthroughs have also tended to emphasize the center circle of the proposed model. Even when other aspects are invoked, it is hard to measure them, and less impressive to present, when the lure of brain images and neurological studies appear to offer profound new insights into this aspect of addictive behavior. The "bio" is sleek and new, and the "-psychosocial" is old and imprecise. This may not be the intent of these researchers, but it is often the result.

For many others, however, there is a far vaguer idea of the "disease" of addiction, one which includes many of the other factors in the model. When a recovering addict experiencing some cravings is told "that is your addiction talking to you," it is unclear which level of the model is being invoked. Perhaps the "talk" is coming from the biological cravings; more likely, however, the psychological or learned dimensions are being referenced.

It is difficult, as well, to speak of a disease being "existential," or even "social" or "cultural," without veering into the realm of the metaphorical, again undermining the meaning of the term "disease."

This semantic confusion undermines a sense of scientific integrity. It is difficult to come to a consensus on the nature of addiction if the terms that are so central to the discourse are so imprecisely defined. I believe that the observed entity we treat in our clinics and rehab centers includes all levels of the proposed model, and that, for convenience and to recognize the challenges faced by a recovering person, the frame of reference should include all levels of this proposed model.

In this spirit, I propose that we include all levels as part of the disease entity, with an understanding that the biological roots of the disorder are the only aspect directly dependent upon a biological explanation. I believe that this helps us to clarify some of the debate about the biological underpinnings of the disorder, and moves us from a purely biological understanding (rooted in advances in our understanding of brain functioning) to a more truly biopsychosocial conception. When an addict is helped to understand that all of these levels are operating and are all relevant to their recovery, a great deal of the mystification which paralyzes action will be relieved.

Another implication of this model is that there is considerable dynamic interaction among the levels of the model. The existential difficulty of "accepting surrender" and the cultural image of a hopeless drunk feed into the level of defensiveness about accepting the presence and nature of the illness. The biological reinforcement provided by the drugs of abuse goes a long way to explain why this habit is particularly pernicious and resistant to extinction. The social factors interplay with psychological factors in conceptions of identity and social interaction. It is helpful to remember that the levels identified are abstractions from the workings of the disorder, as it exists in nature.

Finally, a model such as this one provides some clarity in terms of developing treatment planning efforts. An assessment of the patient's functioning at each level will help clinicians to determine where input is needed. A patient with a high level of family dysfunction may require more immediate attention to that dimension than one whose family is supportive and understanding of recovery. A person with a greater ability to face his or her addiction honestly, without defensive reactions, may require less strenuous intervention on that level. The level of acceptance of the existential dimensions provides a forum for discussion of spirituality, and the possible role of pastoral care. All patients, of course, require a good assessment of their biological functioning, both in terms of pharmacological intervention for withdrawal and for the possibility of anticraving medications.

By coming to an integrative perspective on the disease of addiction, and by utilizing this approach consistently, we are in a better position to understand and manage this crippling disorder in a manner that is both effective and holistic.

References

Adler, A., (1929). *The Practice and Theory of Individual Psychology*. London: Routledge & Kegan Paul.

Alcoholics Anonymous. (2001). *Alcoholics Anonymous*, 4th Edition. New York: AA World Services.

American Psychiatric Association. (1968). *Diagnostic and Statistical Manual of Mental Disorders*, 2nd Edition. Washington, DC: American Psychiatric Association.

American Psychiatric Association. (2005). *Diagnostic and Statistical Manual of Mental Disorders*, 4th Edition, Text Revision. Washington, DC: American Psychiatric Association.

Baler, R. D. & Volkow, N. D. (2006). Drug addiction: The neurobiology of disrupted self-control. *Trends in Molecular Medicine*, **12**, 559–66.

Bateson, G. (1972). The cybernetics of "self": A theory of alcoholism. In Bateson, G. *Steps To An Ecology of Mind*. New York: Ballantine Books.

Brown, S. A., Goleman, M. S., Inn, A. Anderson, L. R. (1980). Expectations of reinforcement from alcohol. *Journal of Consulting and Clinical Psychology*, **48**, 419–26.

Dodes, L. (2002). *The Heart of Addiction*. New York: HarperCollins.

Erickson, C. (2007). *The Science of Addiction*. New York: WW Norton.

Fingarette, H. (1988). *Heavy Drinking: The Myth of Alcoholism as a Disease*. Berkeley: University of California.

Goodwin, D. W. (1994). *Alcoholism: The Facts*. Oxford, U.K.: Oxford University Press.

Humphreys, K. & Rappaport, J. (1993). From the community mental health movement to the war on drugs: A study in the definition of social problems. *American Psychologist*, **48**, 892–901.

Jellinek, E. M. (1960). *The Disease Concept of Alcoholism*. New Haven, Ct.; College and University Press.

Kurtz, E. (1982). Why AA works: The intellectual significance of Alcoholics Anonymous. *Journal of Studies on Alcohol*, **43**, 38–80.

Kurtz, E. & Ketcham, K. (1992). *The Spirituality of Imperfection: Storytelling and the Journey to Wholeness*. New York: Bantam Books.

Marlatt, G. A., Demming, B. & Reid, J. B. (1973). Loss of control drinking. in Alcoholics: an experimental analogue. *Journal of Abnormal Psychology*, **81**(3) 233–41.

Melzack, R. (1990). The tragedy of needless pain. *Scientific American*, **262**, 27–33.

Milam, J. R. & Ketcham, K. (1983). *Under The Influence*. New York: Bantam Books.

Peele, S. (1989). *Diseasing of America: Addiction Treatment Out of Control.* Lexington, MA: Lexington Books.

Rogers, R. L. & McMillin, C. S. (1989). *Don't Help: A Positive Guide to Working with the Alcoholic.* New York: Bantam Books.

Schenker, M. D. (2009). *A Clinician's Guide to 12-Step Recovery.* New York: WW Norton.

Schuckit, M. A. (1988). Reactions to alcohol in the sons of alcoholics and controls. *Alcoholism: Clinical and Experimental Research*, **12**, 465–70.

Schuckit, M. A. (1994). Low level response to alcohol as a predictor of future alcoholism. *American Journal of Psychiatry*, **151**, 184–9.

Slater, P. (1970). *The Pursuit of Loneliness.* Boston: Beacon Press.

Stanton, M. D. (1976). Drugs, Vietnam, and the Vietnam veteran: An overview. *American Journal of Drug and Alcohol Abuse*, **3**, 557–70.

Stanton, M. D. Todd, T. C. *et al.* (1982). *The Family Therapy of Drug Abuse and Addiction.* New York: Guilford.

Tiebout, H. M. (1949). The act of surrender in the therapeutic process. *Quarterly Journal of Studies on Alcohol*, **10**, 48–58.

Tiebout, H. M. (1953). Surrender versus compliance in therapy. *Quarterly Journal of Studies on Alcohol*, **14**, 58–68.

Vaillant, G. (1995). *The Natural History of Alcoholism Revisited.* Cambridge, MA: Harvard University Press.

Vaillant, G. (2003). A 60-year follow-up of alcoholic men. *Addiction*, **98**, 1043–51.

White, W. L. (1998). *Slaying The Dragon: The History of Addiction Treatment and Recovery in America.* Bloomington, IL: Chestnut Health Systems.

Medical sequelae of addiction

Michael Weaver

Introduction

The use of alcohol or drugs may result in many different medical sequelae. Some effects are acute and may be transient, while others may only manifest after long-term use. Withdrawal syndromes differ significantly between classes of drugs, but symptoms within a class are identical regardless of the specific drug in that class (although shorter-acting drugs have a shorter time to onset of withdrawal symptoms). The route of administration also accounts for the severity of potential sequelae (i.e. different complications of smoking compared to injection compared to oral or nasal routes). This chapter reviews and compares notable medical complications as a result of the use and abuse of different classes of drugs, including withdrawal syndromes where applicable.

Alcohol and sedatives

In the US, 90% of men and 70% of women consume alcohol (Johnston *et al.*, 2002) in the form of beer, wine, or liquor. Alcohol is commonly used to the point of mild intoxication, often without serious medical sequelae. Sedatives include benzodiazepines such as diazepam (Valium) and alprazolam (Xanax), barbiturates such as butalbital (in Fiorinal), and benzodiazepine subtype receptor agonists such as zolpidem (Ambien) and eszopiclone (Lunesta). These are prescribed for insomnia or anxiety, but may be abused and are available on the black market.

Acute complications

Acute alcohol intoxication may occur after ingestion of as little as one standard drink (12 g, 1–1.5 fluid ounces of ethanol). Ingestion of sedatives in amounts that exceed the tolerance of the individual also leads to intoxication. As the amount consumed increases, especially beyond the established tolerance of an individual, progressively more impairment occurs

in judgment and other brain functions. Initial signs include slurred speech, mood lability, and inappropriate behavior, followed by incoordination (especially with complex tasks such as driving), ataxia, impaired attention and memory impairment, or "blackouts" (Weaver *et al.*, 1999). High levels result in suppression of the autonomic respiratory drive and may result in coma or death from anoxic brain injury.

Physical signs of acute alcohol or sedative intoxication include nystagmus and decreased reflexes. A benzodiazepine antagonist, flumazenil (Romazicon), is available for treatment of benzodiazepine intoxication. It should be used with caution because it can cause several withdrawal reactions, including seizures in patients with physical dependence (Seger, 2004). Flumazenil is a short-acting agent, so there may be re-sedation after an initial awakening. This can be treated by repeating doses at 20-minute intervals as necessary (Weaver *et al.*, 1999).

Withdrawal syndrome

The clinical features of the acute withdrawal syndrome are identical for all sedatives, including alcohol (which may be considered a short-acting sedative), owing to cross-tolerance among these agents. Abrupt reduction or cessation of sedative use results in a characteristic set of signs and symptoms which can include tremor, anxiety, agitation, autonomic hyperactivity (e.g. elevated heart rate, blood pressure, temperature, and sweating), hallucinations, and seizures (APA, 2000). Withdrawal symptoms are essentially the opposite of the symptoms of acute intoxication. Even a cursory neurological evaluation can reveal altered mental status due to intoxication or withdrawal; hyperreflexia and tremulousness should also prompt consideration of withdrawal. The symptoms may appear as soon as 4–8 hours after the last use, and alcohol withdrawal symptoms usually manifest within 48 hours of the last drink; patients using benzodiazepines with long-acting metabolites (chlordiazepoxide, diazepam) may not show signs of withdrawal for up to 7–10 days after stopping chronic use. Patients who meet criteria from the *Diagnostic and Statistical Manual of Mental Disorders* (DSM; APA, 2000) for dependence on alcohol or sedatives will commonly develop a withdrawal syndrome (Turner *et al.*, 1989) upon total cessation of drinking. Only 5% of those with sedative dependence develop severe withdrawal (delirium tremens, or "DTs") with serious altered mental status and severe autonomic dysregulation; development of delirium tremens carries a mortality of 5%, even when adequately treated (Cushman, 1987). Alcohol and sedatives are the only class of abused drugs that have a potentially fatal withdrawal syndrome; withdrawal from substances in other classes may not occur or may be uncomfortable without being fatal. Risk factors for progression to delirium tremens include larger amounts of sedatives taken chronically, a longer period of use, older age, and comorbid medical problems.

A protracted sedative abstinence syndrome may be seen following very long-term use of benzodiazepines. The insomnia and anxiety that accompany this may last for several months. While not life-threatening, withdrawal symptoms may cause sufficient distress to trigger a relapse to drug use. A very long taper (2–3 months) of the original benzodiazepine dose is useful in this situation (Higgitt *et al.*, 1990).

Long-term consequences

Alcohol dependence results in reduction of the individual's lifespan by 10–15 years. There are many medical problems caused by chronic alcohol use

(Table 3.1). Alcohol use disorders result in 25 000 deaths per year from accidents and 175 000 deaths annually from heart disease, cancer, and suicide (Schuckit & Tapert, 2004). Chronic sedative use results in fewer direct medical sequelae, although dementia with memory loss (recent and remote) may be seen (Weaver *et al.*, 1999).

Many of the sequelae of chronic alcohol use are apparent on physical examination or on routine laboratory testing. Signs of acute hepatitis include jaundice and abdominal tenderness in the right upper quadrant. Signs of chronic alcoholic cirrhosis include spider angiomata, palmar erythema, caput medusae, a shrunken and nodular liver edge, and abdominal distension and/or a fluid wave from ascites. Other signs include peripheral sensorimotor neuropathy. Chronic sedative users who have developed tolerance may have recent and remote memory loss apparent on neurological testing. Laboratory findings may also provide indications of chronic alcohol use. The mean corpuscular volume of red blood cells may be elevated owing to bone marrow suppression. Liver transaminases can be elevated by alcohol use with acute hepatitis.

Fetal alcohol syndrome

Alcohol or sedative use during pregnancy may affect the fetus at any stage of development; it is not known what level of exposure may cause specific birth defects, so complete abstinence should be encouraged as soon as a woman suspects she is pregnant (Weaver, 2003). Fetal alcohol syndrome (FAS) is the leading preventable cause of mental retardation in North America (Smith, 1997).

Table 3.1 Long-term effects of alcohol use

Central nervous system	Gastrointestinal	Malignancy
Seizures	Malnutrition	Mouth
Delirium	Gastritis	Pharynx, larynx
Dementia	Peptic ulcer disease	Esophagus
Cerebral atrophy	Gastrointestinal bleeding	Pancreas
Endocrine	Acute hepatitis	Liver
Diuresis	Pancreatitis	**Other**
Hyperglycemia	Fatty liver	Bone marrow suppression
Male feminization	Cirrhosis	Peripheral neuropathy
Cardiovascular	**Obstetric**	Rhabdomyolysis
Hypertension	Sexual dysfunction	
Arrhythmias	Intrauterine growth retardation	
Cardiomyopathy	Fetal alcohol syndrome/fetal alcohol effects	

The criteria for FAS include: prenatal and/or postnatal growth retardation; central nervous system (CNS) involvement (neurologic abnormality, developmental delay, behavioral dysfunction, intellectual impairment, and/or structural abnormalities); and characteristic facial anomalies (short palpebral fissures, elongated midface, long and flattened philtrum, thin upper lip, and flattened maxilla) (Pagliaro & Pagliaro, 2003). The effects of FAS persist throughout life (Cramer & Davidhizar, 1999). Children who exhibit some but not all of the criteria for diagnosis of FAS, but who have intrauterine alcohol exposure, are identified as having "alcohol-related birth defects" or "fetal alcohol effects" or "fetal alcohol spectrum disorder." Sedative use during pregnancy has been associated with specific teratogenic effects, especially cleft palate, as well as a neonatal abstinence syndrome (Pagliaro & Pagliaro, 2003).

Tobacco

Around the world, 57% of men and 10% of women smoke tobacco products, primarily cigarettes (Mackay & Eriksen, 2002). In the US, about 21% of the adult population smokes (CDC, 2005). Other tobacco products include smokeless tobacco (chewing tobacco and snuff), cigars, and tobacco smoked through a water pipe. Smoked tobacco products cause more respiratory problems while smokeless tobacco causes more head and neck malignancies.

Acute complications

Tobacco cigarette smoking is implicated in acute exacerbations of asthma – especially those episodes requiring treatment in an emergency department (Silverman *et al.*, 2003) – and in exacerbations of chronic bronchitis (Wilson & Rayner, 1995). Exposure to tobacco smoke causes coronary artery spasm and thrombosis, and angina in patients with coronary artery disease. This also occurs in non-smokers exposed to secondhand smoke and is caused by carbon monoxide as well as other components of tobacco smoke (Zevin *et al.*, 2001, Otsuka *et al.*, 2001). Smoking increases the risk of venous thrombosis and pulmonary embolism in women on oral contraceptives (Barton *et al.*, 2002).

Withdrawal syndrome

Symptoms of withdrawal are caused by reduced blood levels of nicotine and are similar with all tobacco products, whether cigarettes, chewing tobacco, or snuff. Withdrawal symptoms include irritability, difficulty concentrating, restlessness, anxiety, depression,

and increased appetite (Karan *et al.*, 2003). Impairment in reaction time and attention also occur. Withdrawal symptoms peak around 48 hours after the last use, then gradually diminish over several weeks. Symptoms of dysphoria, anhedonia, and depression may continue for several months after cessation. The withdrawal syndrome from nicotine is somewhat similar to that of other stimulants.

Long-term consequences

Tobacco smoke causes respiratory tract ciliary paralysis, which reduces resistance to respiratory tract infections and results in recurrent bronchitis and pneumonia (Agius *et al.*, 1998). A history of smoking (of at least 15 pack-years) is sufficient for implication in the cause of chronic obstructive pulmonary disease (COPD), which, along with lung cancer, is the most prevalent smoking-related lung disease (Kamholz, 2006).

Direct exposure to tobacco smoke or secondhand smoke may cause coronary artery disease from acceleration of development of atherosclerotic lesions (Glantz & Parmley, 1995). Smoking is also linked to cerebrovascular disease (Taylor *et al.*, 1998) and peripheral arterial disease (Criqui, 2001), as well as peripheral venous insufficiency of the lower extremities (Gourgou *et al.*, 2002).

Multiple carcinogens are found in tobacco smoke, including powerful nitrosamines and polycyclic aromatic hydrocarbons that are the major etiologic factors in lung cancer (Deutsch-Wenzel *et al.*, 1983). In developed nations, 90% of lung cancer is attributed to smoking (International Agency for Research on Cancer, 2004). Smoking increases the risk of developing all types of lung cancer; the most common smoking-related cancer is adenocarcinoma (Hecht, 2006). Risk for lung cancer increases with duration of smoking and number of cigarettes smoked (IARC, 2004). Smoking causes many other cancers besides lung cancer. Increased risk for cancer of the lip, tongue, and oral cavity is associated with duration and amount of smoking, and this risk is further increased when tobacco use is combined with alcohol consumption (Hecht, 2006). Tobacco use causes transitional cell carcinomas of the bladder, ureters, and renal pelvis owing to concentration of carcinogens in urine. Smoking is associated with cancer of the pancreas, stomach, and liver as well (International Agency for Research on Cancer, 2004).

In a dose-dependent manner, smoking (including exposure to secondhand smoke) reduces female fertility

(Mallampalli & Guntupalli, 2006). Pregnant women who smoke have a higher incidence of early abortion and adverse pregnancy outcomes (Gocze et al., 1999). Tobacco reduces sperm quality, sperm count, and sperm motility in men (Vine, 1996). Smoking is associated with a higher risk of developing type 2 diabetes mellitus (Eliasson, 2003); the increased risk is nearly double that of non-smokers. A higher risk for Grave's disease (Prummer & Wiersinga, 1993) is associated with smoking. Tobacco is a risk factor for gastroesophageal reflux disease and for both gastric and duodenal ulcers. Smokers have a reduced response to treatment for these conditions (Mallampalli & Guntupalli, 2006).

Marijuana

Marijuana is the most frequently abused drug in the US. Approximately 4% of the adult population uses marijuana regularly; this prevalence rate figure has remained relatively steady since the early 1990s (Compton et al., 2004).

Acute complications

Acute marijuana intoxication begins within minutes of smoking and lasts for 3–4 hours (APA, 2000). Impairment of concentration and motor performance lasts for 12–24 hours as a result of accumulation of marijuana in adipose tissue, with enterohepatic circulation and slow release of tetrahydrocannabinol (THC) from fatty tissue stores (Naditch, 1974). A marijuana user may think that he or she is no longer impaired several hours after use, when the acute mood-altering effects have worn off. However, impairment of cognition, coordination, and judgment lasts much longer than the subjective feeling of being "high." Impairment is intensified by combination with other drugs, especially alcohol. This explains why fatal traffic accidents occur more often among individuals who test positive for marijuana (Laumon et al., 2005).

Withdrawal syndrome

Heavy marijuana use of more than 3 weeks' duration results in a withdrawal syndrome after abrupt cessation (Wiesbeck et al., 1996). Marijuana withdrawal begins within 10 hours of the last dose and consists of irritability, agitation, depression, insomnia, nausea, anorexia, and tremor. Most symptoms peak in 48 hours but symptoms last for up to 5–7 days. Some symptoms, such as unusual dreams and irritability, can persist for weeks (Budney et al., 2004).

Long-term consequences

Chronic marijuana use may result in multiple health problems. Unlike most tobacco cigarettes, marijuana is not smoked with filters, so the amount of particulate matter settling on the mucous membrane lining of the upper airway and entering the lungs is increased compared to tobacco smoking. Marijuana smoke contains nearly four times as much tar and 50% more carcinogens than tobacco (Wu et al., 1988). However, many adults who smoked marijuana when they were younger no longer do so. Thus, the exposure to smoke-borne toxins is often greater among tobacco smokers, which results in less attributable mortality among marijuana compared to tobacco smokers (Sidney, 2003). Most individuals who smoke marijuana also smoke tobacco as well, so determining the relative contribution each substance makes to pathogenesis can be challenging.

As with tobacco, marijuana smoking causes decreased pulmonary function, chronic cough, bronchitis, and decreased exercise tolerance (Tashkin et al., 1976). Those who regularly smoke three to four marijuana cigarettes per day experience cough, wheeze, and sputum production (Tashkin et al., 1987), and exhibit histologic abnormalities equivalent to those who smoke approximately 20 tobacco cigarettes per day (Gong et al., 1987). This disparity may be due in part to the different manner in which marijuana and tobacco cigarettes are smoked. On average, marijuana cigarette inhalation delivers almost twice as much smoke. With marijuana, inhalation is one-third longer, and breath-holding time is four times longer (Wu et al., 1988). A link between marijuana use and COPD is suspected (Johnson et al., 2000). Reduction in pulmonary function with marijuana use may start early in life; an 8-year study of young adults aged 18–26 years found a trend toward a reduced ratio of 1 second forced expiratory volume to vital capacity (FEV_1/VC ratio) with increased smoking of marijuana (Taylor et al., 2002).

Marijuana smokers are at increased risk for lung cancer, although the magnitude of risk has not been well quantified (Sridhar et al., 1994). The absolute risk of lung cancer for an individual smoker depends on the amount and duration of marijuana use, and on concomitant exposure to other carcinogens (such as tobacco smoke). Several reports have documented histologic and molecular changes in the bronchial epithelium of marijuana smokers that resemble the metaplastic premalignant changes seen among tobacco smokers (Barsky et al., 1998). Marijuana impairs the immune system by suppressing the activity of natural killer cells and macrophages (Klein *et al.*, 1998).

Tachycardia results from stimulation of the cardiac pacemaker by marijuana, which may worsen hypertension or underlying heart disease (Beaconsfield *et al.*, 1972). During the 60 minutes following marijuana use, the risk of myocardial infarction is increased almost five times over baseline (Mittleman *et al.*, 2001).

In men, marijuana causes decreased serum testosterone levels, sperm count, and sperm motility (Kolodny *et al.*, 1974). This may lead to decreased libido, impotence, gynecomastia, and an increased risk of infertility. In women, marijuana increases the risk of infertility owing to ovulatory abnormality (Mueller *et al.*, 1990). THC accumulates in breast milk and crosses the placenta (Fernandez-Ruiz *et al.*, 2004), which can lead to intrauterine growth retardation, low birthweight (Zuckerman *et al.*, 1989), and abnormal startle reflex responses in newborns (Chiriboga, 2003). Marijuana use during pregnancy can have long-term effects on children, including reduced memory and verbal skills at 4 years of age (Fried & Watkinson, 1990).

Signs of chronic marijuana use include reduction in activities and relationships not associated with the drug, and impairment in cognitive skills. The association between chronic marijuana exposure and cognitive dysfunction has been extensively studied, but with varying results. A syndrome formerly known as the "amotivational syndrome," now called the "chronic cannabis syndrome," has been described in which chronic heavy users develop cognitive impairment with a reduced ability to establish or attain goals in life, resulting in jobs that require less cognitive challenge or technological acuity (Gold *et al.*, 2004). The evidence is fairly consistent that marijuana use results in cognitive deficits that persist for at least hours, and likely days after acute intoxication. Very heavy use of

marijuana is associated with persistent decrements in neurocognitive performance even after 28 days of abstinence (Bolla *et al.*, 2002). It is not clear whether these decrements persist in the long term if the individual is able to maintain long-term abstinence from marijuana (Iversen, 2003).

Stimulants

Stimulants are drugs that stimulate the CNS to produce increased psychomotor activity. Amphetamines – including methamphetamine – and cocaine are the most prevalent abused stimulants, but this class also includes prescription stimulants such as methylphenidate (Ritalin) and combined dextroamphetamine/levoamphetamine (Adderall), as well as "designer drugs" such as methylenedioxymethamphetamine (MDMA, ecstasy).

Acute complications

The short-term complications of stimulant use, including intoxication (Table 3.2), are caused by increased sympathomimetic effects. Repeated use of low doses of stimulants can result in exaggerated startle reactions, dyskinesias, and postural abnormalities (Weaver & Schnoll, 1999).

Amphetamine and designer drugs can cause severe acute toxicity, including fulminant hyperthermia, seizures, disseminated intravascular coagulation, rhabdomyolysis, acute renal failure, hepatotoxicity, hypertension, tachycardia, and increased myocardial oxygen consumption (Henry *et al.*, 1992). Treatment for acute toxicity includes acute stabilization of the airway, breathing, and circulation; activated charcoal; seizure control with benzodiazepines; aggressive management of hypertension with alpha- and beta-antagonists or vasodilators; management of hyperthermia;

Table 3.2 Stimulant intoxication

Physiological effects	Psychological effects	Toxic effects
Dizziness	Restlessness	Hyperthermia
Tremor	Grandiosity	Seizures
Mydriasis	Hypervigilance	Hepatotoxicity
Hyperreflexia	Impaired judgment	Rhabdomyolysis
Hyperpyrexia	Stereotyped behavior	Acute renal failure
Tachypnea	Aggression	Cardiac ischemia
Hypertension		Disseminated intravascular coagulation
Tachycardia		

and consideration of urine acidification. Treatment of acute cocaine intoxication is rarely necessary since it is such a short-acting drug; the exceptions are cases of acute psychotic reactions.

Withdrawal syndrome

A withdrawal syndrome can occur with chronic stimulant use. The "crash," or drastic reduction in mood and energy, can start 15–30 minutes after cessation of a stimulant binge. The user experiences craving, depression, irritability, anxiety, and paranoia. The craving for stimulants decreases over 1–4 hours and is replaced by a craving for sleep, food, and rejection of further stimulant use. Hypersomnolence lasts between 8 hours and 4 days. Sleep is punctuated by brief awakenings during which the user experiences hyperphagia ("the munchies"). This phase is followed by a protracted dysphoric syndrome consisting of anhedonia, boredom, anxiety, panic attacks, generalized malaise, problems with memory and concentration, and occasional suicidal ideation. This induces severe craving that may lead to resumption of stimulant use and a vicious cycle of recurrent binges. Intermittent conditioned craving can last months to years after the last stimulant use, and is gradually extinguished over time. The severity and duration of withdrawal depends upon the intensity of the preceding months of chronic abuse and the presence of predisposing psychiatric disorders, which amplify withdrawal symptoms (Weaver & Schnoll, 1999).

Stimulant withdrawal syndrome is unlike the withdrawal syndrome from alcohol or opioids because it is not accompanied by obvious physical signs and symptoms. Stimulant users may not recognize the subtle and complex manifestations of acute stimulant withdrawal and may think that they are "not addicted" to stimulants because there are not gross physical symptoms to prompt immediate resumption of use in order to avoid withdrawal. Thus, patterns of use of stimulants may be more often in the form of episodic binges, as opposed to chronic daily use for alcohol, benzodiazepines, or opioids when tolerance has developed. Subjective experiences or symptoms other than physiological discomfort are crucial to stimulant dependence; the absence of a daily use pattern does not indicate less impairment (Weaver & Schnoll, 1999).

Long-term consequences

The clinical features of chronic stimulant use include depression, fatigue, poor concentration, and mild parkinsonian features such as myoclonus (inappropriate, spontaneous muscle contractions), tremor, or bradykinesia (slowing of movements). Patients presenting with these signs should be suspected of stimulant abuse and screened carefully.

Medical sequelae in long-term stimulant users tend to accumulate over time, although any specific complication may occur relatively quickly after initiation of use (Table 3.3). This is in contrast to long-term consequences of alcohol, tobacco, or marijuana, which

Table 3.3 Long-term effects of stimulant use

Central nervous system	Cardiovascular	Obstetric
Transient ischemic attack	Hypertension	Placenta previa
Hyperthermia	Arrhythmia	Placental abruption
Seizure	Cardiomyopathy	Premature rupture of membranes
Cerebral vasospasm	Myocardial ischemia	Intrauterine growth retardation
Cerebral hemorrhage	**Gastrointestinal**	Fetal hypertension
Cerebral vasculitis	Anorexia	Sudden infant death syndrome
Pulmonary	Intestinal ischemia	**Other**
Chronic productive cough	Intestinal perforation	Dental enamel erosion
Asthma exacerbation	**Endocrine**	Nasal septal perforation
Pulmonary edema	Hyperprolactinemia	Rhabdomyolysis
Pneumothorax	Elevated thyroxin level	
Pulmonary hemorrhage		
Bronchiolitis obliterans		

usually require years for development of serious medical problems.

High-dose stimulant use over long periods of time causes neurophysiologic changes in brain systems; CNS effects can take months to resolve, and occasionally do not resolve, after cessation of use. As an example, a study in twins found that after at least 1 year of abstinence, abusing twins had deficits in attention and motor skills compared with non-abusing twins (Toomey *et al.*, 2003). Brain imaging of methamphetamine users has shown structural deficits, including gray-matter deficits in the cingulate, limbic, and paralimbic cortices, and significant reductions in hippocampal volume (Thompson *et al.*, 2004). Long-term methamphetamine dependence can cause neurotoxicity even in patients who are no longer users (Ernst *et al.*, 2000). Several studies suggest that MDMA use can lead to cognitive decline in otherwise healthy young people (Gouzoulis-Mayfrank *et al.*, 2000); this neurotoxicity occurs at typical recreational doses.

Opioids

The most commonly used illicit opioid is heroin, with over 2 million users in the US (SAMHSA, 2006). Prescription opioid analgesic abuse is the fastest growing form of drug abuse in the US (Cicero *et al.*, 2005). Abused prescription opioids include hydrocodone (Vicodin, Lortab), oxycodone (Percocet, OxyContin), hydromorphone (Dilaudid), fentanyl (Duragesic, Fentora), and others.

Acute complications

Acute opioid intoxication is characterized by decreased mental status, substantially decreased respiration, miotic pupils, and absent bowel sounds (Sporer, 1999). Signs of opioid intoxication may include pinpoint pupils, drowsiness, slurred speech, and impaired cognition.

Prescription opioid analgesics may be abused and can lead to intoxication or overdose. OxyContin, an oral controlled-release formulation of oxycodone, has been abused by crushing the tablets and then snorting the powder; when taken in this way by people who have no tolerance to the drug, a single 80 mg dose (the highest strength available in a single tablet) can be fatal. Propoxyphene, meperidine, or tramadol can cause seizures.

Withdrawal syndrome

Signs of acute opioid withdrawal syndrome include watering eyes, runny nose, yawning, muscle twitching, hyperactive bowel sounds, and piloerection. Opioid withdrawal has very apparent physical symptoms and a fairly consistent time to onset from the last use (about 8 hours for short-acting opioids such as heroin or oxycodone), which is a prominent factor in repeated administration after development of tolerance. This is in contrast to delirium tremens from alcohol and sedatives, where minor signs of acute withdrawal often do not progress to severe withdrawal; the onset and severity of opioid withdrawal is consistent and predictable for the vast majority of daily users. Opioid withdrawal is treated with substitution of a long-acting opioid (methadone or buprenorphine) for detoxification over several days to months, or maintenance therapy over years combined with counseling and social services.

Long-term consequences

There are multiple consequences of opioid abuse, both to the abuser and to society. Heroin dependence is associated with increased mortality. In one study, the mortality rate of 115 untreated subjects with heroin dependence was 63 times that expected for a non-using group of the same age and sex distribution, and higher than a group of former heroin users in methadone maintenance programs (Gronbladh *et al.*, 1990). Contaminated drugs and inadequate sterile technique when injecting leads to localized and systemic infections (e.g. cellulitis, localized abscess at the injection site, endocarditis). Intravenous drug use with shared needles or syringes is associated with an increased risk of infection with a bloodborne pathogen, such as HIV, hepatitis B, and hepatitis C. Hepatitis C virus infection may also occur in those who abuse heroin but do not inject it. Transmission has been associated with tattooing (Howe *et al.*, 2005) and sharing of straws for intranasal insufflation (Tortu *et al.*, 2004). Long-term consequences of chronic heroin use may differ in nations such as Great Britain where licensed clinics distribute the drug to addicts and facilitate the use of sterile syringes.

On physical examination, posterior cervical lymphadenopathy may suggest early viral infection, especially with HIV. Hepatic enlargement may indicate acute hepatitis; a small, hard liver is consistent with chronic viral hepatitis, which is common among injection drug users who share needles. A heart murmur may indicate subacute bacterial endocarditis. The nasal septum should be examined for perforation from repeated intranasal insufflation (especially when cocaine is mixed with heroin and snorted).

Costs to society include lost work productivity due to intoxication or complications of use, healthcare costs for uninsured users with medical complications, prosecution and incarceration expenses for criminal offenses, and economic and psychological costs to the victims of crimes. Additional costs arise from transmission of diseases such as HIV and hepatitis to sexual contacts who are not themselves drug users.

Chronic use of opioid agonists can result in hyperalgesia, or development of abnormal sensitivity to pain (Ballantyne & Mao, 2003). This manifests clinically as the need for increased doses of opioids to maintain the same level of pain relief, and may explain the failure to achieve pain relief in some patients despite repeated increases of opioid dose (Weaver & Schnoll, 2007a). A possible form of hyperalgesia that has been proposed is narcotic bowel syndrome (Grunkemeier et al., 2007). Affected patients have chronic or recurring abdominal pain that worsens with continued or escalating dosages of opioids. Treatment involves early recognition, an effective physician–patient relationship, and tapering of the opioid (Grunkemeier et al., 2007).

Hallucinogens

Drugs considered hallucinogens are a diverse group of compounds, including lysergic acid diethylamide (LSD), designer drugs, and many others (phencyclidine, ketamine) that produce perceptual distortions. Hallucinogens produce perceptual distortions and cognitive changes with a clear sensorium and without impairment in level of consciousness or attention (Abraham et al., 1996). Use of LSD dropped off in the 1980s, but has increased in the 2000s with a lifetime prevalence of use of 13% among young adults (Wu et al., 2006).

Acute complications

Acute physiologic complications of hallucinogen intoxication rarely require medical treatment (Table 3.4). Ketamine can induce a state of virtual helplessness and pronounced lack of coordination. This is known to users as "being in a K-hole" and can be problematic if the user is in a public setting (Jansen, 1993).

In low-dose intoxication with phencyclidine (PCP, Angel Dust), the patient presents with nystagmus, confusion, ataxia, and sensory impairment. This is the only drug of abuse that causes a characteristic vertical nystagmus (it can also cause horizontal or rotatory nystagmus), which helps to identify it as the cause when a patient presents with intoxication by an unknown drug (Weaver & Schnoll, 2007b). Moderate phencyclidine intake may lead to a catatonic-like picture, with the patient staring blankly and not responding to stimuli; the eyes remain open, even though the patient is comatose. In high doses, it produces seizures and severe hypertension. The hypertension should be treated vigorously since it may cause hypertensive encephalopathy or intracerebral bleeding; intravenous antihypertensive medications should be administered to reduce blood pressure.

Table 3.4 Hallucinogen intoxication

Physiological effects	Psychological effects	Perceptual distortions
Pupillary dilatation	Anxiety	Intensification of perceptions
Tachycardia	Depression	Light trails behind moving objects
Diaphoresis	Paranoia	Micropsia (the sensation that the user is very small in relation to the surroundings)
Incoordination	Hallucinations	Macropsia (the sensation that the user is very large in relation to the surroundings)
Vomiting	Impaired judgment	Synesthesias (cross-linking of the five senses, e.g. "see the sounds, taste the colors")
Tremulousness	Ideas of reference (getting personal messages from the television or radio)	
Hyperreflexia	Depersonalization ("I am not real")	
Hyperthermia	Derealization ("this environment is not real")	
Seizures		

Malignant hyperthermia and seizures may occur with hallucinogen intoxication. Agitation, dry skin, and increased muscle tension are warning signs for hallucinogen hyperthermia. Phencyclidine can also cause life-threatening hyperthermia, with temperatures over 106° Fahrenheit, which may occur many hours after use.

The most effective treatment of phencyclidine intoxication is increasing its urinary excretion by acidifying the urine with ascorbic acid (Weaver & Schnoll, 2007b). Urine acidification should only be performed after it has been determined that the patient does not have myoglobinuria (indicating rhabdomyolysis) to prevent the development of acute renal failure. Some practitioners feel that the benefits of urine acidification are outweighed by the risks, especially in patients with hepatic or renal impairment. Phencyclidine can be deposited in adipose tissue and released over time, which may result in a prolonged state of confusion that can last for weeks; urine acidification may be helpful to deplete the drug.

Long-term consequences

The long-term consequence most commonly associated with hallucinogen use is flashbacks. A flashback is an episode in which certain aspects of a previous hallucinogen experience are re-experienced unexpectedly. The content varies widely and may include emotional or somatic components, but perceptual effects are re-experienced most commonly. This may consist of after-images, trails behind moving objects, flashes of color, or lights in the peripheral visual fields. These episodes last several seconds to several minutes and are self-limiting. Triggers include stress, exercise, use of other drugs (especially marijuana), or entering a situation similar to the original drug experience; they may also occur spontaneously. The unpredictability of flashbacks often provokes anxiety when they occur. Flashbacks are fairly rare and tend to decrease over time in frequency, duration, and intensity, as long as no additional hallucinogen is taken (Strassman, 1984). Flashbacks are unlikely to occur more than 1 year after the original hallucinogen experience. Treatment of flashbacks consists of supportive care, including reassurance that the episode will be brief. Benzodiazepines help reduce anxiety, but haloperidol can worsen flashbacks (Moskowitz, 1971).

Inhalants

Inhalants are volatile substances which produce chemical vapors that can be inhaled for psychoactive effects. Inhalants are second only to marijuana in likelihood of use by adolescents in the US (Johnson *et al.*, 2003) and inhalant abuse can persist into adulthood. Examples of abused inhalants include glue, drycleaning fluids (carbon tetrachloride), gasoline, aerosol propellants from whipped cream cans or deodorant sprays, amyl nitrite, butyl nitrite, nitrous oxide, and ether.

Acute complications

The most severe consequence from abuse of these substances is hypoxia or anoxia, and even a single use can cause death. Many of the solvents are similar to general anesthetics and sensitize the myocardium to catecholamines; fatal arrhythmias have been reported due to solvent abuse (Shepherd, 1989).

Treatment of short-term effects of these drugs involves clearing the drug through the respiratory system. Supplemental oxygen is administered for hypoxia and to enhance clearance of the inhalant. Antiarrhythmic medications can be given as needed.

Long-term consequences

Chronic use by industrial workers has caused peripheral neuropathies (Lolin, 1989), as well as hepatic, renal, and bone marrow damage (Marjot & McLeod, 1989). Cases of methemoglobinemia have been reported secondary to butyl nitrite abuse (Bogart *et al.*, 1986). Chronic complications of abuse usually clear if the person can be kept drug-free, though impairment of working memory and executive cognitive function has been reported.

Conclusion

Abuse of any psychoactive substance can result in medical consequences. Some classes of substances manifest noticeable difficulties, such as tachycardia and anxiety, immediately with stimulants at low doses. Some substances, such as tobacco and alcohol, may take years before long-term medical consequences are diagnosed. More direct routes of administration, such as intravenous injection, may also result in more severe medical consequences. Despite differences in timing of medical sequelae, all abused substances can result in significant medical problems for the individual user. Withdrawal syndromes also vary widely among the classes of abused substances, from unpredictable and potentially fatal alcohol withdrawal to a subtle stimulant withdrawal syndrome that results in depression and craving. A thorough history and physical examination may pick up findings consistent with medical sequelae of substance abuse. A clinician can then use this information appropriately to diagnose a substance use disorder and motivate the patient to address the addiction before additional medical sequelae develop.

References

Abraham, H. D., Aldridge, A. M. & Gogia, P. (1996). The psychopharmacology of hallucinogens. *Neuropsychopharmacology*, **14**, 285–98.

Agius, A. M., Smallman, L. A. & Pahor, A. L. (1998). Age, smoking, and nasal ciliary beat frequency. *Clinical Otolaryngology*, **23**, 227–30.

American Psychiatric Association (APA). (2000). *Diagnostic and Statistical Manual of Mental Disorders*, 4th edn, text revision. Washington DC: American Psychiatric Association.

Ballantyne, J. C. & Mao, J. (2003). Opioid therapy for chronic pain. *New England Journal of Medicine*, **349**, 1943–53.

Barsky, S. H., Roth, M. D., Kleerup, E. C. *et al.* (1998). Histopathologic and molecular alterations in bronchial epithelium in habitual smokers of marijuana, cocaine, and/or tobacco. *Journal of the National Cancer Institute*, **90**, 1198–1205.

Barton, M., Dubey, R. K. & Traupe, T. (2002). Oral contraceptives and the risk of thrombosis and atherosclerosis. *Expert Opinion on Investigational Drugs*, **11**, 329–32.

Beaconsfield, P., Ginsburg, J. & Rainsbury, R. (1972). Marihuana smoking. Cardiovascular effects in man and possible mechanisms. *New England Journal of Medicine*, **287**, 209–12.

Bogart, L., Bonsignore, J. & Carvalho, A. (1986). Massive hemolysis following inhalation of volatile nitrites. *American Journal of Hematology*, **22**, 327.

Bolla, K. I., Brown, K., Eldreth, D. *et al.* (2002). Dose-related neurocognitive effects of marijuana use. *Neurology*, **59**, 1337–43.

Budney, A. J., Hughes, J. R., Moore, B. A. & Vandrey, R. (2004). Review of the validity and significance of cannabis withdrawal syndrome. *American Journal of Psychiatry*, **161**, 1967–77.

Centers for Disease Control. (2005). Cigarette smoking among adults – United States, 2004. *Morbidity and Mortality Weekly Report*, **54**, 1121–4.

Chiriboga, C. A. (2003). Fetal alcohol and drug effects. *Neurologist*, **9**, 267–79.

Cicero, T. J., Inciardi, J. A. & Munoz, A. (2005). Trends in abuse of Oxycontin and other opioid analgesics in the United States: 2002–2004. *Journal of Pain*, **6**, 662.

Compton, W. M., Grant, B. F., Colliver, J. D. *et al.* (2004). Prevalence of marijuana use disorders in the United States: 1991–1992 and 2001–2002. *Journal of the American Medical Association*, **291**, 2114–21.

Cramer, C. & Davidhizar, R. (1999). FAS/FAE: impact on children. *Journal of Child Health Care*, **3**, 31–4.

Criqui, M. H. (2001). Peripheral arterial disease: epidemiologic aspects. *Vascular Medicine* **6**(Suppl. 3), 3–7.

Cushman, P. Jr. (1987). Delirium tremens: update on an old disorder. *Postgraduate Medicine*, **82**, 117–22.

Deutsch-Wenzel, R., Brune, H. & Grimmer, G. (1983). Experimental studies in rat lungs on the carcinogenicity and dose-response relationships of eight frequently occurring environmental polycyclic aromatic hydrocarbons. *Journal of the National Cancer Institute*, **71**, 539–44.

Eliasson, B. (2003). Cigarette smoking and diabetes. *Progress in Cardiovascular Diseases*, **45**, 405–13.

Ernst, T., Chang, L., Leonido-Yee, M. & Speck, O. (2000). Evidence for long-term neurotoxicity associated with methamphetamine abuse: a 1H MRS study. *Neurology*, **54**, 1344.

Fernandez-Ruiz, J., Gomez, M., Hernandez, M. *et al.* (2004). Cannabinoids and gene expression during brain development. *Neurotoxicity Research*, **6**, 389–401.

Fried, P. A. & Watkinson, B. (1990). 36- and 48-month neurobehavioral followup of children prenatally exposed to marijuana, cigarettes, and alcohol. *Journal of Developmental and Behavioral Pediatrics*, **11**, 49–58.

Glantz, S. A. & Parmley, W. W. (1995). Passive smoking and heart disease: mechanisms and risk. *Journal of the American Medical Association*, **273**, 1047–53.

Gocze, P. M., Szabo, I. & Freeman, D. A. (1999). Influence of nicotine, cotinine, anabasine and cigarette smoke extract on human granulosa cell progesterone and estradiol synthesis. *Gynecological Endocrinology*, **13**, 266–72.

Gold, M. S., Frost-Pineda, K. & Jacobs, W. S. (2004). Cannabis. In *Textbook of Substance Abuse Treatment*, 3rd edn, eds. M. Galanter & H. Kleber. Washington DC: American Psychiatric Publishing, pp. 167–88.

Gong, H. Jr, Fligiel, S., Tashkin, D. P. & Barbers, R. G. (1987). Tracheobronchial changes in habitual, heavy smokers of marijuana with and without tobacco. *American Review of Respiratory Diseases*, **136**, 142–9.

Gourgou, S., Dedieu, F. & Sancho-Garnier, H. (2002). Lower limb venous insufficiency and tobacco smoking. *American Journal of Epidemiology*, **155**, 1007–15.

Gouzoulis-Mayfrank, E., Daumann, J., Tuchtenhagen, F. *et al.* (2000). Impaired cognitive performance in drug free users of recreational ecstasy (MDMA). *Journal of Neurology, Neurosurgery and Psychiatry*, **68**, 719.

Gronbladh, L., Ohlund, L. S. & Gunne, L. M. (1990). Mortality in heroin addiction: impact of methadone treatment. *Acta Psychiatrica Scandinavica*, **82**, 223.

Grunkemeier, D. M., Cassara, J. E., Dalton, C. B. & Drossman, D. A. (2007). The narcotic bowel syndrome: clinical features, pathophysiology, and management. *Clinical Gastroenterology and Hepatology*, **5**, 1126.

Hecht, S. S. (2006). Cigarette smoking: cancer risks, carcinogens, and mechanisms. *Langenbeck's Archives of Surgery*, **391**, 603–13.

Henry, J. A., Jeffreys, K. J. & Dawling, S. (1992). Toxicity and deaths from 3,4-methylenedioxymethamphetamine ("ecstasy"). *Lancet*, **340**, 384.

Higgitt, A., Fonagy, P., Toone, B. & Shine, P. (1990). The prolonged benzodiazepine withdrawal syndrome: anxiety or hysteria? *Acta Psychiatrica Scandinavica*, **82**, 165.

Howe, C. J., Fuller, C. M., Ompad, D. C. *et al.* (2005). Association of sex, hygiene and drug equipment sharing with hepatitis C virus infection among non-injecting drug users in New York City. *Drug and Alcohol Dependence*, **79**, 389.

International Agency for Research on Cancer (IARC). (2004). *Tobacco Smoke and Involuntary Smoking. IARC Monographs on the Evaluation of Carcinogenic Risks to Humans*, vol. **83**. Lyon, France: IARC, pp. 1179–87.

Iversen, L. (2003). Cannabis and the brain. *Brain*, **126**, 1252–70.

Jansen, K. L. R. (1993). Non-medical use of ketamine. *British Medical Journal*, **306**, 601–2.

Johnson, M. K., Smith, R. P., Morrison, D. *et al.* (2000). Large lung bullae in marijuana smokers. *Thorax*, **55**, 340–2.

Johnston, L. D., O'Malley, P. M. & Bachman, J. G. (2003). *Monitoring the Future National Results on Adolescent Drug Use: Overview of Key Findings, NIH Pub. No. 03–5374*. Bethesda, MD: National Institute on Drug Abuse.

Johnston, L. D., O'Malley, P. M. & Bachman, J. G. (2002). *Monitoring the Future National Survey Results on Drug Use, 1975–2001, Vol. 1: Secondary School Students*. Rockville, Maryland: National Institute on Drug Abuse.

Kamholz, S. L. (2006). Pulmonary and cardiovascular consequences of smoking. *Clinics in Occupational and Environmental Medicine*, **5**, 157–71.

Karan, L. D., Dani, J. A. & Benowitz, N. (2003). The pharmacology of nicotine and tobacco. In *Principles of Addiction Medicine*, 3rd edn, eds. A. W. Graham & T. K. Shultz. Chevy Chase, MD: American Society of Addiction Medicine, Inc., pp. 225–48.

Klein, T. W., Friedman, H. & Specter, S. (1998). Marijuana, immunity and infection. *Journal of Neuroimmunology*, **83**, 102–15.

Kolodny, R. C., Masters, W. H., Kolodner, R. M. & Toro, G. (1974). Depression of plasma testosterone levels after chronic intensive marihuana use. *New England Journal of Medicine*, **290**, 872–4.

Laumon, B., Gadegbeku, B., Martin, J. L. *et al.* (2005). Cannabis intoxication and fatal road crashes in France: population based case-control study. *British Medical Journal*, **331**, 1371–6.

Lolin, Y. (1989). Chronic neurological toxicity associated with exposure to volatile substances. *Human Toxicology*, **8**, 293.

Mackay, J. & Eriksen, M. (2002). *The Tobacco Atlas*. Geneva: World Health Organization, pp. 24–7.

Mallampalli, A. & Guntupalli, K. K. (2006). Smoking and systemic disease. *Clinics in Occupational and Environmental Medicine*, **5**, 173–92.

Marjot, R. & McLeod, A. A. (1989). Chronic non-neurological toxicity from volatile substance abuse. *Human Toxicology*, **8**, 301.

Mittleman, M. A., Lewis, R. A., Maclure, M. *et al.* (2001). Triggering myocardial infarction by marijuana. *Circulation*, **103**, 2805–9.

Moskowitz, D. (1971). Use of haloperidol to reduce LSD flashbacks. *Military Medicine*, **136**, 754–6.

Mueller, B. A., Daling, J. R., Weiss, N. S. & Moore, D. E. (1990). Recreational drug use and the risk of primary infertility. *Epidemiology*, **1**, 195–200.

Naditch, M. P. (1974). Acute adverse reactions to psychoactive drugs, drug usage, and psychopathology. *Journal of Abnormal Psychology*, **83**, 394–403.

Otsuka, R., Watanabe, H., Hirata, K. *et al.* (2001). Acute effects of passive smoking on the coronary circulation in healthy young adults. *Journal of the American Medical Association*, **286**, 436–41.

Pagliaro, A. M. & Pagliaro, L. A. (2003). Alcohol and other drug use during pregnancy: effect on the developing fetus, neonate, and infant. In *Principles of Addiction Medicine*, 3rd edn, eds. A. W. Graham & T. K. Shultz.

Chevy Chase, MD: American Society of Addiction Medicine, Inc., pp. 1247–58.

Prummer, M. F. & Wiersinga, W. M. (1993). Smoking and risk of Grave's disease. *Journal of the American Medical Association*, **269**, 479–82.

Schuckit, M. A. & Tapert, S. (2004). Alcohol. In *Textbook of Substance Abuse Treatment*, 3rd edn, eds. M. Galanter & H. Kleber. Washington DC: American Psychiatric Publishing, pp. 151–66.

Seger, D. L. (2004). Flumazenil – treatment or toxin. *Journal of Toxicology – Clinical Toxicology*, **42**, 209–16.

Shepherd, R. T. (1989). Mechanism of sudden death associated with volatile substance abuse. *Human Toxicology*, **8**, 287.

Silverman, R. A., Boudreaux, E. D., Woodruff, P. G. *et al.* (2003). Cigarette smoking among asthmatic adults presenting to 64 emergency departments. *Chest*, **123**, 1472–9.

Sidney, S. (2003). Comparing cannabis with tobacco – again. *British Medical Journal*, **327**, 635–6.

Smith, S. M. (1997). Alcohol-induced cell death in the embryo. *Alcohol Health & Research World*, **21**, 287–97.

Sporer, K. A. (1999). Acute heroin overdose. *Annals of Internal Medicine*, **130**, 584–90.

Sridhar, K. S., Raub, W. A. Jr, Weatherby, N. L. *et al.* (1994). Possible role of marijuana smoking as a carcinogen in the development of lung cancer at a young age. *Journal of Psychoactive Drugs*, **26**, 285–8.

Strassman, R. J. (1984). Adverse reactions to psychedelic drugs: a review of the literature. *Journal of Nervous and Mental Disease*, **172**, 577–95.

Substance Abuse and Mental Health Services Administration. (2006). *Results from the 2005 National Survey on Drug Use and Health: National Findings (Office of Applied Studies, NSDUH Series H-30. Rockville*, MD: DHHS Publication No. SMA 06–4194).

Tashkin, D. P., Shapiro, B. J., Lee, Y. E. & Harper, C. E. (1976). Subacute effects of heavy marihuana smoking on pulmonary function in healthy men. *New England Journal of Medicine*, **294**, 125–9.

Tashkin, D. P., Coulson, A. H., Clark, V. A. *et al.* (1987). Respiratory symptoms and lung function in habitual heavy smokers of marijuana alone, smokers of marijuana and tobacco, smokers of tobacco alone, and nonsmokers. *American Review of Respiratory Diseases*, **135**, 209–16.

Taylor, B. V., Oudit, G. Y., Kalman, P. G. *et al.* (1998). Clinical and pathophysiological effects of active and passive smoking on the cardiovascular system. *Canadian Journal of Cardiology*, **14**, 1129–39.

Taylor, D. R., Fergusson, D. M., Milne, B. J. *et al.* (2002). A longitudinal study of the effects of tobacco and cannabis exposure on lung function in young adults. *Addiction*, **97**, 1055–61.

Thompson, P. M., Hayashi, K. M., Simon, S. L. *et al.* (2004). Structural abnormalities in the brains of human subjects who use methamphetamine. *Journal of Neuroscience*, **24**, 6028.

Toomey, R., Lyons, M. J., Eisen, S. A. *et al.* (2003). A twin study of the neuropsychological consequences of stimulant abuse. *Archives of General Psychiatry*, **60**, 303.

Tortu, S., McMahon, J. M., Pouget, E. R. & Hamid, R. (2004). Sharing of noninjection drug-use implements as a risk factor for hepatitis C. *Substance Use & Misuse*, **39**, 211.

Turner, R. C., Lichstein, P. R., Peden, J. G. Jr, Busher, J. T. & Waivers, L. E. (1989). Alcohol withdrawal syndromes: a review of pathophysiology, clinical presentation, and treatment. *Journal of General Internal Medicine*, **4**, 432–44.

Vine, M. F. (1996). Smoking and male reproduction: a review. *International Journal of Andrology*, **19**, 323–37.

Weaver, M. F. (2003). Perinatal addiction. In *Principles of Addiction Medicine*, 3rd edn, eds. A. W. Graham & T. K. Shultz. Chevy Chase, MD: American Society of Addiction Medicine, Inc., pp. 1231–46.

Weaver, M. F. & Schnoll, S. H. (1999). Stimulants – amphetamines, cocaine. In *Addictions: A Comprehensive Guidebook*, eds. B. S. McCrady & E. E. Epstein. New York: Oxford University Press, p. 105.

Weaver, M. F. & Schnoll, S. H. (2007a). Addiction issues in prescribing opioids for chronic nonmalignant pain. *Journal of Addiction Medicine*, **1**, 2–10.

Weaver, M. F. & Schnoll, S. H. (2007b). Phencyclidine and ketamine. In *Treatments of Psychiatric Disorders*, 4th edn, ed. G. O. Gabbard. Washington DC: American Psychiatric Publishing, Inc., pp. 271–80.

Weaver, M. F., Jarvis, M. A. E. & Schnoll, S. H. (1999). Role of the primary care physician in problems of substance abuse. *Archives of Internal Medicine*, **159**, 913–24.

Wiesbeck, G. A., Schuckit, M. A., Kalmijn, J. A. *et al.* (1996). An evaluation of the history of a marijuana withdrawal syndrome in a large population. *Addiction*, **1**, 1469–78.

Wilson, R. & Rayner, C. F. (1995). Bronchitis. *Current Opinion in Pulmonary Medicine*, **1**, 177–82.

Wu, L. T., Schlenger, W. E. & Galvin, D. M. (2006). Concurrent use of methamphetamine, MDMA, LSD, ketamine, GHB, and flunitrazepam among American youths. *Drug and Alcohol Dependence*, **84**, 102–13.

Wu, T. C., Tashkin, D. P., Djahed, B. & Rose, J. E. (1988). Pulmonary hazards of smoking marijuana as compared with tobacco. *New England Journal of Medicine*, **318**, 347–51.

Zevin, S., Saunders, S., Gourlay, S. G. *et al.* (2001). Cardiovascular effects of carbon monoxide and cigarette smoking. *Journal of the American College of Cardiology*, **38**, 1633–8.

Zuckerman, B., Frank, D. A., Hingson, R. *et al.* (1989). Effects of maternal marijuana and cocaine on fetal growth. *New England Journal of Medicine*, **320**, 762–68.

Theory

Suicide and substance abuse

Samoon Ahmad

To be, or not to be.
(*Shakespeare: Hamlet*)

That is, to live or not to live. This is one of the most famous lines in the English language, spoken by Hamlet when he examines the moral ramifications of living and dying and whether to commit suicide. Many patients with mental illness and substance abuse, who so often wonder whether it is nobler to suffer or actively seek to end their suffering, share this quandary. Menninger (1938) conceived of addiction to drugs as a protracted form of suicide.

This chapter will address this issue in the context of the epidemiology and phenomenology of self-destructive (suicidal) behavior. Suicide is the leading cause of premature death among the mentally ill, particularly those with substance abuse disorders. Despite this very high association, a majority of this population does not receive mental health or substance abuse treatment. In recent times, much attention has been paid to the prevention of suicide among those with mental illness alone, while those with substance abuse disorders have had far less consideration.

Epidemiology

The mind is its own place, and in itself can make a heaven of hell, a hell of heaven.

(*John Milton*)

Suicide is the eleventh leading cause of death in the general population and the third among adolescents. A review of the literature suggests that more than 80% of the people who commit suicide have some form of mental illness or substance abuse disorder, and approximately more than 30 000 lives are lost annually to suicide. According to the CDC (Centers for Disease Control and Prevention), there is a suicide every 16 minutes; in 2005, suicide accounted for 32 637 deaths among people of all ages. The total lifetime economic cost of self-injurious behavior approaches 33 billion dollars. In the US, 12 out of every 100 000 people kill themselves every year and, according to several studies, alcohol abuse is an associated factor in at least one-quarter of all suicides. Several studies suggest that alcohol is second only to affective illness among the psychiatric disorders associated with suicide.

Suicide remains the leading cause of death among teenagers, young adults, and those over age 65, bypassing all other diseases, including heart disease, AIDS, cancer, stroke, and diabetes. There are variations in suicide rates by age, gender, and ethnicity. Non-white women attempt suicide more frequently than men while in general white men commit suicide more. Caucasians commit suicide more than blacks. Native American/Alaskan adolescents in the age group 15–24 have a suicide rate of twice the national average. Among Native American women, suicide rates are two to three times higher than women in the general population.

Rates among men of all ages are four times higher than women and are the eighth leading cause of death. Suicide is the third leading cause of death among 15–24-year-olds, and in the age range 15–19, four times as many men as women die by suicide (CDC, 2006); among the 20–24-year age group, more than six times as many men as women committed suicide (CDC, 2006), and for every completed suicide in the 15–24-year age group, there were 100–200 attempted suicides.

The suicide rates are also high among the older age group. There are about 15 suicides per 100 000 people aged 65 and older. This is in contrast to the national average of 11 suicides per 100 000 people in the general population (CDC, 2006). In those aged 75 and older, rates are three times higher than average and risk factors include being divorced, widowed, or suffering from a physical ailment.

Clinical Addiction Psychiatry, ed. D. Brizer and R. Castaneda. Published by Cambridge University Press. © Cambridge University Press 2010.

The most common methods used to commit suicide are firearms, poison, and suffocation, although men and women employ different methods.

Role of substance abuse

Substance abuse disorder remains the second leading cause of suicide after depression and carries a six times greater than average risk. Though actual numbers vary, some reports suggest that 60% of completed suicides occur among substance abusers. The most likely drug identified among the victims is alcohol, affecting one-third of the tested victims and found in as many as 25–45% of people who commit suicide. According to one study (NIMH, 2000), 20% of all non-traffic injury deaths associated with alcohol intoxication were suicides.

A review of the literature shows that alcohol is indeed a significant risk factor for suicide, and disinhibition may be the primary reason. A recent report suggests that drinking within 3 hours of a suicide attempt is the most important alcohol-related risk factor for nearly lethal suicide attempts. Many of these alcoholics kill themselves accidentally and alcohol intoxication may increase the chances of a suicide attempt becoming successful. Other studies suggest that alcohol may induce depression, cognitive impairment and aggressive tendencies, and hence increase suicidal behavior.

Heroin addicts commit suicide at an earlier age than alcoholics and the general population. The rates of suicide in heroin addicts range from 82 per 100 000 to 350 per 100 000.

These data identify substance abuse as a major contributor to completed suicide. In the US, approximately 100 lives are lost daily to suicide alone, bypassing HIV and homicide combined. The DAWN data for 2001 showed that in drug-related visits to the emergency room, 30% of the respondents reported suicide as the motive for taking drugs.

The high rates of suicide among substance abusers can be attributed to the fact that, of the 23 million people in need of substance abuse treatment, only 2–3 million actually receive treatment. There are major gaps in recognizing and understanding the relationship between substance abuse and suicide.

Despite medical, psychiatric, and social understanding, the rates of suicide have remained stable for the past 50 years. Suicide impacts friends, family, and the community in general. Many people are reluctant to ask for help as there is significant stigma associated with suicide, including the comorbid conditions of mental and substance abuse disorders.

Co-occurring disorders

There is a strong association between alcohol use and depression. This comorbidity suggests that 50–70% of the people who commit suicide suffer from both depression and alcohol abuse. The rate of major depression among alcoholics varies from 8 to 98%. This wide variation in range is secondary to the method of diagnosis and the type of population studied. However, current substance abuse alone remains a risk factor and predictor for both suicidal ideation and unplanned attempts. Drug overdoses and most frequently alcohol ingestion account for 80% of all unsuccessful suicide attempts. Research shows that the number of drugs used is more predictive of suicidal gestures than the type of substances used. However, the impact of different drug categories and drug combinations remains unclear. According to Moscicki (1997), addictive disorders and actual intoxication are among the greatest predictors of suicide.

According to Goldston's (2004) review, substance abuse and suicide share some risk factors, including depression, impulsivity, and thrill-seeking behavior. It should also be pointed out that the comorbidity of mental illness and substance abuse leads to significantly higher risk of suicide than each of the conditions alone. A co-occurrence may also promote increased drug use in depression and that may ultimately contribute to depression or other mood disorders. Patients with bipolar disorder and alcohol abuse compared to bipolar alone had a 39% lifetime rate of attempted suicide versus 22%, respectively. According to one estimate, approximately 17 million adults experienced depression and 10% attempted suicide. The rates for suicide climbed to 20% when illicit drugs were added to this equation, highlighting the magnitude of the co-occurring disorders.

A study by Roy (2003) showed that, of the 175 attempted suicides among 449 drug-dependent patients, those who attempted suicide had greater lifetime comorbidity with major depression. Data from the National Survey on Drug Use and Health suggest that patients with major depressive disorder use significantly more illicit drugs, cigarettes, and alcohol. Many people who struggle with suicidal thoughts use drugs to suppress their thoughts and resulting shame. These findings highlight that these subjects may be self-medicating their mood disorders, and in fact suicide risk remains higher even in those who are in remission from alcohol use.

Suicide risk factors

- Recent loss of close interpersonal relationship
- Recent loss of socioeconomic status or occupational role
- White
- Within 45–65 age group
- Male
- Acute intoxication
- Co-occurring mental and substance use disorder
- Prior history of suicide attempt
- Hopelessness
- Lack of social support
- Family history of suicide
- Difficulty in accessing healthcare and drug treatment
- Impulsive behavior
- History of abuse

High risk population

It has been observed that alcoholics kill themselves more often than do non-alcoholics. The suicide rate among alcoholics is 7–20% higher than the general population. The relationship between alcohol and suicide shows that 37% of people who commit suicide have a measurable blood alcohol level at the time of death versus 47% of people who attempt suicide.

Alcohol- and drug-related suicide attempts remain a major reason for emergency room visits, particularly among those aged 12–17 years. According to the Substance Abuse and Mental Health Services Administration (SAMHSA, 2008), in 2005 there were 132 500 visits to the emergency room for alcohol- or drug-related suicide attempts, while in 2004 there were 15 000 drug-related suicide attempts, of which 75% required hospitalization. Alcohol is the most frequently identified substance, and is present in about one-third of those tested. According to a 2005 survey, approximately 17% of US high school students contemplated suicide in the previous 12 months and 8% attempted suicide. According to a SAMHSA 2003 national survey, 8–15% adolescents who died by suicide had received mental health treatment within the past month and 25% had received treatment within the previous year. Rates of depression among youth tend to be higher, yet are underestimated and may also lead to suicide ideation, gesture, or attempts.

Adolescents and youth remain at a very high risk for suicide. According to Curley (1994), for every eight teenagers, one has considered suicide and 35% cited drug abuse as the main reason. Adolescents and college students who use marijuana are three times more likely to consider suicide and 10% have contemplated suicide.

Students who drink alcohol, use illicit drugs, or smoke cigarettes are more likely to consider suicide when compared to those who do not use illicit drugs. In a study by Yuen (2000), the greatest predictors of suicide attempt were depression, substance abuse, grade level, cultural affiliation, and household wage earners' education level. According to the CDC (SAMHSA, 2008), Alaskan Natives and Native Americans are also considered high-risk populations for suicide attempts and this is related to drug and alcohol consumption. According to Taylor (2002), alcohol and other drugs may be abused to suppress suicidal thoughts and the resulting shame.

The rates of suicide among youth in the criminal justice system remain high. According to one study done between 1996 and 1999 (http://health.utah.gov/vipp/suicide/suicideData.html, accessed 10 June 2010), among 151 consecutive suicides (age 13–21), 63% had some contact with juvenile justice and 54% had one or more referral for substance abuse, possession, or use.

Passive suicidal behavior is as dangerous as a gesture or an active act. Many of these individuals indulge in risky behaviors, including needle sharing, accidents, impulsive and reckless behavior, and, more commonly, overdoses. It is only in recent times that suicide has attracted much attention and has been recognized as a complex phenomenon with interplay of genetic, social, and biological factors. Apart from these factors, culture plays an important role, some considering suicide immoral while others consider it honorable.

Phenomenology and conditioning model

As alcoholics tend to have higher suicide rates, it is important to understand the model for addictive behaviors.

Many addicted persons are lucid and realistic in assessing many situations and are not suffering from major mental illnesses or psychotic disorders. They also do not engage purposefully in self-harmful behavior while not abusing drugs. On the flip side, while under the influence of drugs the same people cause a great deal of self-harm by engaging in risky behaviors and exposing themselves to fatal accidents or mortal illness. These individuals employ the defense of denial and engage in self-destructive behaviors in response to a complex sequence of conditioned behaviors.

According to Wikler (1973), the emergence of craving behavior despite any physiologic withdrawal may be precipitated by certain stimuli that evoke the phenomenon of withdrawal. According to him, addictive drugs exert direct effects on the CNS while also producing contrary responses. It is these responses that may lead to physiologic events/withdrawals. This behavior is based on classic conditioning as in Pavlov's experiments where food (unconditioned stimulus) is presented to the dog to evoke salivation and then paired with another conditioned stimulus (bell) repeatedly. Eventually the bell (conditioned stimulus) will alone evoke the original response (salivation), which is now the conditioned response.

Many psychological states, such as anxiety and depression, may serve as precipitant factors for administering drugs and after repeated administration the resulting dysphoria may then become the conditioned stimulus. This conditioned response is then experienced as craving for the addictive drug. The conditioned stimulus serves to elicit the behavioral response before the addict experiences withdrawal feelings and seeks out drugs. These conditioned responses could vary and include going to a bar or a party, a known drug neighborhood or upon experiencing anxiety or depression.

Assessment, prevention and treatment

> Even one death by suicide is one death too many.
>
> *Charles G. Curie, SAMHSA Administrator, July 14, 2002*

Suicide is a major public health concern, affecting people of all ages and ethnicities; it requires a tailored approach to screening and intervention. Concern about suicide is also increasing, both on an individual basis and at a community level. It is essential that key factors implicated in suicide be identified. According to Loebel (2005), suicide is the product of multiple causes and requires a multifaceted approach.

> A focus on the primary prevention of alcohol and drug use disorders and other psychopathological disorders associated with suicide, as well as intervention for those showing early indication of such disorder, are needed in order to have a meaningful impact on the population rate of suicide.
>
> *Wilcox et al. (2004)*

> A skillful doctor cures illness when there is no sign of disease, and thus the disease never comes.
>
> *Liu An, second century Chinese Philosopher*

Since the dawn of civilization, the topic of suicide has been a taboo, hence frequently ignored and, until recently, it has received little attention. As public awareness has increased about the devastating effects of suicide on families and communities, suicide has become more visible on the public health radar screen (US Public Health Service, 1999; 2001; New Freedom Commission on Mental Health, 2003). Despite all of the attention over the past decade, it is still a poorly understood phenomenon and is recognized as the product of the complex interaction of numerous factors, including biological, environmental, sociocultural, interpersonal, psychological, genetic, and neurological spectra (US Public Health Service, 2001; Goldsmith *et al.*, 2002). To add to this complexity, many healthcare providers do not properly recognize the symptoms of mental health disorders and subtle signs that signify suicidal thoughts, ideations or impending attempts.

Over the past decade, numerous programs and agencies have been set up for suicide prevention initiatives. As youth are particularly vulnerable to suicide, the Garret Lee Smith Memorial Act was established to set up a program that addresses youth suicide. SAMHSA has set up a toll-free hotline (the National Suicide Prevention Lifeline), a suicide prevention resource center, and screening for comorbid mental illness. A protocol to devise best practices has been established and, in addition, SAMHSA has developed a treatment improvement protocol specifically to address substance abuse and suicide prevention.

In recent years, there has been a tremendous push by various organizations to transform the healthcare system to better recognize the risk factors for suicide and its prevention. The Surgeon General's Call for Action on Suicide was a major initiative. The National Strategy on Suicide Prevention and New Freedom Commission on Mental Health Report also supported this. There has been a push to identify specific risk factors and implement protective factors.

Gould (2003) identified protective factors that include:

- Strong family and community support
- Restricting access to lethal means of suicide
- Improving access to support and clinical intervention

- Effective treatment for comorbid disorders (substance abuse and mental health)
- Religious and cultural beliefs that discourage suicide (Suicide Prevention Resource Center, 2008).

Moscicki has highlighted the importance of significant environmental interventions to prevent suicide by reducing psychiatric and substance abuse morbidity (in Goldsmith, 2001). An "upstream approach" has been suggested by the US Department of Health and Human Services. This approach focuses on bringing prevention to people in an integrative model to assess, diagnose, and treat. It further suggests identifying, adapting, and advancing evidence-based programs tailored to the cultural, community, and developmental norms of program participants. As youth are more vulnerable to suicide, it is imperative to intervene early to prevent alcohol and drug abuse and reduce the increased risk of suicide. According to Kessler *et al.* (2005), there is a 5-year window of opportunity to intervene early by identification and treatment of mental health problems that can delay subsequent substance abuse and suicide risk. The American Academy of Pediatrics (AAP) has taken steps in urging the greater involvement by pediatricians in assessing the suicide risk and intervening early, thereby reducing suicide among adolescents.

More recently, much attention is being paid to the role of primary care providers to screen for suicide risk. According to the Institute of Medicine (2002), 40% of people who died by suicide had seen a clinician within the month before the suicide. Other studies suggest that more than 80% of those who died by suicide had seen a primary care provider within a year before committing suicide (Mann *et al.*, 2005). A report by Loebel in 2005 highlights even more grim statistics. In one study, 41% had contacted a healthcare professional within a month of death, 47% within a week, and 18% on the day of death. This suggests that clinicians often neglect to ask, discuss, or diagnose suicidal intent among patients, specifically in elderly and older adults.

To reduce suicide effectively, it is important to collaborate on treatment for substance abuse as well as advance suicide prevention programs. A report by SAMHSA shows that there was a 25% decrease in the frequency of substance abuse among the high-risk youth population, highlighting the effectiveness of prevention programs. This suggests more overlap and partnership is successful in helping to solve these problems. Some examples of community-based, state and federal groups and agencies that have helped to identify, screen, diagnose, and reduce suicide include:

- The Surgeon General's Call to Action to Prevent Suicide in 1999
- Federal Steering Group
- National Council for Suicide Prevention
- Association for Education and Research in Substance Abuse (AMERSA)
- National Institute on Drug Abuse (NIDA).

The recommendations of these agencies include:

- A full-time suicide prevention representative designated within the federal steering group
- Establishing a public/private partnership to implement national strategy for suicide prevention
- Design mass media campaigns that highlight associations between smoking, drug use, and suicide.

Future activities to enhance suicide prevention should include:

- Collaborate with Alcoholics Anonymous (AA) and Narcotics Anonymous (NA) to discuss suicide prevention strategies among the members
- Increase awareness regarding the link between substance abuse and suicide
- Train substance abuse healthcare professionals in identifying at-risk populations
- Provide ongoing continuing education, and establish suicide prevention-related exams
- Each and every person suffering from substance abuse disorder should be offered an awareness and education package regarding suicide risk.

The National Strategy for Suicide Prevention established goals and objectives for action that are outlined below:

- Integration of suicide prevention into mental health and substance abuse programs
- Promote support through faith-based groups to destigmatize mental illness, substance abuse and suicide
- Equal reimbursement for mental health/substance abuse disorders
- Develop community-based suicide prevention programs
- Integrate suicide prevention programs into Employee Assistance Programs (EAPs)

- Educate teachers, school staff, school health personnel, clergy, police officers, correctional personnel, and emergency healthcare providers to recognize at-risk behaviors and effective intervention strategies
- Increase substance abuse centers and mental health clinics throughout the country.

There has been a push to implement programs that are more evidence-based and demonstrate effectiveness in reaching desired outcomes. According to SAMHSA, from 50 such programs only 10 have relevance to the prevention of suicide and substance abuse. Some of the evidence-based programs, especially those targeted at the high-risk elderly, adolescent, and youth population, are listed below.

- Dialectical behavior therapy
- American Indian life skills development
- Coping and support training
- Emergency room intervention for adolescent females
- Prevention of suicide in primary care elderly
- Signs of suicide.

It is necessary to reduce the stigma of mental illness, increase awareness about substance abuse and suicide, and implement effective prevention programs. This requires coordinated efforts on the part of the treatment providers, state and federal agencies, as well as a broad-based campaign to educate patients, families, and communities. Despite all the progress made so far, a great deal of work remains to be done.

References

Goldsmith, S. K., (ed.) (2001). *Risk Factors for Suicide: Summary of a Workshop*. Washington, DC: National Academies Press.

Goldsmith S. K., Pellmar, T. C., Kleinman, A. M., Bunny, W. E. (eds) (2002). *Reducing Suicide: A National Imperative*. Washington, DC: National Academies Press.

Goldston, D. B. (2004). Conceptual issues in understanding the relationship between suicidal behavior and substance use during adolescence. *Drug and Alcohol Dependence*, 76(1), S79–91.

Gould, M. S., Greenberg, T., Velting, D. M. & Shaffer, D. (2003). Youth suicide risk and preventive interventions: a review. *Journal of the American Academy of Child and Adolescent Psychiatry*, 42, 386–405.

Institute of Medicine (2002). *Reducing Suicide: A National Imperative*. Washington, DC: National Academy Press.

Kessler, R. C., Borges, G. & Walters, E. E. (1999). Prevalence of and risk factors for lifetime suicide attempts in the national co-morbidity survey. *Archives of General Psychiatry*, 56, 617–26.

Loebel, J. P. (2005). Completed suicide in late life. *Psychiatric Services*, 56(3), 260–2.

Mann, J. J., Apter, A., Pertolote, J. *et al.*(2005). Suicide prevention strategies: a systematic review. *Journal of the American Medical Association*, 284(16), 2064–74.

Menninger, K. (1938) *Man Against Himself*. New York: Harcourt Brace and Company.

Moscicki, E. K. (1997). Identification of suicide risk factors using epidemiological studies. *Psychiatric Clinics of North America*, 20, 499–517.

New Freedom Commission on Mental Health (2003). *Achieving the Promise: Transforming Mental Health Care in America*. Final Report. DHHS Pub. No. SMA-03-3832. Rockville, MD: U.S. Department of Health and Human Services.

Roy, A. (2003). Characteristics of drug addicts who attempt suicide. *Psychiatry Research*, 121, 99–103.

Substance Abuse and Mental Health Services Administration. (2002). *Report to Congress on the Prevention and Treatment of Co-occurring Substance Abus Disorder*. Rockville, MD: US Department of Health and Human Services.

Substance Abuse and Mental Health Services Administration. (2008). *Substance Abuse and Suicide Prevention: Evidence and Implications. A White Papter*. U.S. Department of Health and Human Services. Rockville, MD: SAMHSA.

Suicide Prevention Resource Center. (2008). Risk and protective factors for suicide. www.sprc.org/library/srisk.pdf. Ref taken from: *Substance Abuse and Suicide Prevention: Evidence and Implications–A White Paper*. Rockville, MD: US Department of Health and Human Services Substance Abuse and Mental Health Services Administration.

Taylor, K. (2002). *Seduction of Suicide: Understanding and Recovering from Addiction to Suicide*. Bloomington, IN: 1st Books Library.

USDHHS, US Public Health Service [PHS] (1999). *The Surgeon General's Call to Action to Prevent Suicide 1999*. Washington DC: Public Health Service.

USDHHS, US Public Health Service [PHS] (2001). *National Strategy for Suicide Prevention: Goals and Objectives for Action*. Rockville, MD: Public Health Service.

Wikler, A. (1973). Dynamics of drug-dependence. *Archives of General Psychiatry*, 28, 611–16.

Wilcox, H. C., Conner, K. R. & Caine, E. D. (2004). Association of alcohol and drug use disorders and completed suicide: an empirical review of cohort studies. *Drug and Alcohol Dependence*, **76S**, S11–S19.

Yuen, N. Y. C. (2000). Cultural identification and attempted suicide in native Hawaiian adolescents. *Journal of the American Academy of Child and Adolescent Psychiatry*, **3**, 360–7.

Bibliography

American Association of Suicidology [AAS] (2001). Alcohol consumption and nearly lethal suicide attempts. Supplement to suicide and life-threatening behavior. *The Official Journal of the American Association of Suicidology*, **32**, 30–41.

American College Health Association (2007). *American College Health Association – National College Health Assessment: Reference Group Data Report – Fall 2006.* Baltimore, MD: American College Health Association.

Arias, E., Anderson, R. N., Kung, H. C., Murphy, S. L. & Kochanek, K. D. (2003). Deaths: final data for 2001. *National Vital Statistics Reports,* **52**(3). Hyattsville MD: National Center for Health Statistics.

Borges, G., Walter, E. E. & Kessler, R. C. (2000). Associations of substance use, abuse and dependence with subsequent suicidal behavior. *American Journal of Epidemiology*, **151**(8), 781–9.

Bronisch, T. & Wittchen, H. (1994). Suicidal ideation and suicide attempts: comorbidity with depression, anxiety disorders, and substance abuse disorder. *European Archives of Psychiatry and Clinical Neurosciences*, **244**, 93–8.

Bunker, J. P., Frazier, H. S. & Mosteller, F. (1994). Improving health: measuring effects of medical care. *Milbank Quarterly*, **72**, 225–58.

Caine, E. D. (2004). *Population Based Approaches to Suicide Prevention in Later Life.* Presented at the annual meeting of the American Association of Geriatric Psychiatry, Baltimore, MD: February 22–26, 2004.

Center for Mental Health Services (2007). *Promotion and Prevention in Mental Health: Strengthening Parenting and Enhancing Child Resilience, DHHS Publication No. CMHS-SVP-0175.* Rockville, MD: US Department of Health and Human Services.

Center for School Mental Health Assistance [CSMHA] (2001/2002). The interface between expanded school mental health and substance-related services for youth. *On the Move With School-Based Mental Health*, **6**(3), 1.

Centers for Disease Control and Prevention, National Center for Injury Prevention and Control (2006a). Web-based injury statistics query and reporting system (WISQARS): leading causes of death reports, 1999–2005. From http://webappacdc.gov/sasweb/ncipe/leadcaus10.html (accessed March 5, 2008).

Centers for Disease Control and Prevention, National Center for Injury Prevention and Control (2006b). Substance abuse and suicide prevention: evidence and implications; a white paper; Center for Substance Abuse and Mental Health Services Administration, U.S. Department of Health and Human Services.

Centers for Disease Control and Prevention, National Center for Injury Prevention and Control (2007). Suicide: facts at a glance. From http://www.cdc.gov/ncipc/dvp/Suicide/SuicideDataSheet.pdf. last accessed 10/20/09

Chambliss, J. W. (2001). *Saving Lives in Georgia: Together We Can. The Georgia Suicide Prevention Plan.* Atlanta: SPANUSA.

Cherpitel, C. J., Borges, G. L. G. & Wilcox, H. C. (2004). Acute alcohol use and suicidal behavior: A review of the literature. *Alcoholism: Clinical and Experimental Research*, **28**(5), 18S–28S.

Conner, K. R. & Chiapella, P. (2004). Alcohol and suicidal behavior: Overview of a research workshop. *Alcoholism: Clinical and Experimental Research*, **28**(5), 2S–5S.

Conner, K. R., Duberstein, P. R., Conwell, Y. *et al.* (2000). After the drinking stops: completed suicide in individuals with remitted alcohol use disorders. *Journal of Psychoactive Drugs*, **32**(3), 333–7.

Cornelius, J., Salloum, I. *et al.* (1995). Disproportionate suicidality in patients with comorbid major depression and alcoholism. *American Journal of Psychiatry*, **152**, 358–64.

Elliott, A. J. (1995). Profile of medically serious parasuicide: importance of substance induced mood disorder. *American Psychiatric Association Annual Meeting*, **10**.

Elliott, A., Pages, K., Russo, J. *et al.* (1996). A profile of medically serious suicide attempts. *Journal of Clinical Psychiatry*, **57**, 567–71.

Evangelical Lutheran Church in America [ELCA] (1999). *A Message on Suicide Prevention.* Chicago: Department for Studies, Division of Church in Society.

Frances, A., Fyer, M. & Clarkin, J. (1986). Personality and suicide. *Annals of the New York Academy of Sciences*, **487**, 281–93.

Georgia Council on Substance Abuse (2001). *The Courage to Change: A Report on Substance Abuse in Georgia.* Atlanta: GA Power and Accenture for Georgia Council on Substance Abuse.

Hanson, G. R. (2002). New vistas in drug abuse prevention. *NIDA Notes*, **16**(6), 3–7.

Harris, E. D. & Barraclough, B. (1997). Suicide as an outcome for mental disorders. *British Journal of*

Psychiatry, **170**, 205–28. http://health.utah.gov/vipp/suicide/suicideData.html

Henriksson, M. M., Aro, H. M., Marttunen, M. J. *et al.* (1993). Mental disorders and comorbidity in suicide. *American Journal of Psychiatry*, **150**(6), 935–40.

Inskip, H. M., Harris, E. C. & Barraclough, B. (1998). Lifetime risk of suicide for affective disorder, alcoholism, and schizophrenia. *British Journal of Psychiatry*, **172**, 35–7.

Jones, G. D. (1997). The role of drugs and alcohol in urban minority adolescent suicide attempts. *Death Studies*, **21**, 189–202.

Murphy, G. (1992). *Suicide in Alcoholism.* New York: Oxford University Press.

Murphy, G. & Wetzel, R. (1990). The lifetime risk of suicide in alcoholism. *Archives of General Psychiatry*, **47**, 383–92.

Murphy, G., Wetzel, R., Robins, E. & McEvoy, L. (1992). Multiple risk factors predict suicide in alcoholism. *Archives of General Psychiatry*, **49**, 459–63.

Murphy, S. L., Rounsaville, B. J., Eyre, S. & Kleber, H. D. (1983). Suicide attempts in treated opiate addicts. *Comprehensive Psychiatry*, **24**(1), 79–89.

Nevada Legislative Commission's Subcommittee to Study Suicide Prevention (2002). *Subcommittee Meeting Minutes for February 2, 2002.* Las Vegas: Nevada Legislative Commission.

Nielsen, D., Virkkunen, M. *et al.* (1998). A tryptophan hydroxylase gene marker for suicidality and alcoholism. *Archives of General Psychiatry*, **55**, 593–602.

Norstrom, R. (1995). Alcohol and suicide: a comparative analysis of France and Sweden. *Addiction*, **90**, 1463–9.

Office of National Drug Control Policy [ONDCP] (2000). Year 2000 emergency department data from the drug abuse warning network. From http://www.whitehouse drugpolicy.gov/news/yearend2000/dawn.html (accessed March 22, 2002).

Ohberg, A. (1996). Alcohol and drugs in suicides. *British Journal of Psychiatry*, **169**, 75–80.

Pages, K., Russo, J. *et al.* (1997). Determinants of suicidal ideation: the role of substance use disorders. *Journal of Clinical Psychiatry*, **58**, 510–15.

Potash, J. B. (2000). Attempted suicide and alcoholism in bipolar disorder: clinical and familial relationships. *American Journal of Psychiatry*, **157**, 2048–50.

Rossow, I. (1994). Suicide among drug addicts in Norway. *Addiction*, **89**, 1667–73.

Rossow, I. & Amundsen, A. (1995). Alcohol abuse and suicide: a 40 year prospective study of Norwegian conscripts. *Addiction*, **90**, 685–91.

Roy, A. (2001). Characteristics of cocaine dependent patients who attempt suicide. *American Journal of Psychiatry*, **158**, 1215–19.

Roy, A. (2002). Characteristics of opiate dependent patients who attempt suicide. *Journal of Clinical Psychiatry*, **63**, 403–7.

Suominen, K., Henriksson, M., Suokas, J. *et al.* (1996). Mental disorders and comorbidity in attempted suicide. *Acta Psychiatrica Scandinavica*, **94**(4), 234–40.

Tanney, B. L. (2000). Psychiatric diagnoses and suicidal acts. In *Comprehensive Textbook of Suicidology*, eds. R. W. Maris, A. L. Berman & M. M. Silverman. New York: Guilford Press, pp. 311–41.

US Department of Health and Human Services [USDHHS], Substance Abuse and Mental Health Services Administration, Center for Mental Health Services, National Institutes of Health, & National Institute of Mental Health (1999). *Mental Health: A Report of the Surgeon General.* Rockville, MD: USDHHS.

USDHHS & Centers for Disease Control and Prevention [CDC] (2001). *Suicide Prevention Now: Linking Research to Practice.* Atlanta: CDC.

USDHHS, SAMHSA, & Center for Substance Abuse Treatment [CSAT] (2000a). *Improving Substance Abuse Treatment. The National Treatment Plan Initiative. Changing the Conversation.* Rockville, MD: USDHHS.

USDHHS, SAMHSA, & CSAT (2000b). Improving substance abuse treatment. *The National Treatment Plan Initiative: Panel Reports, Public Hearings, and Participant Acknowledgements. Changing the Conversation.* Rockville, MD: USDHHS.

USDHHS, Substance Abuse and Mental Health Services Administration [SAMHSA] (2001). *Summary of Findings from the 2000 National Household Survey on Drug Abuse (NHSDA Series: H-13, DHHS Publication No. SMA 01–3549).* Rockville, MD: USDHHS.

Web-based Injury Statistics Query and Reporting System (WISQARS): Nonfatal injury reports. From http://web appa.cdc.gov/sasweb/ncipc/nfirates2001.html (accessed February 10, 2010).

Abstinence as a goal

Laurence M. Westreich

Introduction

Abstinence: 1. Denial of the appetites. 2. Habitual abstention from alcoholic beverages.

Webster's II New Riverside University Dictionary (1994)

The word "abstinence" in the context of addiction is freighted with multiple meanings and connotations, not the least of which is the moral imperative to avoid bad or at least disreputable behavior. Most often used regarding sex education, teenagers are advised, logically enough, that "abstinence" is the only sure method for avoiding pregnancy, sexually transmitted diseases (http://www.choosingthebest.org/, accessed November 9, 2008), and, by implication, immoral behavior. Like "sobriety," the word "abstinence" suggests religious (Warner, 2008) and other meanings well beyond the intentions or control of most addiction treaters. Although most clinicians avoid the moral model of addiction which attributes substance use to a bad attitude or lack of willpower, the word "abstinence" is firmly entrenched in addiction's lexicon, and understanding the concept and its implications is necessary for the clinician who has any hope of communicating with an addicted person.

The example of sexual abstinence illustrates, by analogy, an important aspect of the problem for addiction treaters. Although it is undeniably true that sexual abstinence will prevent pregnancy and sexually transmitted disease, sexual abstinence is simply not adhered to by the vast majority of those eligible to practise it. Also, the definition of abstinence is blurry in this context: does oral sex break abstinence? Masturbation? These questions correlate with the multiple questions which can be asked about abstinence from substances: does using another substance break abstinence? Does tobacco? Does switching to compulsive eating or shopping constitute a breach of abstinence?

Those who have found recovery using Alcoholics Anonymous (AA) sometimes denigrate the very concept of "abstinence," making the point that mere cessation of substance use without changing other life patterns is hardly much of a benefit. This state of being is called being a "dry drunk," and necessitates (according to some) embracing AA and living a healthy life, as opposed to simply stopping the substance use.

A bright line exists between those addictions where a true abstinence is theoretically possible (cocaine, alcohol) and those addictions where a true abstinence is either impossible (food) or undesirable (sex, shopping). For the "spectrum addictions" like food or sex, abstinence is usually defined as cessation of *compulsive* participation in the activity, with the acknowledgement that a healthy relationship with the activity is necessary or desirable, and a goal of treatment.

Despite these differences, recent data show that addictive behaviors involving sex (Childress *et al.* 2008), food (News Release, 2002), and gambling (Campbell-Meiklejohn *et al.*, 2008) share biological mechanisms with addiction to substances. Given these similarities, the history, theoretical underpinnings, and practical implications of using abstinence as a goal of addiction treatment deserve scrutiny.

History of abstinence

The Oxford Group, a spiritual movement of the 1920s and 1930s which was an important progenitor of AA, focused more on personal spiritual change than recovery from addiction and, not surprisingly, did not demand total abstinence from alcohol. When AA split from the Oxford Group in the late 1930s, AA published the *Big Book* and began its support of the abstinence ideal in phrases like "don't drink" (White, 1998).

Jellinek's *The Disease Concept of Alcoholism,* which was published in 1960 and is a seminal text in the movement towards conceptualizing alcoholism as a biological condition, characterized the dilemma that the traditional temperance societies faced regarding abstinence:

In the view of most American temperance societies, the idea that alcoholism is an illness is a threat to their educational efforts, which aim at total abstinence and the disappearance of alcoholic beverages. Such an interference is by no means a necessary development; but it must be admitted that in America, the "scientific literature" has concentrated to such a degree on the true alcohol addict and the problem drinker that other important problems arising from the use of alcoholic beverages have been neglected. The reluctance of other temperance societies to accept alcoholism as an illness also stems from their fear that such a conception might serve as an excuse for the "alcoholic."

One standard modern textbook of addiction expresses the surprisingly blasé viewpoint that:

A small minority of alcoholics are (sic) eventually able to drink in moderation but for several months after a heavy drinking bout total abstinence is desirable, for two reasons. First, the physician must follow the patient, sober, for a considerable period to diagnose a coexistent psychiatric problem. Second, it is important for the patient to learn that he or she can cope with ordinary life problems without alcohol.

Goodwin & Gabrielli (1997)

A more common, wide-ranging (and stringent) concept of abstinence has been formally approved (and implicitly encouraged) by the Board of the American Society of Addiction Medicine (1998):

Abstinence is "Non-use of a specific substance. In recovery, non-use of any addictive psychoactive substance. May also denote cessation of addictive behaviors, such as gambling, over-eating, etc."

Alcoholics Anonymous

Although AA promotes abstinence from alcohol and other mind-altering substances – the "first step" is acknowledging that one is powerless over alcohol (Alcoholics Anonymous World Services, 2002) – members lovingly support those who struggle with achieving that abstinence. In fact, one of the AA movement's main strengths is the non-judgmental attitude the active drinker experiences on entering the rooms. AA lore has it that the active drinker is the most important person in the room, and even intoxicated people are told that they are welcome in the meeting "as long as you can sit down and shut up!" So, while abstinence is clearly a goal in AA, the alcoholic is conceived of as a person struggling to achieve that abstinence, and having eventually achieved that state, always vigilant for threats to abstinence.

Of course, the viewpoints of different AA meetings can differ widely: commonly those who are not abstinent from alcohol and other mind-altering substances are expected to listen rather than participate actively in the meeting. Those who take maintenance opioid medications such as methadone and buprenorphine are often – though not always – similarly expected to remain silent during meetings. Appropriately prescribed psychotropic medications like fluoxetine (Prozac) have become so widely accepted that most AA meetings allow the person who is taking those medications to speak without any constraint. Official AA literature (Alcoholics Anonymous World Services, 1984), while warning the reader about the potential for addiction to medications, asserts that "No AA member plays doctor," and notes that "… just as it is wrong to enable or support any alcoholic to become readdicted to any drug, it's equally wrong to deprive any alcoholic of medication which can alleviate or control other disabling physical and/or emotional problems."

Moderation management

By contrast with AA, the much smaller program of moderation management (MM) suggests that some of those who evidence a problem with alcohol can avoid abstinence and return to social drinking. The program suggests that the "problem drinker" carefully assess his or her drinking behaviors, and then choose from a variety of behavior change choices. The MM program lays out a protocol for assuring that one's drinking is safe, and acknowledges that some may need to return to an abstinence-based program like AA.

Despite extensive publicity about MM founder Audrey Kishline's drunk driving incident which resulted in two fatalities (Heckman, 2000), MM actually provides an alternative for those who are unwilling or unable to try for full abstinence. In addition, as a prominent website about MM notes (http://www.moderation.org/faq/rightforme_full.shtml#faq13, accessed November 9, 2008), the MM program is perfectly compatible with those who are or wish to be abstinent from alcohol, but can also support those who have no desire to maintain abstinence.

Despite MM's common sense approach, the very idea of challenging an across-the-board need for abstinence can be highly provocative for those who have internalized the need for abstinence from alcohol as the only path back to a healthy lifestyle. In a notorious incident in 2000, the then-director of a well known addiction treatment program in New York City was dismissed from his position after inviting an MM group to become part of the therapeutic milieu at the facility (Szalavitz, 2000).

Harm reduction

The thematic focus of the harm reduction model differs from MM in a small but significant way – harm reduction proponents focus on reducing damage to those people using substances, and engaging those people in the development of treatment programs, thereby soft-pedaling abstinence as the goal in favor of the necessary strategies in the mean time. One well known organization, the Harm Reduction Coalition (http://www.harmreduction.org/article.php?list=type&;type=62m, accessed November 23, 2008) defines one of its primary goals as "… Accept(ing), for better and for worse, that licit and illicit drug use is part of our world and choos(ing) to work to minimize its harmful effects rather than simply ignore or condemn them…"

A classic harm reduction strategy is the needle exchange program (Sinding, 2005), in which intravenous drug users are offered clean needles in the hope that they will use their drugs as safely as possible. Although needle exchanges and other harm reduction programs have attracted their share of controversy, harm reduction's compatibility with the desire for abstinence has spared it the derision often directed towards MM. Perhaps this is because most addiction treaters of necessity recommend a sort of harm reduction policy as they guide their clients toward health and, yes, abstinence.

Overeaters Anonymous

Although total abstinence from substances like drugs and alcohol is at least possible, no such blanket abstinence is healthy for spectrum addictions like compulsive eating or compulsive sexuality. The 12-step program of Overeaters Anonymous (OA) promotes abstinence from those compulsive eating habits which promote weight gain and, more importantly for OA, an unhealthy self-conception. Rozanne S., OA's founder, came to a revelation while sitting in an AA meeting in 1962 which discussed the concept of abstinence:

> I thought to myself: that's what's wrong with all of us in OA. We're not abstaining from food at any time of the day. We have to close our mouths from the end of one

meal to the beginning of the next. Sometime during the day, we must "abstain" from eating: otherwise we're feeding our compulsion.

Overeaters Anonymous (1994)

In a later clear statement of purpose, an explication of OA's first step (we admitted we were powerless over food – that our lives had become unmanageable) reads: "Clearly, if we are to live free of the bondage of compulsive eating, we must abstain from all foods and eating behaviors which cause us problems" (Overeaters Anonymous, 1990).

Sexual Compulsives Anonymous

A variety of 12-step peer-led groups exist for the sexually compulsive, such as Sexual Compulsives Anonymous (http://www.sca-recovery.org/index.htm, accessed November 23, 2008), Sex Addicts Anonymous (http://www.saa-recovery.org/, accessed November 23, 2008), Sexaholics Anonymous (http://www.sa.org/, accessed November 23, 2008), Sexual Recovery Anonymous (http://www.sexualrecovery.org/, accessed November 23, 2008), and Sex and Love Addicts Anonymous (http://www.slaafws.org/, accessed November 23, 2008). Although none of these groups promote total abstinence from sexual behavior, they espouse varying views on what sort of sexuality is healthy and appropriate. Sexaholics Anonymous recommends sexual relationships only between married partners, and "(f)or the unmarried sexaholic, sexual sobriety means freedom from sex of any kind" (http://www.sa.org/, accessed November 23, 2008).

On the more liberal end of the spectrum, Sexual Compulsives Anonymous promotes a clearly defined sort of sexual abstinence from inappropriate sexuality: "We believe we are not meant to repress our God-given sexuality, but to learn how to express it in ways that will not make unreasonable demands on our time and energy, place us in legal jeopardy, or endanger our mental, physical or spiritual health" (http://www.sca-recovery.org/index.htm, accessed November 23, 2008).

Whatever the philosophical difference among the various peer-led compulsive sexuality groups, all acknowledge that sexuality – like eating – can be healthy and life-affirming rather than destructive. Although the strictness of the control may be different, all advocate a control of sexual behavior rather than total abstinence from it. One popular book on the subject puts that philosophy succinctly:

The myth that controlling our sexuality is against nature is a sad mistake. In order to live with other members of society, we must be able to modify our behaviors…It's natural to control ourselves in order to live peacefully with others and to live peacefully within ourselves.

Sbraga & Donohue (2003)

Abstinence as a therapeutic concept

Abstinence from all potentially addictive substances is the default recommendation for most of those who treat addiction, and for good reason. Clinical observation, common sense, and research data (Witkiewitz, 2008; Self & Nestler, 1998; Milkman *et al.*, 1983) support the proposition that anyone who has had a problem with a substance is vulnerable to becoming addicted again, or becoming addicted to another substance. That said, thinking of what is of most benefit to those suffering from addiction, the clinician should present abstinence as a goal of treatment, rather than demanding that the addicted person immediately become abstinent (ludicrous) or commit to a lifetime of abstinence (not too likely at the beginning of treatment). For those addicts who will not countenance the idea of abstinence, the harm reduction model can provide a healthier alternative to simply abandoning oneself to ongoing addiction, and can keep the user alive until (and if) he or she gets to an abstinent state.

However, those of us who promote abstinence as a first choice must carefully avoid overly concrete interpretations of the concept, which risk sabotaging the efforts of those addicted people we treat. In addition to discouraging people in early recovery, a too-zealous focus on abstinence can demoralize even those in strong recovery. Termed the abstinence violation effect (AVE) by psychologists (Stephens *et al.*, 1994) and, a bit more pungently, "getting a case of the fuck-its" by AA members, an illogical over-attribution of value to abstinence itself can produce guilt and feelings of loss of control in the lapser, thereby promoting more substance use.

Conclusions

Although the term "abstinence" has unfortunate moral and sexual connotations, it is in fact the goal towards which most addiction treaters direct their clients. Cleansed of its historical overtones, the idea of eschewing all use of the addictive substance is undeniably an important treatment goal, but the effective clinician will decide judiciously on how hard to push this concept with a particular individual. Many in early recovery cannot even think about the possibility of committing to a lifetime without their substance – a problem which AA intelligently approaches with its "one day at a time" dictum. Some addicted people may insist on a lifetime of researching the possibilities of using addictive substances in the hopes that their lives will not be destroyed. For others, however, a goal of abstinence will serve as the rock of their improved circumstances of physical and emotional health, work engagement, and relationships. It is up to the thoughtful clinician to choose an approach to abstinence which works best for the suffering addict.

References

Alcoholics Anonymous World Services, Inc. (1984). *The A.A. Member – Medications and Other Drugs*. New York, NY: AA Service.

Alcoholics Anonymous World Services, Inc. (2002). *The Big Book*, 4th edn.

American Society of Addiction Medicine (1998). *Principles of Addiction Medicine*, 2nd edn. Appendix B. Chevy Chase: American Society of Addiction Medicine.

Campbell-Meiklejohn, D. K., Woolrich, M. W., Passingham, R. E. & Rogers, R. D. (2008). Knowing when to stop: the brain mechanisms of chasing losses. *Biological Psychiatry*, **63**(3), 293–300.

Childress, A. R., Ehrman, R. N., Wang, Z. et al. (2008). Prelude to passion: limbic activation by "unseen" drug and sexual cues. *PLoS ONE*, **3**(1), e1506. doi:10.1371/journal.pone.0001506, accessed November 9, 2008.

Goodwin, D. W. & Gabrielli, W. F. (1997). Alcohol: clinical aspects. In *Substance Abuse, A Comprehensive Textbook*, 3rd edn, eds. J. H. Lowinson, P. Ruiz, R. B. Millman & J. C. Langrod. Baltimore, MD: Williams & Wilkins, p. 146.

Heckman, C. (2000). *Seattle Post-intelligencer Reporter*: arrest trips up 'moderate drinking' crusader's cause: movement's founder sent to prison for two DUI fatalities. *Friday*, August 11, 2000.

Milkman, H., Weiner, S. E. & Sunderwirth, S. (1983). Addiction relapse. *Advances in Alcohol & Alcohol Substance Abuse*, **3**(1–2), 119–34.

News Release (2002). New food-addiction link found, mere sight/smell of food spikes levels of brain "pleasure" chemical. *Brookhaven National Laboratory*, 02–40, 5/20/02.

Overeaters Anonymous (1990). *The Twelve Steps and Twelve Traditions of Overeaters Anonymous*. Rio Rancho, NM: Overeaters Anonymous, Inc.

Overeaters Anonymous (1994). *Abstinence, Members of Overeaters Anonymous Share Their Experience, Strength, and Hope*. Rio Rancho, NM: Overeaters Anonymous, Inc.

Sbraga, T. P. & O'Donohue, W. T. (2003). *The Sex Addiction Workbook*. Oakland, CA: New Harbinger Publications, Inc.

Self, D. W. & Nestler, E. J. (1998). Relapse to drug-seeking: neural and molecular mechanisms. *Drug and Alcohol Dependence*, **51**(1–2), 49–60.

Sinding, S. W. (2005). Does 'CNN' (condoms, needles and negotiation) work better than 'ABC' (abstinence, being faithful and condom use) in attacking the AIDS epidemic? *International Family Planning Perspectives*, **31**(1), 38–40.

Stephens, R. S., Curtin, L., Simpson, E. E. & Roffman, R. A. (1994). Testing the abstinence violation effect construct with marijuana cessation. *Addictive Behaviors*, **19**(1), 23–32.

Szalavitz, M. (2000). Drink Your Medicine. The Smithers rehab center stuns the AA faithful by cutting out a few steps. *New York Magazine*, 1 Comment Add Yours 00 Comments |Add Yours Jul 3, 2000.

Warner, J. (2008). *The Day George Bush Stopped Drinking: Why Abstinence Matters to the Religious Right*. McClelland & Stewart.

Websters's II New Riverside University Dictionary (1994). Boston, MA: The Riverside Publishing Company/ Houghton Mifflin.

White, W. L. (1998). The birth of Alcoholics Anonymous: a brief history. In *Slaying the Dragon, The History of Addiction Treatment and Recovery in America*, ed. W. L. White. Bloomington, IL: Chestnut Health Systems.

Witkiewitz, K. (2008). Lapses following alcohol treatment: modeling the falls from the wagon. *Journal of Studies on Alcohol*, **69**(4), 594–604.

6 Ibogaine therapy for substance abuse disorders

Deborah C. Mash

Introduction

Ibogaine is a naturally occurring psychoactive indole alkaloid derived from the roots of the rainforest shrub *Tabernanthe iboga*. Ibogaine is used by indigenous peoples of Western Africa in low doses to combat fatigue, hunger, and thirst, and in higher doses as a sacrament in religious rituals (Goutarel *et al.*, 1991).

The use of ibogaine for the treatment of drug dependence was based on anecdotal reports by groups of self-treating addicts that the drug blocked opiate withdrawal and reduced craving for opiates, cocaine, and other illicit drugs for extended time periods (Shepard, 1994; Alper *et al.*, 1999). Preclinical studies supported these early claims and provided proof-of-concept in animal models (Dzoljic *et al.*, 1988; Glick *et al.*, 1992).

Addiction is a behavioral pattern of drug abuse characterized by compulsive use, loss of behavioral control, and a high tendency to relapse. An integrated medical, psychosocial, and spiritual treatment is often needed to achieve recovery in addicted patients. Ibogaine is a unique pharmacotherapy for the treatment of substance abuse disorders because it fosters a life change or may work as a transition-based therapy similar to the goals set in the 12-step fellowship programs. While ibogaine's effects on behavior are complex, the beneficial actions of the drug on withdrawal symptoms and cravings are because of an interaction of the active metabolite noribogaine with neurotransmitters in the brain reward and addiction circuit.

Historical overview

Ibogaine is an indole alkaloid found in the root bark of *Tabernanthe iboga* (Apocynaceae family), a shrub that grows in West Central Africa. The forest-dwelling pygmy populations attribute the discovery of the plant to the warthogs (Barabe, 1982). *Tabernanthe iboga* or Iboga is a perennial rainforest shrub and hallucinogen. In parts of Africa where the plant grows, the bark of the root is chewed for various pharmacological or ritualistic purposes.

Iboga stimulates the central nervous system (CNS) when taken in small doses and induces visions in larger doses. Discussion of the CNS and cardiovascular actions of ibogaine has appeared in the literature since the early 1900s (Popik *et al.*, 1995). In the 1950s, CIBA investigated ibogaine as an antihypertensive agent, but were unconvinced of its commercial potential. The general interest in the Apocynaceae family (of which *Tabernanthe iboga* is a member) led scientists to pursue chemical, pharmacological, and behavioral studies of ibogaine (Pouchet & Chevalier, 1905; Lambert & Heckel, 1901; Phisalix, 1901). The French pharmacologists Lambert, Heckel, and Pouchet studied the pharmacology of ibogaine early in the 20th century (Hoffer & Osmond, 1967). Ibogaine was marketed in France under the tradename *Lambarene* until 1970.

The putative anti-addictive properties of ibogaine were first described by Howard Lotsof (1995). He reported that ibogaine administration led to an active period of visualizations that were described as a "waking dream state," followed by an intense cognitive phase of "deep introspection." Drug-dependent individuals who received ibogaine treatment reported that the visions usually center on early childhood, traumas, or other significant life events. Some reported that the experience gave them insights into their addictive and self-destructive behaviors. Opiate- and cocaine-dependent subjects reported an alleviation or, in some cases, a complete cessation of drug "craving" for extended periods of time, and some addicts remained drug-free for several years thereafter. Most astounding were the reports of opiate-dependent patients who stated that ibogaine completely blocked the symptoms of opiate withdrawal.

An informal self-help network provided ibogaine treatments from 1987 until 1993 to addicts in Europe (Shepard, 1994). Based on his own experience and that of six of his friends, Howard Lotsof formed a

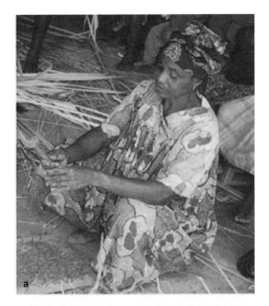

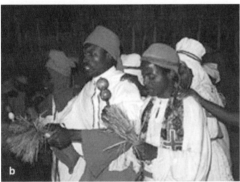

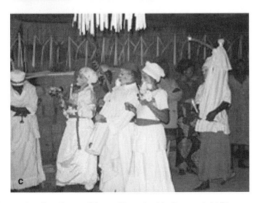

Figure 6.1 Ritual use of iboga (ibogaine) in Equatorial Africa. Ibogaine is considered a "sacred" plant substance by the Fang Bwiti religious movement. The Bwiti take the plant extract in the hope that they will discover the path of life and death, a discovery that saves one from a confused and wandering state within the deep equatorial forest. (a) Woman preparing *Tabernanthe iboga* root. The roots are scraped, dried, and powdered. The iboga plant is considered "mature" after 4 years. Parts (b) and (c) illustrate the traditional ceremony. The Bwiti priest is joined by initiates dressed in white who are followed by a woman carrying sacred iboga to be placed on the altar. Photographs courtesy of Eneka Onono (BBC London).

company and filed a series of US patents describing a method for treating narcotic, psychostimulant, nicotine, alcohol, and polydrug dependence with ibogaine (US Patents 4 499 096; 4 587 243; 4 857 523). In 1993, the Drug Abuse Advisory Panel of the US FDA reviewed and granted us a phase 1 pharmacokinetic and safety trial in male subjects (IND 39 680). This clinical protocol was initially limited to include only ibogaine veterans. In April of 1995, the FDA approved a revised clinical protocol to conduct these studies in cocaine-dependent male volunteers. A dose run-up and safety evaluation of ibogaine hydrochloride in human volunteers was never completed owing to a lack of funds to support US clinical trials.

Varieties of human ibogaine experience

Ibogaine has been used in equatorial Africa in a ritual context associated with the Fang Bwiti religion. The Bwiti are a Central African religious group whose usage of *Tabernanthe iboga*, the plant source of ibogaine, forms an integral part of their society. There are estimated to be approximately 2–3 million members of the Bwiti religion scattered in groups throughout the countries of the Gabon, Zaire, and Cameroun. Most are from the two principal tribal groups of the region, the Fang and the Mitsogho. The origins of the religion are obscure, but most writers seem to believe Bwiti is essentially derived from pygmy religious traditions.

The rootbark of the *Tabernanthe iboga* plant, usually referred to as 'iboga' or 'eboka', is taken in large doses for the Bwiti initiation ritual, a powerful 'rebirth' ceremony that group members typically undergo before the commencement of their teenage years (Fig. 6.1). Both sexes are initiated and the ceremony typically lasts 3 days, beginning on a Thursday afternoon and ending on Sunday morning. The consumption of iboga is supervised by the "nganga," a senior priest of the religion whose knowledge of iboga's effects on the body and mind is such that he or she is aware of when the initiate has had a sufficient, non-toxic dose of the root bark. The overall objective of the ritual is to allow the initiate to enter deeply into the subconscious mind with the intent of emerging "reborn." The initiate is expected to actually meet the original Bwiti, the founders of the religion, in the form of primordial male and female figures, but only after the terrors that lurk before them have been overcome. The Bwiti take the plant extract in the hope that they will discover the path of life and death, a discovery that saves one from a confused and wandering state within the deep equatorial forest (Fermandez & Fernendez, 2001).

Ibogaine has had a variety of uses, ranging from a trypanocide (antiparasitic) to an adjunct for psychotherapy (Naranjo, 1969; 1973). The psychotropic effects of oral ibogaine administration to drug-dependent patient volunteers has been observed in offshore studies (Mash *et al.*, 1998; 2001). Guidance was provided to prepare patients and to provide psychological support during and after the ibogaine experience. A semi-structured elicitation narrative was used to capture perceptual changes and subjective interpretation of the effects of ibogaine. Patients that met DSM-IV criteria for dependence on cocaine (n = 30; 10 females, 20 males) or opiates (n = 30; 11 females, 19 males) were included. Subjects narrated their subjective experience of oral dose ibogaine HCl administration, including changes in sensation and perceptions. The interviewer, trained in open-ended elicitation techniques, obtained descriptions of the acute drug effects. After an initial stimulus question, the interviewer used a guided questionnaire to obtain specific content areas. The main content areas were sensations, perceptions, and interpretations of the experience. A content coding scheme was developed to capture key elements from the narrative. Cross-coding was repeated until the coders achieved greater than 90% agreement.

Ibogaine administered in a single *po* dose in the range of 10 mg/kg resulted in active visualizations similar to a waking dream state lasting between 4 and 8 hours. After this time, subjects reported that the major drug effects had subsided, but subjects remained introspective and in a calm and quiet state for the remaining 20–24 hours post-dose medical monitoring period. Only 61% of the subjects reported the experience of visual effects (Table 6.1). Visual images or hallucinations were reported by 55% of the subjects. There were common elements to the subjective experiences of drug-dependent patients treated with ibogaine. Table 6.2 lists commonly cited perceptual content (self-reports). A common perception was that the experience was "dream-like" or that the subject felt that he or she was observing a film or movie. Often, the content centered on early childhood or critical life events. Unlike opiate-dependent patients, the cocaine

Table 6.1 Sensory and perceptual changes

Visual effects/dimensionality	61.7%
Visual images, hallucinations	55.0%
Feeling of being "high"	50.0%
Change in quality of thinking	50.0%
Change in rate of thinking	46.7%

Using the hallucinogen rating scale (Strassman *et al.*, 1994). $n = 60$, $P < 0.05$.

Table 6.2 Self-reports of ibogaine experience

Dreamlike state	45.0%
Able to resist/control experience[a]	
Cocaine-dependent subjects	40.0%
Opiate-dependent subjects	16.7%
As film or movie	36.7%
Passive/outside observer	28.3%
Life review	16.7%
Unaware of reality/immersed in experience	11.7%

Semi-structured elicitation narrative and coding of content were used to obtain common areas of content. [a]Categories with significant differences between opiate- and cocaine-dependent groups. $n = 60$, $P < 0.05$.

Table 6.3 Frequently reported interpretations of the ibogaine experience

Given insight	86.7%
Need to become sober/abstinent now	68.3%
Cleansed/healed/reborn	50.0%
Second chance at life	40.0%
Increased self-confidence	33.3%
Impending self-destruction if drug use continued	18.3%

Semi-structured elicitation narrative. $n = 60$, $P < 0.05$.

abusers more frequently reported a desire to resist or control the experience. Clients' interpretation of the benefit of the experience is summarized in Table 6.3. The most common elements were a renewed sense of self and insight into destructive behaviors. These observations support early investigations into the purported therapeutic uses of ibogaine by psychiatrist Claudio Naranjo (1969). Although further studies in controlled environments are undoubtedly necessary, these initial findings suggest that ibogaine may have therapeutic benefit when used as an adjunct to brief intervention to promote abstinence in drug-dependent populations.

Opiate detoxification with ibogaine

Early, albeit anecdotal, observations suggested that ibogaine was effective in blocking opiate withdrawal symptoms after only a single dose administration. These claims were supported by preclinical studies in animals, providing proof-of-concept. Ibogaine decreased naloxone-precipitated withdrawal in morphine-dependent rats (Glick *et al.*, 1991), and reduced or interrupted morphine self-administration in rats for several days after a single drug administration (Popik *et al.*, 1995). These effects were dose-dependent. These seminal observations suggested that ibogaine or an unidentified metabolite blocked opiate withdrawal, but the pharmacologic mechanisms of action were unknown.

Physical dependence on opiates is characterized by a distinctive pattern of signs and symptoms that make up the opiate/opioid withdrawal syndrome. The physical dependence produced by an opiate usually emerges following discontinuation of medication (spontaneous withdrawal) or by antagonist-precipitated withdrawal. We reviewed a case series of opiate-dependent clients who were seeking ibogaine treatment and who demonstrated active dependence by clinical evaluation, objective observations, and positive urine toxicology screens (Mash *et al.*, 2000; 2001). Utilizing the objective opiate withdrawal scale (OOWS), two physicians rated (as present or absent) physical signs typically associated with opiate withdrawal during a 10-minute period of observation (Mash *et al.*, 2000; 2001). The pre-ibogaine assessment was performed by the attending physician approximately 1 hour before ibogaine administration and 12 hours after the last dose of opiate. The next assessment was performed 24 hours following ibogaine administration and at 36 hours after the last opiate dose. Objective physician ratings were subjected to repeated measures analysis of variance (ANOVA) with the treatment phase as the within-subjects factor.

The physical dependence produced by an opiate was assessed by discontinuation of opioid treatment (spontaneous withdrawal). Ibogaine was administered in oral doses in a range of 10–12 mg/kg. Physician ratings demonstrated that ibogaine administration can facilitate rapid detoxification from heroin, methadone, and prescription opiates. The 36-hour post-ibogaine OOWS was significantly lower than at entry

(prior to ibogaine administration)(Mash *et al.*, 2000; 2001). These investigations suggest that ibogaine may be effective in reducing signs and symptoms of opiate withdrawal. Objective signs of opiate withdrawal were rarely seen and none became more severe at later time points (Mash *et al.*, 2000; 2001). The results suggest that ibogaine provides a safe and effective treatment for withdrawal from heroin, prescribed opiates, and methadone.

Self-report measures of withdrawal, cravings, and depression

The acute withdrawal syndrome in addicts deprived of heroin or methadone begins approximately 8 hours after the last heroin dose, peaks in intensity at 1–2 days and subjective symptoms subside within 7–10 days. The opiate-symptom check list (OP-SCL) was used to assess withdrawal symptoms, since many subjects' verbal reports about withdrawal experience are exaggerated both in number and severity of symptoms (Mash *et al.*, 2000; 2001). Subjects completed a series of standardized self-report instruments relating to mood and craving at three different time points and between 7 and 10 days after the last dose of opiate or cocaine (Mash *et al.*, 2000; 2001). Self-reported depressive symptoms were determined by the Beck Depression Inventory (BDI; Beck *et al.*, 1961). Scores were subjected to repeated measures analyses of variance across treatment phase (pre-ibogaine, post-ibogaine, and discharge) as the within-subjects factor for the total score from the OP-SCL and BDI.

Ibogaine was effective in reducing patients' self-reports of withdrawal symptoms in the dose range tested. Opiate craving increases during the early stages of withdrawal (Martin & Jasinski, 1969). Ibogaine subjects undergoing opiate detoxification reported significantly decreased drug craving for opiates on five measures taken from the heroin (HCQN-29) craving questionnaire at 36 hours post-treatment (Table 6.4). These measures inquired about specific aspects of drug craving, including urges, as well as thoughts about drug of choice or plans to use drug, the positive reinforcing effects of the drug, or the expectation of the outcome from using a drug of choice for the alleviation of withdrawal states. Perceived lack of control over drug use is a common feature of substance abuse disorders and is most operative under conditions of active use, relapse, or for subjects at high risk. Opiate-dependent

Table 6.4 Opiate craving in ibogaine-detoxified patients

Subscale	Pre-ibogaine	Post-ibogaine	Discharge at 1 month	Follow-up	$F_{(3, 24)}$	P
Desire to use	3.48	1.89	1.29	1.29	17.61	0.0001
Intention to use	2.79	1.51	1.20	1.20	26.63	0.0001
Expect positive outcomes	4.30	2.28	1.80	1.87	37.42	0.0001
Relief of negative states	4.63	3.38	2.78	2.31	9.99	0.0002
Lack of control	3.87	3.00	2.70	2.31	7.13	0.0014

Heroin craving questionnaire NOW (HCQN) was used to measure drug craving before and at 36 hours and 5–7 days after ibogaine detoxification from opiates. Lower means indicate less craving. A 1-month follow-up assessment demonstrates reduced cravings across all measures. For each subscale, all post-ibogaine means differ from pre-ibogaine at $P < 0.05$.

patients undergoing detoxification demonstrated that across these five craving measures, the mean scores were significantly decreased at program discharge (Mash *et al.*, 2001). Cocaine-dependent patients reported reduced craving using cocaine (CCNQ-29) craving questionnaires (Mash *et al.*, 2000), providing independent support for initial claims that ibogaine effectively blocks cocaine craving in the days to weeks after oral administration.

Depression, anxiety, and anergia are part of the postacute withdrawal syndrome that frequently leads to an early relapse in detoxified opiate patients. Post-acute withdrawal symptoms are caused by persistent physiological adaptation and disturbances in neurotransmitters, and are also caused by the hyperexcitability of specific neuronal pathways which results from chronic and long-term abuse. Ibogaine was effective in alleviating depression and anxiety, in diminishing anger and in improving vigor (Fig. 6.2). Ibogaine promotes appreciable shortening of the time course of both post and acute withdrawal symptoms when compared with self-reports from heroin- or methadone-dependent individuals undergoing sudden withdrawal; few to no adverse events were noted among the ibogaine subjects (Mash *et al.*, 2000; 2001). These results suggest that ibogaine is an effective drug for opiate detoxification and may be an alternative therapy for patients wishing to withdraw from opiates.

Identification of a primary metabolite of ibogaine

Ibogaine demonstrated long-lasting effects on withdrawal symptoms and drug craving in humans following a single dose and also showed persistent effects on drug self-administration in rodents (Glick *et al.*, 1991; Cappendijk & Dzoljik, 1993). These observations led us and others to search for a possible active metabolite of ibogaine. Our group developed an analytic method for quantifying ibogaine in blood samples from rats, primates, and humans (Hearn *et al.*, 1995b; Mash *et al.*, 1995a). Using full scan electron impact gas chromatography/mass spectrometry (GC/MS), a primary metabolite, 12-hydroxyibogamine (noribogaine), was detected for the first time in blood and urine samples. The analytic procedure involved a solvent extraction under basic conditions with D3-ibogaine as an internal standard. Urine taken from dosed monkeys and humans was extracted under strongly basic conditions and analyzed by GC/MS in full scan electron impact ionization mode (Hearn *et al.*, 1995a).

All samples were found to contain a second major component eluting after ibogaine. Similar spectral characteristics of this peak to ibogaine's spectrum defined it as an ibogaine metabolite, formed by loss of a methyl group (Fig. 6.3). The site for metabolic demethylation of ibogaine was the methoxy group, resulting in the compound 12-hydroxyibogamine (noribogaine). The identity of the desmethyl metabolite was confirmed using an authentic standard of noribogaine (OmniChem S.A., Belgium); this metabolite gave a single peak at the same retention time and with the same electron impact fragmentation pattern as the endogenous compound isolated from monkey and human urine (Hearn *et al.*, 1995b).

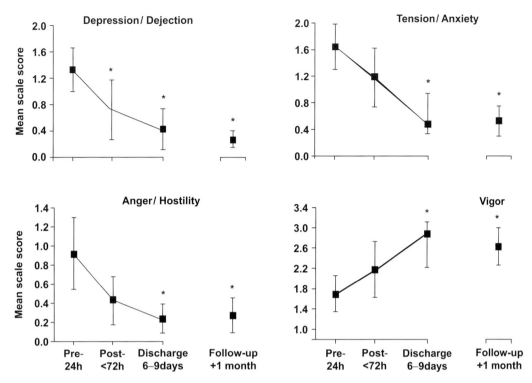

Figure 6.2 Profile of mood ratings in recently detoxified opiate addicts. Four profile of mood states (POMS) factors are shown (three negative valence; one positive valence). Subjects reported being less depressed, less anxious, less angry (or hostile), and feeling more vigorous post-ibogaine administration. The early trends become significant at program discharge. Subjects continued to report improved mood and increased vigor at the 1-month follow-up (mean values ± 1 s.d; n = 25).

Figure 6.3 Biotransformation of ibogaine to noribogaine. Ibogaine undergoes O-demethylation at the 12-position by the activity of liver enzymes. The gut wall metabolism of ibogaine contributes to the pre-systemic metabolism in humans.

Cytochrome P450 metabolism, genetic polymorphisms and pharmacokinetics

Like most CNS drugs, ibogaine is a highly lipophilic compound and is subject to extensive biotransformation. Ibogaine is metabolized to noribogaine in the gut wall and liver (Fig. 6.4). Ibogaine is O-demethylated to noribogaine primarily by cytochrome P4502D6 (CYP2D6). Ibogaine O-demethylase activity examined in pooled human liver microsomes suggested that two (or more) enzymes are involved in this reaction (Obach

et al., 1998). The enzyme CYP2D6 showed the highest activity toward the formation of 12-hydroxyibogamine (noribogaine), followed by CYP2C9 and CYP3A4 (Obach *et al.*, 1998).

Depending on whether a particular isoenzyme is present or absent, individuals are classified as extensive or poor metabolizers. The influence of genetic polymorphisms on the biotransformation of ibogaine under in-vivo conditions demonstrated that there are statistically significant differences in the two populations with regard to C_{max} and $t_{1/2}$ (elim)

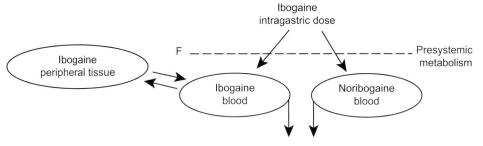

Figure 6.4 First-pass metabolism to noribogaine following oral administration. Ibogaine undergoes extensive first-pass metabolism in the liver and gut wall.

and area under the plasma concentration–time curve (AUC) of the parent drug and metabolite, indicating that the disposition of ibogaine is dependent on polymorphic CYP2D6 distribution (Mash *et al.*, 2000). Pharmacokinetic measurements were obtained from drug-dependent patient volunteers who had received single oral doses of ibogaine. Figure 6.5 illustrates the complex pharmacokinetic profiles of ibogaine and the metabolite following oral doses. CYP2D6 mediated metabolism of ibogaine, resulting in high levels of noribogaine in the blood, with C_{max} values in the same range as the parent drug. The time required to eliminate the majority of absorbed ibogaine (> 90%) was 24 hours post-dose (Fig. 6.5). The pharmacokinetic profiles measured in whole blood demonstrate that the concentrations of 12-hydroxyibogamine (noribogaine) measured at 24 hours remained elevated, which is in agreement with previous findings (Hearn *et al.*, 1995a). Elevated concentrations of noribogaine were measured in blood at 24 hours after drug administration, which limited the quantification of the terminal half-life of the metabolite. Noribogaine was measured in CYP2D6-deficient subjects, but at concentrations that were markedly lower than for the extensive metabolizers (Fig. 6.5). Conversion of the parent to noribogaine in CYP2D6-deficient subjects likely reflects the metabolic contribution of the other minor cytochromes (CYP2C9, CYP3A4). Pharmacokinetic measurements in human volunteers administered oral doses of ibogaine showed that the AUC for the parent compound was approximately threefold less than that of the active metabolite (Mash *et al.*, 2000). Thus, the active metabolite reach sustained high levels in blood after single administration of the parent drug with an extended terminal half-life.

Mechanisms underlying beneficial effects of ibogaine: role of the metabolite

Ibogaine's ability to alter drug-taking behavior may be caused by combined actions of either the parent drug and/or its active metabolite at key pharmacological targets that modulate the addiction circuit (Popik *et al.*, 1995; Staley *et al.*, 1996; Pablo & Mash, 1998). The active metabolite noribogaine has multi-target pharmacologic activities different from ibogaine. Noribogaine has selectivity for mu receptors and shows intrinsic activity at mu opioid receptors not seen with the parent drug. The affinity for mu receptors of the CNS is orders of magnitude lower than that of morphine. Noribogaine's efficacy as a mu opioid agonist most likely accounts for ibogaine's ability to block the acute signs of opiate withdrawal and its suppressive effects on morphine self-administration in rodent studies (Pablo & Mash, 1998).

Noribogaine also has significant monoaminergic activity that inhibits serotonin (5-hydroxytryptamine; 5-HT) reuptake (Mash *et al.*, 1995a; Staley *et al.*, 1996; Baumann *et al.*, 2000). Preclinical evaluation of noribogaine's anti-cocaine effects in rat models demonstrates that noribogaine antagonizes cocaine-induced locomotor stimulation and reinforcement (Mash & Schenk, 1996). Chronic cocaine increases kappa opioid receptor density, striatal dynorphin, and dynorphin gene expression in the striatum (Spangler *et al.*, 1996). The upregulation of kappa opioid receptors after cocaine treatment occurs predominantly in brain regions that are highly innervated by serotonin. The affinity of noribogaine for mu and kappa opioid and 5-HT transporter may underlie noribogaine's ability to antagonize the effects of cocaine in rodent models.

Ibogaine's effects on NMDA receptor-coupled cation channels accounts for the psychotropic (PCP-like

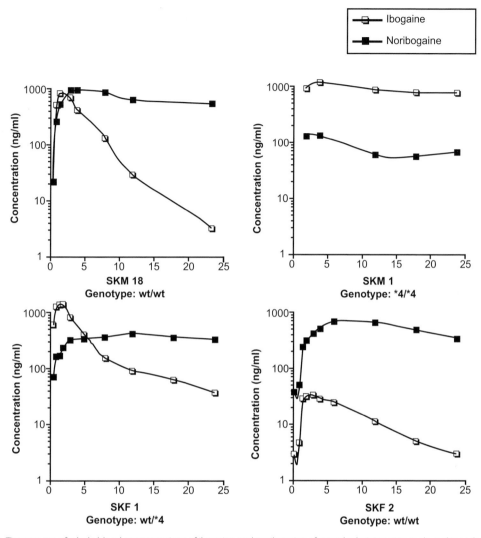

Figure 6.5 Time course of whole blood concentrations of ibogaine and noribogaine after oral administration to drug-dependent volunteers. Pharmacokinetics of ibogaine and noribogaine after oral doses in human subjects. Data shown are from representative male and female subjects. Values for parent drug and desmethyl metabolite were measured in whole blood samples at the times indicated. Males are shown in the top panels; females are shown in the lower panels. CYP2D6 genotypes illustrate fast, wt/wt; intermediate, wt/*4; and slow, *4/*4 metabolizers. SKF 2 was a CYP2D6 ultrarapid metabolizer genotype who had blockade of opiate withdrawal symptoms, but reported no visual changes or hallucinations. SK, St. Kitts, W.I.

actions) (Staley *et al.*, 1996; Mash *et al.*, 1995b). Noribogaine, unlike the parent drug, does not interact with this site, providing evidence for its lack of psychotropic effects at therapeutic blood levels. This suggestion is in keeping with metabolic and pharmacokinetic studies in human volunteers, which show that the time course and subjective reports of visual phenomena and hallucinations is directly correlated with blood levels of ibogaine, but not with blood levels of noribogaine (Mash *et al.*, 2001). Since ibogaine is cleared rapidly after oral administration, the observed after effects of ibogaine treatment on drug craving, mood, and cognition may be related to the targeted actions of the metabolite noribogaine.

Noribogaine as pharmacotherapy for drug dependence

Clinical and preclinical investigations are determining how psychological symptoms associated with drug withdrawal, including depressed mood states and drug cravings, maintain chronic patterns of drug use (Gawin, 1991; Kenna *et al.*, 2007). Studies of cocaine and opiate dependence in animal models provide a rationale for pharmacotherapeutic agents with potential to attenuate withdrawal symptoms, to decrease drug craving, and to reduce relapse to previous patterns of drug use (O'Brien, 1997). Drug treatments that re-establish pre-dependence "set points" in these neural systems may alleviate drug craving and diminish the possibility for relapse. Ibogaine shows promise as a pharmacotherapy for these indications, but the psychotropic effects limit the likelihood of further development.

Interventions with specific pharmacological agents are guided by an understanding of the neurochemical derangements that underlie clinical phases of drug abstinence (Dackis & Gold, 1985; Gawin & Ellinwood, 1988). A rational approach to pharmacotherapy includes the development of agents to: a) initiate and facilitate the acute phase of abstinence; b) diminish drug-specific withdrawal symptoms; and c) prevent cue-associated relapse to previous patterns of drug-taking behavior. Ibogaine is a prodrug that is converted to an active metabolite (Mash *et al.*, 1998; 2000; 2001). As such, it works as a medication that facilitates the first phase of abstinence by reversing the neurochemical alterations that are induced by chronic psychostimulant or opiate use. Noribogaine has actions that are targeted to multiple neurotransmitter systems; its actions most likely underlie the beneficial effects of ibogaine on craving and depression associated with withdrawal from opiates and cocaine (Staley *et al.*, 1996; Pablo & Mash, 1998; Baumann *et al.*, 2001a, b).

Noribogaine's pharmacology as a mu opioid agonist with an apparently long duration of action offers potential advantages over existing treatments for opioid dependence. Noribogaine may have a lower potential for abuse than full mu opioid agonists: this may reduce regulatory burdens. Some efficacy of noribogaine is mediated by mechanisms other than its opioid agonist effects, which may help facilitate acceptance of noribogaine as a treatment for opioid dependence in some countries where the resources, regulatory culture, and the perception of substitution treatment as "substituting one drug for another" have combined to make implementation of harm reduction programs extremely difficult. The existing human data on ibogaine significantly limit the risks that: a) pharmacological findings will not translate into clinical effects; or b) unexpected acute toxicities will emerge to limit development of noribogaine. Noribogaine may have potential for development as an atypical analgesic agent, providing an alternative for chronic pain sufferers other than opiates with high abuse liability.

Conclusion

The discovery that ibogaine eliminates the signs and symptoms of opioid withdrawal and diminishes craving for opioids was first made in the 1960s by a group of self-treating heroin addicts (Shepard, 1994). A single oral dose of ibogaine (6–19 mg/kg) was associated with a disruption of five addicts' use of opiates for up to 6 months. Ibogaine has since been administered to thousands of opiate and cocaine addicts, but it has never been proven effective in a controlled clinical trial. Despite this gap between anecdotal report and valid evidence, open-label observations support the conclusion that ibogaine therapy appears safe and efficacious for patients seeking detoxification from opiates and cocaine.

Ibogaine treatment for opiate dependence demonstrates the reduction in duration of clinical detoxification and the reduction in subjective reports of persistent dysphoria and drug craving. Ibogaine therapy is a novel approach that has similarities with other detoxification pharmacotherapies, including substitution with longer acting opiates (e.g. methadone or buprenorphine). However, ibogaine appears to be a prodrug, with the beneficial effects residing in the active metabolite noribogaine.

Addiction affects physical, psychological, and spiritual domains with serious consequences for the individual and society. William James suggested "the greatest revolution of our generation is the discovery that human beings, by changing the inner attitudes of their minds, can change the outer aspects of their lives" (James, 1890). Ibogaine may help addicts to establish a substance-free recovery because the ibogaine experience itself has benefit or meaning, providing an adjuvant to psychotherapy. Noribogaine, an atypical opiate with low abuse liability, could be developed as an alternative pharmacotherapy to help addicts make the transition from illicit drug use to a drug-free life.

Acknowledgements

The author acknowledges the contribution of Frank Ervin, M.D., Professor of Psychiatry, McGill University, who served as the Clinical Director of the Healing Visions Institute for Addiction Recovery, St. Kitts, W.I. We are grateful to the staff of the Healing Visions Institute for Addiction Recovery Ltd, and Holistic Counseling Inc., Miami FL, for their collaborative support of the Ibogaine Research Project. Rachel Tyndale, Ph.D., Ewa Hoffman, M.S., John Pablo, Ph.D.,

Julie Staley, Ph.D., Linda Duque, M.A., and Margaret J. Basile M.S. contributed to many of the studies presented here. This work was funded in part by the Addiction Research Fund, University of Miami Miller School of Medicine, Miami, FL, and the National Institute on Drug Abuse.

References

Alper, K. R., Lotsof, H. S., Frenken, G. M., Luciano, D. J. & Bastiaans, J. (1999). Treatment of acute opioid withdrawal with ibogaine. *American Journal of Addiction*, **8**, 234–42.

Barabe, P. (1982). Religion of Eboga or the Bwiti of the Fangs. *Medecine Tropicale (Marseilles)*, **42**(3), 251–7.

Baumann, M. H., Pablo, J. P., Ali, S. F., Rothman, R. B. & Mash, D. C. (2000). Noribogaine (12-hydroxyibogamine): a biologically active metabolite of the antiaddictive drug ibogaine. *Annals of the New York Academy of Sciences*, **914**, 354–68.

Baumann, M. H., Pablo, J., Ali, S. F., Rothman, R. B. & Mash, D. C. (2001a). Comparative neuropharmacology of ibogaine and its O-desmethyl metabolite, noribogaine. *Alkaloids: Chemical and Biological Perspectives*, **56**, 79–113.

Baumann, M. H., Rothman, R. B., Pablo, J. P. & Mash, D. C. (2001b). In vivo neurobiological effects of ibogaine and its O-desmethyl metabolite, 12-hydroxyibogamine (noribogaine), in rats. *Journal of Pharmacological and Experimental Therapy*, **297**(2), 531–9.

Beck, A. T., Ward, C. H., Mendelson, M., Mock, J. & Erbaugh, J. (1961). An interview for measuring depression. *Archives of General Psychiatry*, **4**, 561–71.

Cappendijk, S. L. T. & Dzoljic, M. R. (1993). Inhibitory effects of ibogaine on cocaine self-administration in rats. *European Journal of Pharmacology*, **241**, 261–5.

Dackis, C. A. & Gold, M. S. (1985). Pharmacological approaches to cocaine addiction. *Journal of Substance Abuse Treatment*, **2**, 139–45.

Dzoljic, E. D., Kaplan, C. D. & Dzoljic, M. R. (1988). Effect of ibogaine on naloxone-precipitated withdrawal syndrome in chronic morphine dependent rats. *Archives Internationales de Pharmacodynamie et de Therapie*, **294**, 64–70.

Fermandez, J. W. & Fernendez, R. L. (2001). "Returning to the path": the use of iboga[ine] in an equatorial African ritual context and the binding of time, space, and social relationships. The Alkaloids. *Chemistry and Biology*, **56**, 235–47.

Gawin, F. H. (1991). Cocaine addiction: psychology and neurophysiology. *Science*, **251**, 1580–6.

Gawin, F. H. & Ellinwood, E. H. (1988). Cocaine and other stimulants: actions, abuse and treatment. *New England Journal of Medicine*, **318**, 1173–82.

Glick, S. D., Rossman, K., Steindorf, S., Maisonneuve, I. M. & Carlson, J. N. (1991). Effects and aftereffects of ibogaine on morphine self-administration in rats. *European Journal of Pharmacology*, **195**(3), 341–5.

Glick, S. D., Rossman, K., Rao, N. C., Maisonneuve, I. M. & Carlson, J. N. (1992). Effects of ibogaine on acute signs of morphine withdrawal in rats: independence from tremor. *Neuropharmacology*, **31**, 497–500.

Goutarel, R., Gollnhofer, O. & Sillans, R. (1991). Pharmacodynamics and therapeutic applications of iboga and ibogaine. *Psychedelic Monographs and Essays*, **6**, 71–111.

Hearn, W. L., Mash, D. C., Pablo, J. et al. (1995a). Pharmacokinetics of ibogaine: analytical method, animal–human comparisons, and the identification of a primary metabolite. *Proceedings of the TIAFT-SOFT Joint Congress*, October 21–November 4, 1994, ed. V. Spiehler. Ann Arbor, MI: Omnipress, pp. 325–34.

Hearn, W. L., Pablo, J., Hime, G. & Mash, D. C. (1995b). Identification and quantitation of ibogaine and an O-demethylated metabolite in brain and biological fluids using gas chromatography/mass spectrometry. *Journal of Analytical Toxicology*, **19**, 427–34.

Hoffer, A. & Osmond, H. (1967). *The Hallucinogens*. New York: Academic Press.

James, W. (1890). *The Principles of Psychology*. New York, NY: Dover, Inc.

Kenna, G. A., Nielsen, D. M., Mello, P., Sciesl, A. & Swift, R. M. (2007). Pharmacotherapy of dual substance abuse and dependence. *CNS Drugs*, **21**(3), 213–37.

Lambert, M. & Heckel, E. (1901). Sur la racine d'iboga et sur l'ibogaine. *Comptes Rendus*, **133**, 1236.

Martin, W. R. & Jasinski, D. R. (1969). Physiological parameters of morphine dependence in man – tolerance, early abstinence, protracted abstinence. *Journal of Psychiatric Research*, **7**, 9–17.

Mash, D. C. & Schenk, S. (1996). Preclinical screening of an ibogaine metabolite (noribogaine) on cocaine-induced hyperlocomotion and cocaine self-administration. *Society for Neuroscience Abstracts*, **22**, 1929.

Mash, D. C., Staley, J. K., Baumann, M. H., Rothman, R. B. & Hearn, W. L. (1995a). Identification of a primary metabolite of ibogaine that targets serotonin transporters and elevates serotonin. *Life Science*, **57**, PL45–50.

Mash, D. C., Pablo, J., Staley, J. K. et al. (1995b). Properties of ibogaine and a principal metabolite (12-hydroxyibogamine at the MK-801 binding site on the NMDA- receptor complex. *Neuroscience Letters*, **192**, 53–6.

Mash, D. C., Kovera, C. A., Buck, B. E. et al. (1998). Medication development of ibogaine as a pharmacotherapy for drug dependence. *Annals of the New York Academy of Sciences*, **844**, 274–92.

Mash, D. C., Kovera, C. A., Pablo, J. *et al.* (2000). Ibogaine: complex pharmacokinetics, concerns for safety, and preliminary efficacy measures. *Annals of the New York Academy of Sciences*, **914**, 394–401.

Mash, D. C., Kovera, C. A., Pablo, J. *et al.* (2001). Ibogaine in the treatment of heroin withdrawal. *Alkaloids: Chemical and Biological Perspectives*, **56**, 155–71.

Naranjo, C. (1969). Psychotherapeutic possibilities: new fantasy enhancing drugs. *Clinical Toxicology*, **2**, 209–24.

Naranjo, C. (1973). *The Healing Journey. New Approaches to Consciousness*. New York, NY: Pantheon.

Obach, R. S., Pablo, J. & Mash, D. C. (1998). Cytochrome P4502D6 catalyzes the O-demethylation of the psychoactive alkaloid ibogaine to 12-hydroxyibogamine. *Drug Metabolism and Disposition*, **25**(12), 1359–69.

O'Brien, C. P. (1997). A range of research-based pharmacotherapies for addiction. *Science*, **278**, 66–9.

Pablo, J. & Mash, D. C. (1998). Noribogaine stimulates naloxone-sensitive [35S]GTPgS binding. *NeuroReport*, **9**, 109–114.

Phisalix, M. C. (1901). Action physiologique de l'ibogaine. *Comptes Rendus Societe de Biologie*, **53**, 1077.

Popik, P., Layer, R. T. & Sholnick, P. (1995). 100 Years of ibogaine: neurochemical and pharmacological actions

of a putative anti-addictive drug. *Pharmacological Reviews*, **47**, 235–53.

Pouchet, G. & Chevalier, J. (1905). Les nouveaux remedes. Sur l'action pharmacodynamique de l'ibogaine. *Bulletin Géneral de Thérapeutique*, **149**, 211.

Shepard, S. G. (1994). A preliminary investigation of ibogaine: case reports and recommendations for further study. *Journal of Substance Abuse Treatment*, **11**(4), 379–85.

Spangler, R., Ho, A., Zhou, Y. *et al.* (1996). Regulation of kappa opioid receptor mRNA in the rat brain by 'binge' pattern cocaine administration and correlation with preprodynorphin mRNA. *Brain Research – Molecular Brain Research*, **38**, 71–6.

Staley, J. K., Ouyang, Q., Pablo, J. *et al.* (1996). Pharmacological screen for activities of 12-hydroxyibogamine: a primary metabolite of the indole alkaloid ibogaine. *Psychopharmacology*, **127**, 10–18.

Strassman, R. J., Qualls, C. R., Uhlenhuth, E. H. & Kellner, R. (1994). Dose-response study of N, N-dimethyltryptamine in humans. II. Subjective effects and preliminary results of a new rating scale. *Archives of General Psychiatry*, **51**(2), 98–108.

Vocci, F. J., Acri, J. & Elkashef, A. (2005). Medication development for addictive disorders: the state of the science. *American Journal of Psychiatry*, **162**(8), 1432–40.

7

Therapeutic communities in the new millennium

George De Leon

Residential therapeutic community (TC) programs for substance abuse appeared a generation after TCs in psychiatric hospitals, pioneered by Jones (1953) and others in the UK. Today, the term *therapeutic community* is generic, describing a variety of short- and long-term residential programs, as well as day treatment and ambulatory programs that serve a wide spectrum of drug- and alcohol-abusing patients. Although the TC model has been widely adapted for different populations and settings, it is the traditional long-term residential prototype for adults with serious substance abuse problems and has documented effectiveness. The initial sections of this chapter provide a description of the TC approach and summarize the research on efficacy. The remaining sections review adaptations of the traditional TC model for various special populations and briefly outline challenges to the TC in the new millennium.

The therapeutic community approach

The TC for addictions and related disorders can be understood as a unique social psychological treatment approach for substance abuse and related disorders that can be distinguished from other major drug treatment modalities in two general ways. First, the primary "therapist" in the TC is the community itself, consisting of peers who serve as role models of successful personal change and staff members who serve as rational authorities and guides in the recovery process. Second, the TC approach is based on an explicit perspective of the substance use disorder, the person, the recovery process, and healthy living. It is this perspective that guides its method and shapes the program model.

The therapeutic community perspective

The TC perspective consists of four interrelated views, each of which is briefly outlined here. Detailed expositions of the TC perspective are contained elsewhere (De Leon, 2000; 2008).

View of the disorder

Drug abuse is viewed as a disorder of the whole person, affecting some or all areas of functioning. Cognitive and behavioral problems are evident, as are mood disturbances. Thinking may be unrealistic or disorganized; values are confused, non-existent, or antisocial. Frequently there are deficits in verbal, reading, writing, and marketable skills. Moral, or even spiritual issues, whether expressed in existential or psychological terms, are apparent. The problem is the individual, not the drug. Addiction is a symptom, not the essence of the disorder.

View of the person

Although TCs originally attracted individuals addicted to narcotics, most of the current TC patient populations are non-opioid-abusing persons with different lifestyles, and various social, economic, and ethnic or cultural backgrounds. Notwithstanding these demographic and social differences, substance abusers in TCs share clinical characteristics that center around immaturity or antisocial dimensions (see De Leon, 2000, Chapter 3). For example, they include low tolerance for all forms of discomfort and delay of gratification; problems with authority; inability to manage feelings (particularly hostility, guilt, and anxiety); poor impulse control (particularly sexual or aggressive impulses); poor judgment and reality testing concerning consequences of actions; unrealistic self-appraisal regarding discrepancies between personal resources and aspirations; prominence of lying, manipulation, and deception as coping behaviors; and personal and social irresponsibility (e.g. inconsistency or failures in meeting obligations). In addition, many TC residents have marked deficits in learning and in marketable and communication skills.

Whether they are antecedent or consequent to serious involvement with drugs, these characteristics are commonly observed to be correlated with chemical dependency. More important, in TCs, a positive change in these characteristics is considered to be essential for stable recovery.

View of recovery

In the view of recovery employed in the TC, the aim of rehabilitation is global, involving both a change in lifestyle and a change in personal identity. The primary psychological goal is to change the negative patterns of behavior, thinking, and feeling that predispose the individual to drug use; the main social goal is to develop the skills, attitudes, and values of a responsible drug-free lifestyle. Stable recovery, however, depends on a successful integration of these social and psychological goals. Behavioral change is unstable without insight, and insight is insufficient without felt experience. Several assumptions underlie the recovery process itself which are grounded in the TC approach: developmental learning, motivation, mutual self-help, and social learning.

Recovery as developmental learning

Multidimensional change unfolds as a developmental process of social learning, which occurs through mutual self-help in a social context. This is the basis for the stage/phase format of TC programs (see page 66).

Motivation

Recovery depends on pressures to change – positive and negative. Some patients seek help, driven by stressful external pressures; others are moved by more intrinsic factors. For all, however, remaining in treatment requires continued motivation to change. Therefore, elements of the rehabilitation approach are designed to sustain motivation or to enable detection of early signs of premature termination.

Self-help and mutual self-help

Strictly speaking, treatment is not provided; rather, it is made available to the individual in the TC through its staff and peers and the daily regimen of work, groups, meetings, seminars, and recreation. However, the effectiveness of these elements depends on the individual, who must constantly and fully engage in the treatment regimen. In self-help recovery, the individual makes the main contribution to the change process. In mutual self-help, individuals assist each other in the self-help process. The principal messages of recovery, personal growth, and "right living" are mediated by peers through confrontation and sharing in groups, by example as role models, and as supportive, encouraging friends in daily interactions.

Social learning

A lifestyle change occurs in a social context. Negative patterns, attitudes, and roles were not acquired in isolation, nor can they be altered in isolation. Thus, recovery depends not only on what has been learned but also on how and where learning occurs. This assumption is the basis for the community's serving collectively as teacher. Learning is active, involving doing and participating. A socially responsible role is acquired by acting the role. What is learned is identified with the individuals involved in the learning process – with supportive peers and staff members serving as credible role models.

View of right living

Sustained recovery requires a perspective on self, society, and life that must be continually affirmed by a positive social network of others within and beyond the TC. This assumption is evident in the TC view of right living. TCs adhere to certain precepts that constitute a view of healthy personal and social living. These precepts concern moral behavior, values, and a social perspective that are intimately related to the TC view of the individual and of recovery. For example, in TCs, unambiguous moral positions are held regarding social and sexual conduct. Explicit right and wrong behaviors are identified for which there are appropriate rewards and sanctions. These include antisocial behaviors and attitudes; the negative values of the street, jails, or negative peers; and irresponsible or exploitative sexual conduct.

Certain values are emphasized as being essential to sustain social learning and personal growth. These values include truth and honesty (in word and deed), a work ethic, self-reliance, earned rewards and achievement, personal accountability, responsible concern (being one's brother's or sister's keeper), social manners, and community involvement. Treatment helps the individual to focus on the importance of the personal present (here and now) versus the historical past (then and when). Past behavior and circumstances are explored only to illustrate the current patterns of dysfunctional behavior, negative attitudes, and outlook. Residents are encouraged and trained to assume personal responsibility for their present reality and future. The view of right living is mediated in the expectations of the community as well as through staff- and peer-led teaching seminars.

The therapeutic community method and model

How the TC facilitates individual change can be summarized in the phrase "community as method" (De Leon, 1997; 2000). The latter can be briefly defined as "the purposive use of the peer–staff community to facilitate social and psychological change in individuals." In this definition, community provides the *context* (social relationships – peers and staff – and the daily therapeutic and educational activities) for learning to occur; community sets the *expectations* or *standards* for how individuals should participate in the context; and community continually *evaluates* and *responds* to whether or not individuals meet community expectations through corrective and affirmative peer feedback, staff-delivered privileges, and disciplinary sanctions. In striving to meet the community's expectations for participation, residents pursue their individual goals of socialization and psychological growth (De Leon, 2000, Chapter 22). In the TC approach, recovery unfolds through the interaction between the individual and the community.

The program model consists of the elements and planned activities that individuals learn to use to change themselves. These can be organized in terms of the TC structure or social organization and the TC process in terms of the individual's passage through stages of change within the context of community life.

TC social structure

The relatively small staff census of the TC is complemented by resident peers at junior, intermediate, and senior levels. These groups constitute the community or family in the residence. This peer-to-community structure strengthens the individual's identification with a perceived ordered network of others. More important, it arranges relationships of mutual responsibility to others at various levels in the program.

The daily operation of the community itself is the task of the residents, who work together under staff supervision. The broad range of resident job assignments illustrates the extent of the self-help process. Residents perform all house services (e.g. cooking, cleaning, kitchen service, minor repair), serve as apprentices, run all departments, and conduct house meetings, certain seminars, and peer encounter groups.

The TC is managed by the staff who monitor and evaluate patient status, supervise resident groups, assign and supervise resident jobs, and oversee house operations. The staff conduct therapeutic groups (other than peer encounter groups), provide individual counseling, organize social and recreational projects, and confer with significant others. They make decisions about resident status, discipline, promotion, transfers, discharges, furloughs, and treatment planning. The social organization of the TC reflects the fundamental aspects of community as a method: work as education and therapy, mutual self-help, peers as role models, and staff members as rational authorities.

Work as education and therapy

Work and job changes have clinical relevance for substance-abusing patients in TCs, most of whom have not successfully negotiated the social and occupational world of the larger society. Vertical job movements carry the obvious rewards of status and privilege. However, in their various work roles and functions, clients also reveal the clinical characteristics of the disorder; continual community feedback facilitates change in these characteristics.

Mutual self-help (peer confrontation and affirmation)

In their jobs, groups, meetings, recreation, personal and social time, residents continually express to one another the main messages and expectations of the community. Prominent examples of mutual self-help are peer verbal correctives and affirmations: these are essential elements of community as method. These verbal interactions illustrate examples of peer confrontation in that they provide "face to face" feedback to members as to whether they are meeting community expectations of program participation, recovery, and right living. Correctives aim to raise the individual's awareness of behaviors and attitudes that require changing. Correctives range in severity from mild reminders ("pull ups") to stern conversations ("verbal reprimands"). Affirmations aim to encourage or reinforce positive clinical change or personal growth. Except as part of certain rituals (e.g. closing group sessions or meetings), affirmations are usually spontaneously offered as supportive expressions or "push ups" (e.g. "Yes, you can do it," "You're doing great," "You're my role model") or specific acknowledgments (e.g. "You have really changed"). Affirmations provide the crucial balance to verbal correctives and staff disciplinary sanctions.

Peer confrontations are intended to facilitate learning in those delivering as well as receiving them.

Observing, affirming, reminding, and correcting others reciprocally reinforces self-learning through practice, rehearsal, or role modeling. Thus, verbal affirmations and correctives are quintessential examples of the principle of mutual self-help (Center for Substance Abuse Treatment, 2005a, p.169).

Peers as role models

Peers, serving as role models, and staff members, serving as role models and rational authorities, are the primary mediators of the recovery process. TC members who demonstrate the expected behaviors and reflect the values and teachings of the community are viewed as role models. Thus, all members of the community – room-mates, older and younger residents, and junior, senior, and directorial staff – are expected to be role models. TCs require these multiple role models to maintain the integrity of the community and ensure the spread of social learning efforts.

Staff members as rational authorities

Staff members foster the self-help learning process through performance of the managerial and clinical functions described above and through maintenance of psychological relationships with the residents as role models, parental surrogates, and rational authorities. TC residents often had difficulties with authorities who have not been trusted or who have been perceived as guides and teachers. Therefore, residents need a positive experience with an authority figure that is viewed as credible (recovered), supportive, corrective, and protective so that they may gain authority over themselves (personal autonomy). As rational authorities, staff members provide the *reasons* for their decisions and explain the *meaning* of consequences. They exercise their powers to teach, guide, facilitate, and correct rather than to punish, control, or exploit.

Treatment process elements

The treatment process may be defined as the interaction between the treatment interventions and individual change. Unlike other treatment approaches, however, the TC treatment intervention is the daily regimen of planned and unplanned activities and social intercourse occurring in formal and informal settings.

The typical day in a TC is highly structured. It begins at 7:00 A.M. and ends at 11:00 P.M. During this time, residents participate in a variety of meetings, educational, encounter and other therapeutic groups,

and recreational activities; residents perform job functions and receive individual counseling. As interventions these activities may be divided into three main categories: therapeutic–educative activities, community-enhancement activities, and community and clinical management elements.

Therapeutic–educative activities

Therapeutic–educative activities consist of various forms of group processes and individual counseling. These activities provide residents with opportunities to express feelings, divert negative acting-out, and resolve personal and social issues. They increase communication and interpersonal skills, bring about examination and confrontation of behavior and attitudes, and offer instruction in alternative modes of behavior.

The main forms of group activity in the TC are encounters, probes, marathons, and tutorials. These differ somewhat in format, objectives, and method, but all have the goal of fostering trust, personal disclosure, intimacy, and peer solidarity to facilitate therapeutic change. The focus of the encounter is behavioral. Its approach is supportive confrontation, and its objective is to modify negative behavior and attitudes directly. Probes and marathons have as their primary objective substantial emotional change and psychological insight. In tutorials, the learning of concepts and specific skills is emphasized.

Other groups convene regularly or as needed, supplementing the four main groups. These vary in focus, format, and composition. For example, weekly or biweekly "static" (caseload) groups are convened. These home groups consist of the same composition of peers who address and mutually monitor ongoing clinical progress. Special gender, ethnic, or age-specific or health theme groups may use encounter or tutorial formats. Dormitory, room, or departmental encounters may address issues of daily community living.

One-to-one counseling balances the needs of the individual with those of the community. Peer exchange is ongoing and is the most consistent form of informal counseling in TCs. Staff counseling sessions may be formal or informal and are usually conducted as needed. The staff counseling method in the TC is not conventional, as is evident in its main features: transpersonal sharing, direct support, minimal interpretation, didactic instructions, and concerned confrontation. The focus of staff counseling is to address issues that may impede progress, and to facilitate the patient's adjustment to and constructive use of the peer community.

In addition, TC programs incorporate a variety of conventional groups, such as anger management, domestic violence, parenting, as well as other evidence-based strategies, including cognitive restructuring, relapse prevention training, and motivational enhancement. However, these are supplements rather than substitutes for the primary approach, which is community as method.

Community-enhancement activities

Community-enhancement activities include the four main facility-wide meetings: the morning meeting, the seminar, the house meeting (these three meetings are held each day), and the general meeting (which is called when needed). Although different in format, all meetings have the common objective of facilitating the individual's assimilation into the community.

All residents of the facility and the staff on the premises attend the morning meeting, which takes place after breakfast and usually lasts for 30 minutes. The purpose of the meeting is to instil a positive attitude at the beginning of the day, motivate residents, and strengthen unity. This meeting is particularly relevant because most residents of TCs have never adapted to the routine of an ordinary day.

Seminars take place every afternoon and usually last 1 hour. Because it brings all residents together, the seminar in the afternoon complements the daily morning meeting and the house meeting in the evening. A clinical aim of the seminar is to balance the individual's emotional and cognitive experience. Residents lead most seminars, although some are led by staff members or, less frequently, by outside speakers. The seminar is unique among the various meetings and groups in the TC in its emphasis on listening, speaking, and conceptual behavior. Seminar topics directly or indirectly relate to the TC perspective on recovery and right living.

House meetings take place nightly after dinner, usually last up to an hour, and are coordinated by a senior resident. The main aim of these meetings is to transact community business, although they also have a clinical objective. In this forum, social pressure through public acknowledgment of positive or negative behaviors is judiciously applied to facilitate individual change.

General meetings take place only when needed and are usually called so that negative behavior, attitudes, or incidents in the facility can be addressed.

All residents and staff members (including those not on duty) are assembled at any time and for an indefinite duration. These meetings, conducted by multiple staff members, are designed to identify problem individuals or conditions or to reaffirm motivation and reinforce positive behavior and attitudes in the community.

Community and clinical management elements

Community and clinical management elements maintain the physical and psychological safety of the environment and ensure that resident life is orderly and productive. They protect the community as a whole and strengthen it as a setting for social learning. The main elements which are staff managed are privileges, disciplinary sanctions, surveillance, and urine testing.

Privileges

In the TC, privileges are explicit rewards that reinforce the value of achievement. Privileges are accorded concomitant with overall clinical progress in the program. Displays of inappropriate behavior or negative attitude can result in loss of privileges, which can be regained through demonstrated improvement.

Staff members deliver all privileges, which may range from telephone use and letter writing (early in treatment) to overnight furloughs (later in treatment). Successful movement through each stage earns privileges that grant wider personal latitude and increased self-responsibility.

Disciplinary sanctions

TCs have their own specific rules and regulations that guide the behavior of residents and the management of facilities. The explicit purpose of these rules is to ensure the safety and health of the community. However, their implicit aim is to train and teach residents through consequential learning.

In the TC, social and physical safety is a prerequisite for psychological trust. Therefore, sanctions are invoked against any behavior that threatens the physical safety of the therapeutic environment. For example, breaking one of the TC's cardinal rules (such as "no violence or threat of violence") or a house rule (such as the unapproved borrowing of a book) is a threat that must be addressed. Loss of privileges or a speaking ban may be applied for less severe infractions. Job demotion or loss of accrued time may be invoked for more serious infractions. Expulsion may be appropriate for behavior that is incorrigible or dangerous to others. Sanctions may also be delivered for a resident's persistent failure in meeting community expectations. Examples are non-participation in community activities or repeated displays of negative attitudes toward the program.

All sanctions are implemented by staff members, usually as written contracts with the resident. These agreements make explicit the behaviors addressed, and the nature and duration of the consequences. Although contracts are often perceived as punitive, their basic purpose is to create a learning experience by compelling residents to attend to their own conduct, to reflect on their own motivation, and to consider alternative forms of behavior under similar situations.

Surveillance and urine testing

The TC's most comprehensive method for assessing the overall physical and psychological status of the residential community is the house run. Several times a day, staff members and senior residents walk through the entire facility, examining its overall condition. House runs provide global snapshot impressions of the facility: its cleanliness, planned routines, safety procedures, morale, and psychological tone. They also illuminate the psychological and social functioning of individual residents and peer groups.

Most TCs use unannounced random urine testing or incident-related urine testing procedures. When urine tests positive for drugs, the action taken depends on the drug used, the resident's time and status in the program, the resident's history of drug and other infractions, and the locus and condition of use. Actions may involve expulsion, loss of accrued time, radical job demotion, or rescinding of privileges for specific periods. Review of the triggers or reasons for drug use is also essential.

TC process: program stages and phases

Recovery in the TC is a developmental process, which can be understood as a passage through stages of learning. The learning that occurs at each stage facilitates change at the next, and each change reflects movement toward the goals of recovery. Three major program stages characterize change in long-term residential TCs: orientation–induction, primary treatment, and re-entry.

The aim of *orientation* (0–60 days) is to assimilate the individual into the community. Formal seminars and informal peer instruction prepare the individual

to navigate the program. The focus is on teaching the rules and expectations of the program and demonstrating how to participate in the roles, therapeutic groups, and community meetings.

The three phases of *primary treatment* roughly correlate with time spent in the program (2–4, 5–8, and 9–12 months). The daily therapeutic–educational regimen of meetings, groups, job assignments, and peer and staff counseling remains the same throughout the year of primary treatment. However, progress is reflected at the end of each phase in terms of three interrelated dimensions of change: community status, development or maturity, and overall psychological adjustment. After a year, residents are fully trained participants in the group process and often serve as facilitators. A high level of personal disclosure is evident in groups, in peer exchange, and in their increased use of staff counseling.

Re-entry is the stage at which the individual must strengthen skills for autonomous decision-making, solidify the capacity for self-management, and rely less on rational authorities or a well formed peer network. The two phases of the re-entry process are *early re-entry* and *later re-entry*. The main objective of the early re-entry phase (13–18 months) is to prepare patients for separation from the community. During this phase, the development of plans for the individual is a collective task involving the patient, a key staff member, and peers. These plans are comprehensive blueprints for long-term psychological, educational, and vocational efforts, which include goal attainment schedules, methods of improving interpersonal and family relationships, and counseling on social and sexual behavior. Particular emphasis is placed on life skills seminars, which provide training for life outside the community. Attendance is mandated for sessions on budgeting, job-seeking, use of alcohol, sexuality, parenting, use of leisure time, and so on. Patients may be attending school or holding full-time jobs, either within or outside the TC. Still, they are expected to participate in house activities when possible and to have some community responsibilities (e.g. monitoring of the facility at night).

The objective of the later re-entry phase (19–24 months) is successful separation of the client from the community. Patients have a "live-out" status; they hold full-time jobs or attend school full-time, and they maintain their own households, usually with live-out peers. They may participate in Alcoholics Anonymous (AA) or Narcotics Anonymous (NA), or attend family or individual therapy sessions. Contact with the TC is frequent at first and is gradually reduced to weekly telephone calls and monthly visits with a primary counselor.

Completion marks the end of active program involvement. Graduation itself, however, is an annual event conducted in the facility for individuals who have completed the program, usually 1 year after their residence is over. Thus, the TC experience is a preparation rather than a cure. Residence in the program facilitates a process of change that must continue throughout life. What is gained in treatment are tools to guide the individual on a path of continued change. Completion, or graduation, therefore, is not an end but a beginning.

Aftercare

TCs have always acknowledged the patient's efforts to maintain sobriety and a positive lifestyle beyond graduation. Until recently, long-term TCs addressed key clinical and life adjustment issues of aftercare during the re-entry stages of the 2-year program. However, funding pressures have resulted in shorter planned durations of residential treatment. This has underscored the necessity for aftercare resources to address both primary treatment as well as re-entry issues. Thus, many contemporary TCs offer post-residential aftercare treatment and social services within their systems, such as intensive day treatment and step-down outpatient ambulatory treatment, or linkages with outside agencies.

Therapeutic community research and evaluation

Effectiveness

A substantial amount of evaluation literature documents the effectiveness of the TC approach in rehabilitating drug-abusing individuals; see reviews in Anglin & Hser (1990); Condelli & Hubbard (1994); De Leon (1984), (1985), (2004); Gerstein & Harwood (1990); National Institute on Drug Abuse (2002); Simpson & Curry (1997); Simpson & Sells (1982); Tims & Ludford (1984); and Tims *et al.* (1994). The findings of single- and multi-program studies regarding short- and long-term post-treatment outcomes are summarized in this section.

Substantial improvements are noted on separate outcome variables (i.e. drug use, criminality, and employment) and on composite indices for measuring individual success. Maximally to moderately favorable outcomes (in terms of opioid, non-opioid, and alcohol use; arrest rates; re-treatment; and employment) occur in more than half of the sample of patients who have completed programs.

There is a consistent positive relationship between time spent in residential treatment and post-treatment outcome. For example, in long-term TC programs, success rates (on composite indices of no drug use and no criminality) determined 2 years after completion of treatment are approximately 90% for graduates or completers, 50% for dropouts who remain in residential treatment for more than 1 year, and 25% for dropouts who remain in residential treatment for less than 1 year (De Leon *et al.*, 1982). In studies that investigated psychological outcomes, results uniformly showed marked improvement at follow-up (e.g. Biase *et al.*, 1986; De Leon, 1984; Holland, (1983). A direct relationship has been demonstrated between post-treatment behavioral success and psychological adjustment (De Leon, 1984; De Leon & Jainchill, 1981–2).

Retention

Dropout is the general rule for all drug treatment modalities. For TCs, retention is of particular importance because research has established a firm relationship between time spent in treatment and successful outcome. Reviews of the TC retention research are contained in the literature (De Leon, 1985; 1991; Lewis & Ross, 1994; Simpson & Curry, 1997). The key findings from these are summarized here.

Retention rates and predictors of dropout

Dropout rates are highest for the first 30 days of residence but decrease sharply thereafter (De Leon & Schwartz, 1984). This temporal pattern of dropout is uniform across TC programs (and other modalities). Retention rates vary considerably across programs, implicating differences in organizational sophistication and fidelity of treatment delivery (Simpson & Curry, 1997).

No reliable patient characteristics predict retention, with the exceptions of severe criminality and severe psychopathology, which are correlated with earlier dropout. Studies point to the importance of dynamic factors in predicting retention in treatment, such as perceived legal pressure, motivation, and readiness for treatment (Broome *et al.*, 1997; De Leon *et al.*, 2000a).

Enhancing retention in therapeutic communities

Some attempts to enhance retention in TCs have involved supportive individual counseling, improved orientation to treatment by experienced staff members as "senior professors" (De Leon *et al.*, 2000a), and family alliance strategies to reduce early dropout (De Leon, 1991). Other efforts involve providing special facilities and programming for mothers and children (Coletti *et al.*, 1997; Stevens *et al.*, 1997) and teaching curriculum-based relapse prevention methods (Lewis & Ross, 1994) to sustain retention throughout residential treatment. Recent studies in European TCs demonstrate the importance of a social network in sustaining retention in treatment (Soyez *et al.*, 2006). Evidence of progress in TC research includes studies that investigate the role of pharmacotherapy in retention. For example, antidepressant medication for some clients and buprenorphine for opioid abusers appear to decrease early dropout from TCs. Although such findings are promising, they require replication at multiple sites.

Treatment process research

Recent developments have facilitated empirical studies into the underinvestigated area of treatment process. These developments include formulations of the perspective and essential elements of the TC approach and of the stages of recovery in the TC (De Leon, 1995; 2000). Research findings illuminate some of the essential program elements which may serve as active ingredients in the treatment process.

Several examples of process-related research follow. Studies of substance abusers involved in the criminal justice system underline the critical importance of client participation in community activities for treatment effectiveness. Inmates who were highly motivated were more fully engaged in a prison-based TC; they were more likely to enter aftercare and have better post-release outcomes (Melnick & De Leon, 1999; Melnick *et al.*, 2001b). A recent report demonstrates that substance abusers who were more involved in providing verbal affirmations and corrections during their stay in a prison-based TC treatment were significantly less likely to be reincarcerated 2 years after release (Warren *et al.*, 2006). Another prospective study documents that, among substance abusers treated in a prison-based TC, those with greater

self-perceived change at 1 year post-release were significantly less likely to be reincarcerated 3 years later (De Leon *et al.*, 2006). Finally, an investigation of encounter group process in community-based TCs indicates that benefits occur to both those who deliver as well as to those who receive confrontation (Broekaert *et al.*, 2004).

The evolution of the therapeutic community: modifications and application

The traditional TC model described in this chapter is actually the prototype of a variety of TC-orientated programs. Today, the TC modality includes a wide range of programs serving a diverse population of patients who use a variety of drugs and present concomitantly with complex social and psychological problems. Patient differences, as well as clinical requirements and funding realities, have encouraged the development of modified residential TC programs with shorter planned durations of stay (3, 6, and 12 months) as well as TC-orientated day treatment and outpatient ambulatory models. Overwhelmed with alcohol and drug abuse problems, some correctional facilities, medical and mental hospitals, and community residences and shelters have implemented TC programs within their settings.

Examples of these adaptations are more fully described elsewhere (De Leon, 1997; 2000, Chapter 25; Center for Substance Abuse Treatment, 2005a, b). Modifications in practice and in program elements for special populations and settings center upon treatment goals and planned duration of treatment, flexibility of the program structure to accommodate individual differences, and on intensity of peer interactions. Special services and interventions are integrated into the program as complements to the primary TC treatment. Successful implementation of TC program models within special settings requires accommodation to the goals, procedures, personnel, general practices, and restrictions of these settings.

Research provides evidence for the effectiveness of modified TCs for special populations. These study populations include adolescents in various adaptations of the community-based TC (Hubbard *et al.*, 1988; Jainchill, 1997); inmates in prison TCs (Inciardi *et al.*, 1997; Simpson, Wexler and Inciardi., 1999; Wexler *et al.*, 1999a; b); substance abusers with serious and persistent co-occurring psychiatric disorders (De

Leon *et al.*, 2000a; Sacks *et al.*, 1997); addicted mothers and their children (Coletti *et al.*, 1997; Winick & Evans, 1997); and patients receiving methadone in a day-treatment TC (De Leon *et al.*, 1995). The findings and conclusions from the research on TCs for special populations are reviewed elsewhere (Center for Substance Abuse Treatment, 2005a, b).

In general, findings show that drug use and criminality decline and there are improvements in employment and psychological status. Improvements are correlated with length of stay in treatment. Fiscal studies indicate that TC-orientated programs show favorable cost–benefit gains, particularly in reduction of expenditures associated with criminal activity in mental health services.

The therapeutic community: challenges in the new millennium

The modifications of the traditional model and its adaptation for special populations and settings are redefining the TC modality within mainstream human and mental health services. Most contemporary TC programs adhere to the perspective and approaches described in this chapter. However, the basic peer/ social learning framework has been enlarged to include additional social, psychological, and health services. Staff composition has been altered, reflecting the fact that traditional professionals – social workers, case managers, and correctional, mental health, medical, educational, family, and childcare specialists – serve along with experientially trained TC professionals.

These changes in patient populations, services, and staffing have brought to the surface complex issues such as divergence of the modified program from the proven TC model, and impact of staff diversity and integration upon outcomes. Program diversity has led to problems maintaining treatment fidelity and effectiveness. The response to this issue has been the development of national standards of TC programming (Commission on Accreditation of Rehabilitative Facilities, 2000 [cited in De Leon, 2000, p. 390]) and quality assurance models (Kressel *et al.*, 2002) based on theory and clinical practice. Staff issues are related to the TC's philosophy of drug-free living and the TC's self-help perspective; other issues are related to differences in therapeutic concepts and terms, staff members' academic education, staff members' experience with addiction, and staff members' roles and functions within the context of a peer–community model.

The issues of staff integration have been addressed through the development of TC training curricula based on theory and standards (Therapeutic Communities of America, 1999; Center for Substance Abuse Treatment, 2006). Vigorous training and orientation efforts are guided by a common perspective of recovery (Carroll & Sobel, 1986; Deitch & Solit, 1993; De Leon, 1985; Galanter *et al.*, 1991; Talboy, 1998). Indeed, the cross-fertilization of personnel and methods between traditional TCs and mental health and human services portends the evolution of a new TC: a general treatment model applicable to a broad range of populations whose affiliation with a self-help community leads to positive individual change.

References

Anglin, M. D. & Hser, Y. I. (1990). Treatment of drug abuse. In *Crime and Justice: An Annual Review of Research*, vol. **13**, eds. M. Tonry & J. Q. Wilson. Chicago, IL: University of Chicago Press, pp. 393–460.

Biase, D. V., Sullivan, A. P. & Wheeler, B. (1986). Daytop miniversity – phase 2 – college training in a therapeutic community: development of self concept among drug free addict/abusers. In *Therapeutic Communities for Addictions: Readings in Theory, Research, and Practice*, eds. G. De Leon & J. T. Ziegenfuss. Springfield, IL: Charles C. Thomas, pp. 121–30.

Broekaert, E., Vandevelde, S., Schuyten, G., Erauw, K. & Bracke, R. (2004). Evolution of encounter group methods in therapeutic communities for substance abusers. *Addictive Behaviors*, **29**, 231–44.

Broome, K. M., Knight, D. K., Knight, R. *et al.* (1997). Peer, family, and motivational influence on drug treatment process and recidivism for probationers. *Journal of Clinical Psychology*, **53**, 387–97.

Carroll, J. F. X. & Sobel, B. S. (1986). Integrating mental health personnel and practices into a therapeutic community. In *Therapeutic Communities for Addictions: Readings in Theory, Research, and Practice*, eds G. De Leon & J. T. Ziegenfuss. Springfield, IL: Charles C. Thomas, pp. 209–26.

Center for Substance Abuse Treatment (2005a). Substance abuse treatment for persons with co-occurring disorders. *Treatment Improvement Protocol (TIP Series) #42*. DHHS Publication No. (SMA) 05–3992. Rockville, MD: Substance Abuse and Mental Health Services Administration.

Center for Substance Abuse Treatment (2005b). Substance abuse treatment for adults in the criminal justice system. *Treatment Improvement Protocol (TIP Series) #44*. DHHS Publication No. (SMA) 05–4056. Rockville, MD: Substance Abuse and Mental Health Services Administration.

Center for Substance Abuse Treatment (2006). *Therapeutic Community Curriculum: Participant's Manual*. DHHS Publication No. (SMA) 06–4122. Rockville, MD: Substance Abuse and Mental Health Services Administration.

Coletti, S. D., Schinka, J. A., Hughs, P. H. *et al.* (1997). Specialized therapeutic community treatment for chemically dependent women and their children. In *Community as Method: Therapeutic Communities for Special Populations and Special Settings*, ed. G. De Leon. Westport, CT: Greenwood, pp. 115–28.

Commission on Accreditation of Rehabilitative Facilities (2000). *The 2000 Behavioral Health Standards Manual*. Tucson, AZ: Commission on Accreditation of Rehabilitative Facilities. Available from: CARF, 4891 East Grant Rd., Tucson, AZ 85712.

Condelli, W. S. & Hubbard, R. L. (1994). Client outcomes from therapeutic communities. In *Therapeutic Community: Advances in Research and Application*, *(NIH Publ No 94–3633)*, eds F. M. Tims, G. De Leon & N. Jainchill. Rockville, MD: National Institute on Drug Abuse, pp. 80–98.

Deitch, D. A. & Solit, R. (1993). Training drug abuse treatment personnel in therapeutic community methodologies. *Psychotherapy*, **30**(special issue), 305–16.

De Leon, G. (1984). *The Therapeutic Community: Study of Effectiveness* (NIDA Treatment Research Monograph ADM-84–1286). Rockville, MD: National Institute on Drug Abuse.

De Leon, G. (1985). The therapeutic community: status and evolution. *International Journal of Addiction*, **20**, 823–44.

De Leon, G. (1995). Therapeutic communities for addictions: a theoretical framework. *International Journal of Addiction*, **30**, 1603–45.

De Leon, G (ed.). (1997). *Community as Method: Therapeutic Communities for Special Populations and Special Settings*. Westport, CT: Greenwood.

De Leon, G. (2000). *The Therapeutic Community: Theory, Model, and Method*. New York: Springer.

De Leon, G. & Jainchill, N. (1981–1982). Male and female drug abusers: social and psychological status 2 years after treatment in a therapeutic community. *Amercian Journal of Drug & Alcohol Abuse*, **8**, 465–97.

De Leon, G. & Schwartz, S. (1984). The therapeutic community: what are the retention rates? *American Journal of Drug & Alcohol Abuse*, **10**, 267–84.

De Leon, G., Wexler, H. K. & Jainchill, N. (1982). Success and improvement rates 5 years after treatment in a therapeutic community. *International Journal of Addiction*, **17**, 703–42.

De Leon, G., Staines, G. L. *et al.* (1995). Therapeutic community methods in methadone maintenance (passages): an open clinical trial. *Drug and Alcohol Dependence*, **37**(1), 45–57.

De Leon, G., Melnick, G. & Hawke, J. (2000a). The motivation-readiness factor in drug treatment: implications for research and policy. In *Emergent Issues in the Field of Drug Abuse*, Vol. **7**, *Advances in Medical Sociology Series*, ed. J. Levy, R. Stephens & D. McBride. Stamford, CT: JAI Press Inc., pp. 103–29.

De Leon, G., Hawke, J., Jainchill, N. *et al.* (2000b). Therapeutic communities: enhancing retention in treatment using "senior professor" staff. *Journal of Substance Abuse Treatment*, **19**, 375–82.

De Leon, G., Melnick, G., Cao, Y. & Wexler, H. K. (2006). Recovery-oriented perceptions as predictors of reincarceration. *Journal of Substance Abuse Treatment*, **31**, 87–94.

Galanter, M., Egelko, S., De Leon, G. *et al.* (1991). Crack/cocaine abusers in the general hospital: assessment and initiation of care. *American Journal of Psychiatry*, **149**, 810–15.

Gerstein, D. R. & Harwood, H. J. (eds.) (1990). *Treating Drug Problems*, Vol. **1**. *A Study of the Evaluation, Effectiveness, and Financing of Public and Private Drug Treatment Systems*. Institute of Medicine. Washington DC: National Academy Press.

Holland 1983: Holland, S. (1983). Evaluating community based treatment programs: A model for strengthening inferences about effectiveness. *International Journal of Therapeutic Communities*, **4**(4), 285–306.

Hubbard, R. L., Collins, J. J., Rachal, J. V. *et al.* (1988). The criminal justice client in drug abuse treatment. *NIDA Research Monographs*, **86**, 57–80.

Inciardi, J. A., Martin, S. S., Butzin, C. A. *et al.* (1997). An effective model of prison-based treatment for drug-involved offenders. *Journal of Drug Issues*, **27**, 261–78.

Jainchill, N. (1997). Therapeutic communities for adolescents: the same and not the same. In *Community as Method: Therapeutic Communities for Special Populations and Special Settings*, ed. G. De Leon. Westport, CT: Greenwood, pp. 161–78.

Jones, M. (1953). *Therapeutic Community: A New Treatment Method in Psychiatry*. New York: Basic Books.

Kressel, K., Kennedy, C. A. *et al.* (2002). Managing conflict in an urban health care setting: what do 'experts' know? *Health Care Law Policy*, **5**(2), 364–446.

Lewis, B. F. & Ross, R. (1994). Retention in therapeutic communities: challenges for the nineties. *NIDA Research Monographs*, **144**, 99–116.

Melnick and De Leon 1999:Melnick, G., & De Leon, G. (1999). Clarifying the nature of therapeutic community treatment: The survey of essential elements questionnaire (SEEQ). *Journal of Substance Abuse Treatment*, **16**(4): 307–313.

Melnick et al 2001b:Melnick, G., De Leon, G., Thomas, G., Wexler, H. K., & Kressel D. (2001b). Treatment process in therapeutic communities: Motivation, progress and outcomes. *American Journal of Drug and Alcohol Abuse*, **27**(4), 633–650.

Sacks, S., Sacks, J., De Leon, G. *et al.* (1997). Modified therapeutic community for mentally ill chemical "abusers": background; influences; program description; preliminary findings. *Substance Use and Misuse*, **32**, 1217–59.

Simpson, D. D., Wexler, H. K. and Inciardi, J. A. (Eds.) (1999) Drug treatment outcomes for correctional settings, part i. The Prison Journal (special Issue), **79**(3), 291–371.

Simpson, D. D. & Sells, S. B. (1982). Effectiveness of treatment for drug abuse: an overview of the DARP research program. *Advances in Alcohol & Substance Abuse*, **2**, 7–29.

Stevens, S. J., Arbiter, N. & McGrath, R. (1997). Women and children: therapeutic community substance abuse treatment. In *Community as Method: Therapeutic Communities for Special Populations and Special Settings*, eds. G. De Leon. Westport, CT: Greenwood, pp. 129–42.

Soyez, V., De Leon, G., Rosseel, Y. & Broekaert, E. (2006). The impact of a social network intervention on retention in Belgian therapeutic communities: a quasi experimental study. *Addiction*, **101**, 1027–34.

Talboy, E. S. (1998). *Therapeutic Community Experiential Training: Facilitator Guide*. Kansas City, MO: University of Missouri–Kansas City, Mid-America Addiction Technology Transfer Center.

Tims, F. M., De Leon, G. & Jainchill, N. (eds.) (1994).Therapeutic community: advances in research and application. Proceedings of a Meeting, May 16–17, 1991. *NIDA Research Monographs*, **144**, 1–286.

Tims and Ludford 1984: Tims, F. M., & Ludford, J. P. (Eds.). (1984). *Drug abuse treatment evaluation: Strategies, progress and prospects. National Institute on Drug Abuse Research Monograph 51* (DHHS Publication No. [ADM] 84–1329). Rockville, MD: National Institute on Drug Abuse.

Wexler et al 1999a,: Wexler, H.K., De Leon, G., Thomas, G., Kressel, D., & Peters, J. (1999). The Amity prison TC evaluation: Reincarceration outcomes. *Criminal Justice and Behavior*, **26**(2): 144–167.

[a]Wexler et al 1999b, Wexler, H. K. Melnick, J., Lowe, L., et.al: Three year reincarceration outcomes for Amity inpriosn therapeutic community and afrtercare in California. The Prison Journal., 79: 321–336.

Winick, C. & Evans, J. T. (1997). A therapeutic community for mothers and their children. In *Community as Method: Therapeutic Communities for Special Populations and Special Settings*, ed. G. De Leon. Westport, CT: Greenwood, pp. 143–60.

End Reference

The material for this chapter is adapted from a comprehensive account of the therapeutic community theory, model, and method provided elsewhere (De Leon, 2000).

8

Cosmetic psychopharmacology: drugs that enhance wellbeing, performance, and creativity

Richard N. Rosenthal & Laurence M. Westreich

Introduction

The desire to improve oneself, whether in academics, athletics, or even everyday functioning, is a natural human drive. In fact, the push for self-improvement is the base upon which society builds its skyscrapers, literary masterpieces, universities, and initial public offerings.

When modern medicine offered up the barbiturate sedatives which emerged as "Mother's Little Helper" (The Rolling Stones, *Aftermath*, 1966) in the post-World War 2 era, many saw their use as a direct response to the dissolution of traditional family and society structures. But the past 30 years have seen an explosion of psychopharmacologic preparations and their widespread use far beyond anything imaginable in the 1960s drug culture.

The legendary drug use of the 1960s represented wide illegal experimental use of marijuana and hallucinogens for consciousness changing or raising, with only fringe elements of society using harder drugs like heroin and cocaine. Today's legal psychopharmacologic consumer, by contrast, is more likely to use for the sake of a specific and non-recreational purpose. In *The Simpsons* episode, aired October 3, 1999 and titled "Brother's Little Helper," the title (cartoon) character is prescribed "Focusyn," which improves his school performance but makes him paranoid (http://simpsons.wikia.com/wiki/Brother%27s_Little_Helper, accessed November 19, 2008).

Even setting aside the prescription of psychotropic medications for the treatment of diagnosed psychiatric illnesses like attention deficit disorder and depression, our society is remarkably tolerant to the use of psychotropic medications for non-medical use. This "cosmetic psychopharmacology" will be the subject of this chapter. Peter Kramer M. D. (1993) describes the essential questions for the modern user of psychotropic medications:

…psychic steroids for mental gymnastics, medicinal attacks on the humors, antiwallflower compound – these might be hard to resist. Since you only live once, why not do it as a blonde? Why not a peppy blonde? Now that questions of personality and social stance have entered the world of medication, we as a society will have to decide how comfortable we are with using chemicals to modify personality in useful, attractive ways.

In our hyper-competitive academic and work environment, the substantial pressure for improved production, whether of grades or work output, leads to the modification of psychopharmacologic treatments to treat non-disease states like fatigue, poor motivation, or boredom. Of course, the dividing line between "disease" and "non-disease" states is subjective and hotly contested. Similarly, there is a blurring of boundaries between accepted techniques like ingestion of protein supplements, and (officially) unacceptable body sculpting techniques like anabolic steroids or weight-reducing diuretics.

Similarly, debates rage in the world of professional sports regarding the ethics of substance use, the boundaries of that use, and the huge amounts of money tempting athletes and scientists to collaborate in their attempts to improve athletic performance without being caught. The realm of "psycho-exploration," the attempts to promote psychotherapeutic change or dispel anxiety using hallucinogenics, are described. Finally, this chapter will examine the claims and counterclaims about the enhancement of creative, especially musical, production while under the influence of mind altering substances.

"Ramping it up," the improvement of everyday functioning

In *Beyond Therapy: Biotechnology and the Pursuit of Human Improvement*, the President's Council on Bioethics (2003) sought to conduct a "fundamental inquiry into the human and moral significance of developments in biomedical and behavioral science and technology." One of the conclusions they came to was that "…exactly because of their impressive powers to alter the workings of body and mind, the 'dual uses' of the same technologies make them attractive also to people who are not sick but who would use them to look younger, perform better, feel happier, or become more "perfect." As such, it is a reality that people use substances to improve their performance in a range of human endeavors: interpersonal relationships, vocations, schooling, self-awareness, physical competition, and creativity. To better understand the ethical aspects of this usage, it may be useful for clinicians to distinguish the basis upon which these substances are used – therapeutic, medical enhancement, and non-medical enhancement.

Therapy is ethically unquestionable as it "is the use of biotechnical power to treat individuals with known diseases, disabilities, or impairments, in an attempt to restore them to a normal state of health and fitness." More deserving of ethical scrutiny is enhancement, which "is the directed use of biotechnical power to alter, by direct intervention, not disease processes but the 'normal' workings of the human body and psyche, to augment or improve their native capacities and performances" (President's Council on Bioethics, 2003). Examples of the former and latter include surgical reconstruction as compared to augmentation, or psychopharmacology compared to cosmetic psychopharmacology, the topic at hand. Although these are apparently clear ideas, the actual distinctions between remediable non-disease states, sub-threshold disorder states (e.g. poor motivation, indecisiveness), and disease states may be less precise. What is clear is that, although enhancements are not necessarily therapeutic, all therapies are enhancing (Chatterjee, 2004). It is not easy to argue against medications that enhance memory functioning in elderly persons with cognitive changes, but what about drugs blocking memory formation, purportedly to inhibit the consolidation of memories of traumatic events to prevent post-traumatic stress disorder (PTSD)? One can consider prevention of disease states a laudable effort, but what if those drugs were to be used as an enhancement simply to prevent bad memories (Farah et al., 2004)?

Part of the determination of therapy versus performance enhancement may reside in the way in which we ascribe what is normal. Is normality a disease-free state? If the person is not free of disease, then therapy is appropriate. What about someone with an IQ of 100? This is normal by definition. If it were 86, would a theoretical intervention be therapy or enhancement? If normal means healthy, then the definition of health becomes important.

The World Health Organization (WHO) defines health as "a state of complete physical, mental and social well-being" which is beyond a simple disease-free state and allows a broader potential ethical basis for enhancement (preamble to the Constitution of the WHO as adopted by the International Health Conference, New York, June 19–22, 1946; signed on July 22, 1946 by the representatives of 61 states [Official Records of the World Health Organization, no. 2, p. 100] and entered into force on April 7, 1948). There is a range of over-the-counter, prescription medications, and illicit substances available that people use to enhance their cognitive, creative, and physical performance.

One purpose of medicine, in addition to the alleviation of suffering, is to improve the quality of life. A question that arises in this context is: if we could enhance cognition in disease, should we do it in health? Yesavage and colleagues (2002) performed a placebo-controlled study of oral donepezil mg/day (cholinesterase inhibitor) in commercial pilots over a 1-month period. At the end of the study period, pilots receiving the active medication performed better in flight simulation tests compared to controls, especially in emergency situations. So, it is clear that in situations requiring expertise, people who are already competent can be stimulated to perform better with cognitive-enhancing drugs.

In the everyday context of work or school, the use of stimulants is ubiquitous. Caffeine, an adenosine receptor competitive antagonist, is probably the most popular drug on the planet, and is consumed in a variety of ways, including coffee, tea, cola, and other soft drinks, candies, dark chocolate, and energy drinks. Doses of caffeine in typical servings range from 10 to 50 mg in green teas, soft drinks, and energy bars, 70–100 mg in brewed coffee, black teas, caffeine tablets, and energy drinks such as Red Bull®, and greater than 200 mg in a 16 oz. Starbuck's coffee and Jolt Cola (Bramstedt & Katrina, 2007; McCusker et al., 2003; 2006). In healthy adults, moderate daily caffeine intake up to 400 mg (6 mg/kg in a 65-kg person) is not associated with negative effects on behavior, cardiovascular function, bone mineralization and calcium balance, cancer incidence or male fertility (Nawrot et al., 2003). In addition to the gustatory and social pleasures one might experience in the context of using caffeinated products, the principal desired effects are the stimulant and ergogenic properties that allow one more subjective energy, reduced fatigue, better concentration, and increased capacity for mental or physical exertion (Akerstedt & Ficca, 1997; Ivy *et al.*, 1979; Trice &, Haymes, 1995). Caffeine use has significant benefits. Workers who consume more than 220 mg of caffeine/day have about half the risk of frequent/very frequent cognitive failures (memory, attention, choice of action) and a similar reduction in risk for accidents at work (Smith, 2005). With respect to cognitive functioning, regular caffeine increases capacity for information processing, leading to improvements in simple reaction time, choice reaction time, incidental verbal memory, and visuospatial reasoning (Jarvis, 1993). Thus, a large percentage of the population enhances their performance in a real and substantive way through daily use of caffeinated products.

Since glucose priming alone enhances learning and memory (Sunram-Lea *et al.*, 2002), adding glucose to caffeinated drinks, and presumably other caffeine-containing products, enhances speed, accuracy, and sustained selective attention (Rao *et al.*, 2005). This is the rationale for energy drinks. For example, in a double-blind controlled study of a glucose-based energy drink versus a control glucose-based drink without caffeine, taurine, and glucurono-lactone, drivers in the experimental group demonstrated significantly less lane drifting and decreased reaction times in interactive real-car driving simulator tests (Horne & Reyner, 2001). Energy drink sales in the US have increased at an annual rate of 55%, a more than sixfold increase over the 5-year period from 2002 to 2006 (Reissig *et al.*, 2008). Energy drinks are of special public health concern in that the FDA does not regulate them, nor does it require warning labels advising of their caffeine content or proper use. Representative energy drinks currently in the US market offer a range from relatively low caffeine concentrations such as that seen in the top-selling brands similar to that in brewed coffee (5–11 mg/oz), to higher concentration drinks that deliver 20–35 mg/oz caffeine, to ultraconcentrated "shot-type" drinks with 90–170 mg/oz caffeine.

Although there is good evidence for the performance-promoting effects of caffeine, it can cause toxicity at higher doses, with symptoms of anxiety, restlessness, insomnia, nausea, vomiting, and, at higher doses, seizures, and arrhythmia

(Broderick & Benjamin, 2004). Twenty-four ounces of "Wired X505" or 20 oz. of "Fixx" energy drinks offer 500 mg or more of caffeine, which is cause for concern (Reissig *et al.*, 2008). Adolescents and young adults have less mature frontal lobe functioning than adults, and thus as a group are less likely to inhibit risk-taking behavior, or be responsive to negative feedback from the internal or external environment. Adolescents have reduced metabolic capacity for caffeine (likely owing to changes in sex hormones), so they are affected more intensely per unit dose than adults, and there are several reports of severe toxicity and fatalities due to overdoses of caffeine in adolescents and young adults (Bramstedt & Katrina, 2007; Lane & Connor, 1994). Malinauskas *et al.* (2007) recorded energy drink consumption patterns of 496 randomly surveyed state university college students and found that 51% were users typically 1–4 days per month, the majority of whom used one dose to address situations of insufficient sleep (67%), to increase energy (65%), or to drink with alcohol while partying (54%). Of students who used energy drinks, 49% consumed three or more while partying with alcohol. These last data give cause for alarm because, while supporting increased alertness during periods of alcohol consumption, caffeine does not reduce objective effects of alcohol intoxication, such as impairment of motor coordination and visual reaction time, potentially leading to increased activity in the context of impaired judgment and physical control (Ferreira *et al.*, 2006). In a survey of 4237 college students from 10 universities (O'Brien *et al.*, 2008), students who reported consuming alcohol mixed with energy drinks have, even after adjusting for the volume of alcohol consumed, significantly higher rates of alcohol-related consequences, such as being taken advantage of, or taking advantage of another, sexually, riding with an alcohol-impaired driver, being physically hurt or injured, and requiring medical treatment.

In addition to the use of stimulants to improve performance that are available in foodstuffs and over-the-counter preparations, there are also prescription stimulants that are used for reasons other than treatment of disorders for which they are typically prescribed, such as attention deficit hyperactivity disorder (ADHD) or excessive daytime sleepiness associated with narcolepsy. There is a well described indication of stimulant drugs for the treatment of ADHD, but there is also use in populations that are not diagnosed with the disorder, who use the medications in ways not intended by the manufacturer. Among 10 904 randomly selected students from 199 4-year American colleges, the past year prevalence of non-medical prescription stimulant use was estimated at 4% and was as high as 25% at individual schools (McCabe *et al.*, 2005). Adult attitudes may also affect the context within which younger members of society assess the risks and benefits of non-medical use of prescription cognitive enhancers. An internet poll about non-medical use of cognition enhancers such as modafinil and methylphenidate found that 80% of the 1400 respondents favored adult discretion over use of these medications (Maher, 2008).

Recreational use of ADHD medications has increased greatly over the past decade (Dupont *et al.*, 2008). Adolescents and young adults who obtain methylphenidate from classmates, family or friends with legitimate prescriptions frequently abuse the drug by crushing and snorting it to get high. However, there is a subpopulation of non-prescription use that is not recreational. For example, both Babcock & Byrne (2000) and Dupont *et al.* (2008) cite the use of non-prescribed methylphenidate by students, who, instead of taking oral doses, insufflate the medication at higher than standard doses not only for recreational purposes, but also before examinations or to write term papers. Others simply take oral doses to study. Recreational use aside, one can question the fairness of students taking exams in a state of heightened cognitive functioning, not dissimilar to the issues of performance enhancement on the athletic field, where stimulants and many other enhancing methodologies are prohibited.

Methylphenidate is a catecholamine reuptake inhibitor that increases postsynaptic dopaminergic stimulation in the brain through blockade of the DA reuptake transporter, and is used for the treatment of children and adults with ADHD (Wilens, 2008). Methylphenidate improves attention, concentration, working memory, distractibility, and motor hyperactivity in patients with ADHD (Pary *et al.*, 2002). Although approved for use in treatment of ADHD, methylphenidate has been demonstrated to improve executive functioning such as working memory and planning in healthy adults as well, with greater effects on those with lower levels of baseline performance, an effect also seen with mixed amphetamine salts (Adderall) in healthy adults (Elliott

et al., 1997; Mehta *et al.*, 2000; Farah *et al.*, 2008). These effects are not lost on the non-patient community and methylphenidate is well known on college campuses for use as a "study aid" (Maher, 2008).

Modafinil is a wakefulness-promoting drug, approved in the US for the treatment of narcolepsy, daytime sleepiness owing to obstructive sleep apnea, and shift work sleep disorder (Kumar, 2008). Although not approved for use in ADHD, modafinil has been demonstrated to improve short-term memory span, visual memory, spatial planning, and stop-signal motor inhibition in patients with ADHD (Turner *et al.*, 2004). Modafinil has been demonstrated in controlled trials to improve symptoms of ADHD in children and adolescents significantly (Amiri *et al.*, 2008; Biederman *et al.*, 2005). In patients with schizophrenia, modafinil is associated with better executive functioning and attentional performance (Morein-Zamir *et al.*, 2007). There is off-label usage in patients where excessive daytime sleepiness is due to other causes, such as closed-head trauma, as well as use in ADHD, postanesthetic sedation, cocaine dependence and withdrawal, and as an adjunct to antidepressants for depression, even in the absence of convincing evidence from replicated clinical trials (Teitelman, 2001; Ballon & Feifel, 2006). Modafinil increases arousal and reduces attentional deficits due to sleep deprivation (Lagarde *et al.*, 1995; Caldwell *et al.*, 2000; Gill *et al.*, 2006). In addition, modafinil significantly improves fatigue levels, motivation, and vigilance, as well as performance on digit span, visual pattern recognition memory, spatial planning, and reaction time in normal adults (Baranski *et al.*, 2004; Turner *et al.*, 2004). Given these characteristics, it becomes more likely, especially in the face of a relatively safe side-effects profile (headaches, insomnia, anxiety, and palpitations) and in spite of the rare occurrence of severe dermatological reactions such as Stevens–Johnson syndrome and toxic epidermal necrolysis, that this drug will be used to enhance performance, not just to treat approved disorders, or be prescribed off-label by physicians (Kumar, 2008). Newspapers and weblogs have been carrying stories about modafinil for several years. Modafinil "...has been credited with fuelling the rise of the '24-hour society' by helping truckers, students, night-clubbers and international travelers stay awake through the night or cope with jet lag" (Williams *et al.*, 2008). Studies have shown that, in America, about 75% of people taking the pill do so for non-medical reasons, often to skip a few hours' or a night's sleep. It is popular with parents coping with young children, computer gamers, and students facing exams (Leake, 2008). Arrington (2008), in an online technical weblog states, "...the buzz lately is that it's the 'entrepreneur's drug of choice' around Silicon Valley."

Cognitive performance enhancement may be achievable, but there can be negative medical consequences. For medications with abuse liability, there is already scheduling to restrict legitimate use to prescriptions by physicians, since those drugs are more likely to be abused in vulnerable populations. Methylphenidate and amphetamine are dopaminergic, which increases the reward associated with tasks performed under the medicated condition, and can lead to compulsive use and dependence in vulnerable people (Volkow & Swanson, 2008). In spite of the Federal Schedule regulating the prescription of these drugs, even well educated professional people are using these drugs to enhance their cognitive performance. In the informal online poll mentioned above, readers of the journal *Nature* were asked whether they had used any of three medications (modafinil, methylphenidate, β-blockers) for a non-medical, cognition-enhancing purpose. Among the 1400 people from 60 countries who responded, 20% responded positively, of whom 44% had used modafinil, 62% had used methylphenidate, and 15% β-blockers. The most popular reasons for taking these drugs as cognitive enhancers were to improve concentration and focus on a specific task, or to remediate jet lag. The medications used were procured from several sources: the internet (34%), a physician's prescription (52%), and from a pharmacy (14%)(Maher, 2008).

Body sculpting with drugs

Although the use of substances to mold one's body is probably perceived by the user as a purely physical maneuver, in fact the behavior betrays a psychosocial need clearly met by the body sculpting. In the now-common dermatologic practices of acne reduction, hair replacement, and wrinkle reduction, an ever-growing pharmacopeia offers a more youthful appearance to the patient/client. For weight loss medications and surgeries, the line between cosmetic improvement for psychological benefit and the medically necessary procedure is often a bit

blurrier – the obese individual who has a stomach stapling procedure may reap many medical benefits in addition to the enhanced self-esteem that his or her weight loss may bring. Multiple problems – such as the Fen-Phen disaster – have led to heavy scrutiny of both stimulant weight loss agents (Carneiro *et al.*, 2006) and the non-stimulant anorectics (Colman, 2005). Manipulating one's body for non-athletic reasons is a common, if unexamined, fact of modern medical care.

Although the use of performance-enhancing drugs for psychological improvements in athletics is discussed below, the exact same substances can be used for psychological benefit. In the research summarized in his book, *The Adonis Complex* (2000), Harrison Pope, M. D. comments on the purely psychological need many men have for a body which attains a cultural ideal, which has changed over the past 60 years. Dr. Pope quotes a *Psychology Today* survey which found 15% of men dissatisfied with their overall appearance in 1972, which rose to 34% in 1985, and 43% in 1997. This dissatisfaction is translated, according to Dr. Pope, into various body manipulations, including the use of steroids for achieving muscle bulk rather than function – which is, in contrast to performance-enhancing use, a purely cosmetic procedure for psychological benefit.

Athletics
Ethical issues

Before addressing the details of psychopharmacology in sport, one should examine first the philosophical and ethical issues involved: to wit, who cares? That is, if an adult person chooses to take a substance to enhance his or her athletic performance, what difference should that make to anyone or, put the other way, why shouldn't the substance-taking garner the same sort of admiration that a rigorous training regimen elicits? One philosopher in the field, Thomas Murray, writes and speaks about five major arguments against doping control, and the problems he sees with each argument (http://www.wada-ama.org/rtecontent/document/PlayTrue_Issue3_2007_Murray_En.pdf, accessed November 25, 2008; and "Testing for high: ethical considerations," presented at the Growth Hormone Summit (Major League Baseball and The Office of Continuing Medical Education at UCLA) Beverly Hills, California, November 10, 2008).

First, Thomas writes, is the "It's all the same" argument, which suggests that the evolution of sports and sports equipment – faster skis, better swimsuits, improved training methods – should encompass substances also. But Thomas argues that not all improvements are the same, in that some undermine the essential meaning of sport, including, in his estimation, performance-enhancing drugs. (He does mention other improvements which would be similarly rejected by all, such as wheels on the bottom of a runner's shoes.)

Secondly, Thomas says, is "the line-drawing problem," in which skeptics assert that prohibitions on certain substances are hopelessly arbitrary and therefore unfair. Although he concedes the arbitrariness of some such rules, Thomas says that fact does not remove the necessity for making rules to which all competitors must adhere. If the pitcher's mound were not 60 feet 6 inches from the home plate, the game of baseball would be changed for all involved, so no one suggests changing this distance, arbitrary as it is.

The paternalism argument is the third issue that Murray cites as an argument against doping control, best described as the "Hey! You'll put your eye out" argument. Critics point out that athletics entails certain risks, some sports contain grave risks, and elite athletes are both able and very willing to assume those risks. But Murray points out that the obvious coercion the athletes are under to match the dangerous training methods of their peers is patently unfair and dangerous, when those training methods are illegal and dangerous. Only by achieving a "level playing field," where all athletes adhere to the same rules, can this brutal coercion be removed.

The fourth argument against doping control which Murray addresses is the inevitability problem – that resistance is futile. Although Murray acknowledges that control of doping is difficult and imperfect, that fact does not take away from the necessity for controls. He also notes that improvements in technique make testing efforts much better than they have been in the past.

Finally, Murray addresses "transhumanism," the idea that humans should strive for the ultimate in sports performance in the same way that we strive for excellence via science and technology in all other spheres. Here Murray notes that the spirit of sport is to do the best with the bodies we have, and that "..as long as people care about human excellence, natural talents, and the dedication and intelligence required to

perfect those talents, I believe the spirit of sport…can and should survive."

Prescribed medications

Medications that are appropriately prescribed for psychiatric illness can, of course, improve performance when the psychiatric symptoms are lifted. Some of these medications are banned in competitive sports, so the athlete who wants to use these medications must request a "therapeutic use exemption" (TUE). The TUE allows an athlete to use a banned substance after an appropriate diagnostic assessment, a legitimate prescription, and ongoing monitoring. Psychostimulants for the treatment of ADD/ADHD are the most common class of medications for which athletes request a TUE. Despite the acknowledged risks for athletes using stimulants – even those legitimately prescribed (Avois et al., 2006) – the stimulant medications remain a common and well founded treatment for adults with ADD/ADHD (Spencer et al., 2001). So, the addiction psychiatrist working in the sports environment must fashion a plan which allows the ADD/ADHD sufferer to use appropriately prescribed medication, while denying those medications to those who are merely using the medications to improve their athletic performance. Major sports organizations, including the Olympics (http://www.wada-ama.org/en/exemptions.ch2, accessed November 3, 2008), the NCAA (http://www.ncaa.org/wps/ncaa?ContentID=481, accessed November 3, 2008), the National Football League, Major League Baseball (Major League Baseball/Major League Baseball Player Association Press release; MLB, players association modify joint drug agreement. April 11, 2008), and the National Hockey League (http://www.nhl.com/nhlhq/cba/drug_testing072205.html, accessed November 5, 2008), all have appeals processes for granting TUEs.

In addition to using medications for bona fide psychiatric illness, athletes may of course use prescribed medications to improve their performance. One interesting example of this phenomenon is the use of beta-blockers to improve performance. Beta-blockers are an accepted treatment for stage fright in performers, presumably because of their mild anti-anxiety effects (Brantigan et al., 1982). Competitive athletes in some sports may be banned from using beta-blockers because of a perceived unfair advantage (Mottram, 2005): in shooting sports the antitremor effect of the beta-blocker can be an advantage and the induced bradycardia may give the shooter more opportunity to pull the trigger between heartbeats, thereby allowing a shot without the bump of the heartbeat against the chest wall and the stock of the gun. However, the anti-anxiety effects (and elaboration on those effects) are probably more important, regardless of the athlete's perception of any physical effects. A journalist, writing about his own experience playing golf after having taken a beta-blocker he cadged from a friend, wrote: "…I felt strangely calm – oblivious, even. Beta blockers suppress parts of the central nervous system and slow the heart rate, reducing symptoms of anxiety, such as tremors and sweating – and the yips. I hit a sand iron to the front of the green, chipped up, and holed a 10-foot putt…" (Cassidy, 2008).

Supplements

Similarly to prescribed medication, nutritional supplements are used by athletes to improve performance, but their effect is probably more psychological than otherwise. Because of the Dietary Supplement Health and Education Act (DSHEA) of 1994, the supplement industry is able to promote various non-prescription substances for athletic performance as long as there is no claim that the substances treat any medical problem. So, a multi-million dollar industry has arisen which touts amino acids, protein supplements, and other substances as performance-improving, with little peer-reviewed evidence to support those claims, and no legal requirement to present any such evidence of safety or efficacy. Only with the occurrence of a disaster such as multiple deaths related to a particular substance is the industry required to take a particular substance off the shelves (FDA issues regulation prohibiting sale of dietary supplements containing ephedrine alkaloids and reiterates its advice that consumers stop using these products. Food and Drug Administration Press Release, February 6, 2004).

For example, kava kava, a supplement widely thought to have anti-anxiety and anti-insomnia effects (http://www.anxiety-and-depression-solutions.com/articles/complementary_alternative_medicine/herbs_supplements/kava_kava.php, accessed November 29, 2008) has been shown to have significant anti-anxiety effects (van der Watt et al., 2008), but concern over reports of hepatic toxicity has increased in recent years (Escher et al., 2001). This concern about side-effects points out an ongoing and serious problem with nutritional supplements: they are seen by the public as probably effective and natural (read: safe) so are rarely subjected to the same scrutiny as prescription medications. Since the supplements are usually easier to obtain and need no doctor's prescription, those trying to improve their mood are likely to try them long before trying prescription medications. Ideally, those trying these substances should weigh the potential psychological benefits against an accurate list of the substance risks – exactly as they would for a prescription medication.

Anabolic androgenic steroids

The most obvious public discussion about cosmetic pharmacology – if not *psycho*pharmacology – in sports has been about the use of anabolic androgenic steroids (AAS) by athletes and others (Cancesco, 2005; Bryant, 2005). In addition to purportedly enhancing physical performance, AAS have been associated with physical problems like tendon rupture (Laseter & Russell, 1991), as well as reductions in HDL cholesterol, shrunken testes, and liver cysts (Lukas, 2009). However, AAS also cause significant psychiatric pathology, the most distinctive of which is "roid rage." As in the case of World Wrestling Foundation wrestler Chris Benoit, the popular media may exaggerate the effects of steroids on complexly determined human behaviors (CNN Larry King Live Transcript, July 9, 2007). However, peer-reviewed papers have published case series and literature reviews documenting AAS-related hostility, aggression, hallucinations, and delusions (Perry et al., 1990; Pope & Katz, 1988). Although aggressiveness is necessary in all sports, it is hard to imagine that "rage" benefits the athlete under any circumstance: even the physical ferocity necessary at the line of scrimmage must be contained, time-limited, and focused.

Steroid-related affective symptoms are much more common than psychosis, however, and the affective symptoms are generally experienced by unsophisticated AAS users who are taking dosages at the high end of the spectrum, far beyond those that render performance enhancement. Mood symptoms can include depression, hypomania, and frank mania (Trenton & Currier, 2006). One manifestation of withdrawal from AAS can be a profound depression (Brower et al., 1990), which has been implicated in the completed suicide of some users (http://www.taylorhooton.org/, accessed November 1, 2007).

Although the very existence of true physiologic dependence and withdrawal from AAS has been questioned, careful analysis shows that both phenomena occur, usually in the heavy AAS user. An early case study of an AAS user who stopped abruptly revealed typical correlates of withdrawal: the sudden onset of dysphoria, fatigue, psychomotor retardation, impaired concentration, along with suicidal ideation (Brower *et al.*, 1989). This symptom picture disappeared after 4 days. The same group reported a later case series of 49 AAS-using competitive weight lifters (Brower *et al.*, 1991) and found that 94% endorsed at least one symptom of DSM-III-R dependence, with 84% experiencing physiologic withdrawal, 51% using more AAS than intended, and 49% spending more time than they had intended on substance-related activities.

Although true addictive behaviors do follow some AAS use, most users experience little in the way of immediate dependence or withdrawal. Despite this lack of immediate addictive consequences, these users face the same long-term risk of medical and psychiatric sequelae as those who experience short-term negative effects. In addition, the legal consequences of illicit use and the negative effects on an institution condoning or even promoting AAS can be catastrophic. Although AAS use has been widespread in US sport over the past 20 years, better public understanding of the pernicious psychiatric effects of these drugs on individual athletes and sport itself has led to increased vigilance for illicit use, and severe sanctions for the users.

Stimulants

Although the "rage" attributed to AAS users can hardly be particularly useful in any sport, the optimism, enhanced motivation, and self-confidence that stimulants bring can be useful both in training and on the athletic field. Stimulant drugs ranging from amphetamine to caffeine are widely used in the general population, and in the form of legally prescribed medications have some legitimate medical uses, such as the treatment of attention deficit disorder (ADD) and narcolepsy. Although professional athletes have long acknowledged using stimulants for fatigue (Frias, 2006), the substances have effects on mood and motivation also. Athletes sometimes use amphetamines and other stimulants in the form of "greenies," but since these substances are illegal and therefore not monitored by the FDA the user has no idea what is really inside the capsule that a team mate or drug dealer gives to him. The capsule could contain amphetamine, caffeine, sugar, or cyanide for that matter.

Stimulant drugs run the gamut from widely available and relatively harmless to illegal and extremely dangerous. For instance, although caffeine is perfectly legal, drugs like amphetamine and methylphenidate are illegal without a prescription, and are banned by professional and amateur sports.

All stimulant drugs work on dopamine and norepinephrine to increase mental alertness, decrease fatigue, and elevate the mood. These drugs also cause appetite suppression, weight loss, increased sexuality, and an emotional feeling of high self-confidence. However, each of these effects is matched by a corresponding "crash" when the substance wears off: users describe a sense of physical and mental lethargy, hunger, and emotional ups and downs as the stimulants wear off. When athletes use stimulant drugs to improve their performance, they run the risk of many unintended but quite severe side-effects. Although jitteriness and anxiety from too much of a stimulant drug usually resolves on its own, the more serious side-effects do not.

The serious side-effects of stimulant drugs arise from cardiovascular and CNS effects: stimulants which are either very potent or taken in large amounts can cause hypertension and arrhythmias and, in susceptible individuals, can promote severe dehydration (Martinez *et al.*, 2002), cerebrovascular attacks (De Silva *et al.*, 2007), myocardial infarctions (Westover *et al.*, 2008), and burst aneurysms (McEvoy *et al.*, 2000). The stimulants can provoke agitation, impaired judgment, hallucinations, or suspiciousness which can rise to the level of paranoia. Stimulants can also cause an increase in body temperature which, combined with the increased urination caused by the drugs, can lead to fatal consequences for the athlete who is training for long hours. For those who take stimulants over the long term, side-effects include weight loss, chronic heart disease, skin disease, and disturbed thinking processes (Galanter & Kleber, 2004).

Those who take stimulant drugs sometimes take a depressant drug like heroin, alcohol, or marijuana to help them "come down" from the effects of the stimulant. (The actor John Belushi died when he injected himself with cocaine and heroin in an attempt to decrease the crash associated with cocaine alone.) Athletes who use stimulants for performance sometimes use alcohol or marijuana to help themselves relax and get to sleep after the game. Although athletes have popularized the use of stimulant medications to improve their alertness and performance, clearly many adults outside of professional sports use stimulants also. In the years between 1992 and 2002, the admission rate to treatment for methamphetamine/amphetamine rose from 10 persons per 100 000 population to 52 persons per 100 000, demonstrating a massive increase in admissions, most of which were for smokeable methamphetamine (Drug and Alcohol Services Information System Report, 2004).

Of great concern is that, in 2005, 13.1% of twelfth graders admitted they had taken amphetamine illicitly, while 8.0% admitted that they had tried cocaine at some point. Of the twelfth graders surveyed, 37.7% answered that taking amphetamines once or twice was a "great risk," with the others reporting less concern about taking amphetamine (Monitoring the Future, 2005).

Amphetamine (Adderall, Dexedrine, Desoxyn, and others)

Although banned by amateur and professional sports, and illegal without a prescription, these medications have some legitimate uses, most commonly for the treatment of ADD or depression. However, when used inappropriately they can cause all of the side-effects listed above. Although these medications are sometimes prescribed for weight loss, the disastrous effects of overuse and subsequent withdrawal have almost eliminated this indication for the medication.

Methylphenidate (Ritalin, Metadate, Concerta, and others)

Commonly prescribed for ADD, methylphenidate is heavily advertised and available in long-lasting forms such as Concerta. Although less potent than amphetamine, methylphenidate can cause the same side-effects if taken in high enough dosages or for long enough. Like amphetamine, methylphenidate is banned by sports organizations and illegal without a prescription.

Caffeine

Although legal and permitted by most sports authorities, caffeine has its own set of potential side-effects. In addition to the potential for jitteriness and stomach upset possible from caffeine use, withdrawal from caffeine can incite headaches and fatigue.

Nicotine

Nicotine is a stimulant drug which, like other stimulants, causes withdrawal reactions. It is this withdrawal reaction that causes the cigarette smoker to crave nicotine and feel "relaxed" when he smokes a cigarette. He or she has simply treated his withdrawal syndrome and naturally feels better. Some athletes use spit tobacco as a stimulant during competition, but of course become addicted and need to use the substance all the time. (Of course, the stimulant nicotine is neither illegal nor banned by sports, but in the form of tobacco kills more Americans every year than alcohol, cocaine, and heroin combined [CDC, 2002].)

Blood doping and genetic manipulation

Although the use of blood doping agents like erythropoietin (EPO) for endurance sports is likely intended only to improve stamina, there is ample evidence that EPO improves mood – even in those who are not ill. In one study of healthy volunteers (Miskowiak *et al.*, 2008), 3 days after EPO administration the injectees reported improvements in self-reported mood and cognitive function as compared to a control group who had received sham injections. The authors noted that the responses were similar "…to behavioral effects observed with serotonergic antidepressants…" and that EPO might therefore be tried with frankly depressed individuals. Another study – this one of anemic patients – noted that mood was one of many factors improved by the administration of exogenous EPO (Silverberg *et al.*, 2001). Although forward-looking research about genetic manipulation has focused on treating disease states and (theoretically, at least) improving athletic performance, there is no doubt that future scientists will look at psychological benefits to be obtained from genetic manipulation.

Psychotherapeutic exploration using drugs

Dahlsgaard and colleagues (2005) performed an exhaustive search of the core texts of the world's substantial and ancient religious and philosophical traditions for convergent virtues that contribute to a fulfilling, happy life, and found that one of the six overarching virtues was transcendence, supported by strengths that provide meaningful connection to the larger universe. Small wonder, then, that humanity has been attempting for millennia to create contexts through ritualized behavior (e.g. religious and spiritual traditions) and through the use of psychoactive substances within which to expand personal experience to the level of transcendence. Hallucinogens have been used by various cultures for shamanic healing or divination rituals, religious ceremonies, or, in western psychotherapy, to intensify self-analysis or self-understanding (Metzner, 1998). Sessa (2005) reviewed the research of the decades of the 1950s and 1960s and cited more than 2000 papers with positive results of psychedelic-assisted (mostly LSD) psychotherapy for tens of thousands of patients. However, most of the research was of uncontrolled case reports lacking in appropriate follow-up.

In the 1970s and 1980s, prior to becoming illegal in the US, 3, 4-methylenedioxymethamphetamine (MDMA), better known today as the street drug ecstasy, was used by psychotherapists to enhance the therapy process through its purported empathogenic or "relationship-enhancing" properties, but it was placed on Schedule I in 1985 and legitimate research and practice with the drug in the US ceased (Rosenthal & Solhkhah, 2005; Sessa, 2005). The practice of MDMA-assisted psychotherapy was reviewed by Sessa, who found that most of the early research reports suffered from the times in which they were done – that in spite of subjects mostly reporting positive effects, the studies were lacking in adequate controls and follow-up. Most of the reports, however, in contradistinction to the well documented harms associated with street use, found little harm associated with its use in clinical situations (Sessa, 2005).

Currently, there are new studies for treatment of specific disorders. For example, Mithoefer (2008), at the Medical University of South Carolina, recently completed a phase II double-blind placebo-controlled trial of MDMA-assisted immersion psychotherapy for treatment-resistant PTSD in crime victims and combat veterans. Randomized controlled pilot trials of hallucinogens for reducing anxiety and need for analgesia in terminally ill cancer patients are being conducted with psilocybin at Harbor-UCLA Medical Center (Grob *et al.*, 1996) and MDMA at Brigham and Women's Hospital (Halpern *et al.*, 2008). There is, at present, little rationale as to why these medications should not be explored for psychotherapeutic uses under strict research conditions, but also little well supported positive outcome data.

Psilocybin, a mixed 5-HT$_{1A/2A}$ receptor agonist typically found and consumed in *Psilocybe cubensis* mushrooms, has had a role in religious ceremonies in native American cultures for hundreds of years (Wasson, 1980). Similarly, peyote, the cactus in which mescaline is found, is a current sacrament used in healing ceremonies of the Native American Church (Csordas *et al.*, 2008). Typically, in the context of well integrated ritual, expectancy, and social context, the use of psychedelic drugs is not associated with adverse outcomes, and may be beneficial. Ayahuasca is an ancient sacramental and medicinal drug mixture of dimethyltryptamine and various harmala alkaloids (β-carbolines which inhibit monoamine oxidase) used by Amazon Basin tribal members and Mestizos, and ceremonially by several Brazilian churches (e.g. Uniao do Vegetal, Santo Daime). It is capable of inducing self-limited but intense aversive psychological reactions or transient psychotic episodes (Gable, 2007). However, there is no evidence that ayahuasca used within the religious community has substantial abuse or dependence potential and the risk of sustained psychological disturbances is minimal. Grob and colleagues (1996) compared 15 members of a Brazilian church that used ayahuasca with a control group of 15 non-members, and found that all 15 church subjects claimed that their experience with religious ritual use of ayahuasca had a profound positive impact on the course of their lives.

Recently, Griffiths and colleagues (2006) conducted a double-blind trial of psilocybin administered in a comfortable, structured, and supportive environment compared to a methylphenidate control in a crossover design in 36 hallucinogen-naïve subjects; they found that 22 (61%) of the psilocybin-treated group had full mystical experiences compared to four subjects in the methylphenidate group, including statistically significant experiences of unity, intuitive knowledge, and transcendence of time and space. Of the psilocybin group, 79% had moderate or very much increased sense of personal wellbeing or life satisfaction. Both subjects and external raters rated the psilocybin group as having significant changes in positive attitudes, positive mood, altruism, and positive behavior at 2-month follow-up, and more than 50% of subjects rated the experience as among the top five personally meaningful experiences of their lives, yet there were no significant effects on measures of personality. At 14-month follow-up, 58% of subjects rated the psilocybin experience as among the top five personally meaningful experiences of their lives, and 67% counted it as among the five most spiritually significant experiences of their lives (Griffiths *et al.*, 2008). This trial provides strong evidence under controlled scientific conditions that hallucinogens can produce lasting positive changes in healthy individuals.

Given the transformative nature of the peak experiences demonstrated by this study, it raises the question as to whether there is any application for the use of this and related psychedelic (i.e. mind-manifesting) drugs for enhancement of quality of life over and above that of therapeutic application for psychiatric disorders. It also brings into question the age-old moral precept that one cannot achieve spiritual gain without personal effort, as opposed to taking a pill. However, there are also concerns in that in the Griffiths study (2006; 2008), potential subjects with mental illness or a family history of schizophrenia, bipolar I or II disorder were excluded, yet 17% of the subjects who administered psilocybin experienced transient ideas of reference/paranoid ideation and 25% had strong anxiety/dysphoria (dominating the whole session in 13%) – this under controlled supportive conditions in healthy individuals. Thus, we have a risk of adverse consequences in the uncontrolled use of consciousness-expanding substances in the general population, in spite of the potential positive effects. There are negative effects of psychedelics upon measures of attention, learning, memory, and psychomotor performance, which, when coupled with situations requiring normal cognitive or physical competence, may increase the risk of cognitive failures and accidents (Sessa, 2007). For example, psilocybin significantly reduces attentional tracking ability, probably because of a reduced ability to suppress or ignore distracting stimuli (Carter *et al.*, 2005). Casualties of experimentation with hallucinogens have been described for decades; however, to place things in perspective, LSD and MDMA have been ranked well below most street drugs, abused prescription drugs, alcohol, and tobacco as potential sources of harm (Kleber, 1967).

It is clear that the decades-long ban on human research with this class of drugs has been because of political rather than scientific reasons, with the premise that the negative public health impact and criminal aspects of the use of these drugs outweigh any potential therapeutic use. Now there are well constructed safety guidelines for human hallucinogen research (Johnson *et al.*, 2008). It remains for well crafted scientific exploration of these drugs under controlled conditions to reveal whether they can be further harnessed for therapeutic application.

Creative expression

"Any musician who says he is playing better on tea, the needle, or when he is juiced, is a plain, straight liar."– Charlie Parker, quoted in Keepnews (1988).

Part of the problem with understanding the effects of drugs as potential enhancements of creative expression is the difference between subjective evaluation and objective ratings of creativity. When artists are engaged in a creative process that is already intrinsically reinforcing and it is coupled with the additional reinforcing properties of a particular drug, then the synergy that occurs will likely alter the subjective experience of the process toward wanting to be back in that state, especially in vulnerable individuals. This may have an impact on one's interpretation of the quality of the creative output. Kerr and colleagues (1991), comparing groups of writers, artists, and musicians to a control group, found that if a creative artist had the perception that drugs enhanced their performance, then they were likely to use it again, but there also was little actual correlation between creativity and substance use. Drugs that actually enhance creativity by objective standards may still be a pipe dream, but there are some intriguing findings for stimulants and hallucinogens.

Marijuana

There is a long association between the use of marijuana and creative artists, but it is unclear how much of this is cultural, and how much may be due to independent associations of drug use and psychopathology. Although marijuana may enhance the subjective experience of playing music, for example, there is little objective evidence in the research literature to support its use as a creativity-enhancing drug. For example, one component of the creative process is deemed to be the creation of new associations to stimuli presented to the subject. However, in one study, associations to novel stimuli were not enhanced in the subjects under the influence of cannabis (Tinklenberg *et al.*, 1978).

Hallucinogens

Hallucinogens clearly create novel experience as part of the well described subjective effects of mescaline, psilocybin, LSD, dimethyltryptamine (DMT), or related compounds. Common effects are alterations in perception, emotional range and lability, expansion in individual thought and identity, and capacity for transcendence of normative beliefs and values (Sessa, 2007; see erratum, 2008). As such, there is novel substrate for people to act creatively upon, as was demonstrated in the psychedelic art style created in the 1960s, and found on numerous rock concert posters, magazines, comic books, and even fine art of the era. Case study analysis of samples of the comic artist Robert Crumb's work before, during, and after his use of psychedelic drugs suggested his artistic style was significantly altered both during and after his episode of psychedelic drug use (Jones, 2007). There are also several examples of creative artists whose work was directly influenced by psychedelic drugs, including Aldous Huxley, who in 1954 famously documented his experience with mescaline in *The Doors of Perception*. However, providing a new domain for artistic exploration is not in and of itself sufficient to garner creativity. Hallucinogens may enhance the illumination stage of creativity, but it isn't clear if they make people creative (Lanni *et al.*, 2008). It is more likely that creative types will use the method to explore creative output, rather than that LSD might turn one into a musical or artistic prodigy. For example, in a study that, for ethical reasons, couldn't be done at present, Zegans and colleagues in 1967 gave LSD versus a placebo control to unprepared graduate students, testing a range of creativity measures, and found that in the subjects with baseline creative traits, there was an increase in novel thoughts and associations.

Most research studies exploring the effects of psychedelic drugs upon creativity were early, uncontrolled, and anecdotal in nature, but generally positive (Janiger *et al.*, 1989). In an open label pre-post design, Harman and colleagues in 1966 primed 27 subjects working in creative technical fields with the expectancy that mescaline treatment would increase their creativity and demonstrated significantly increased subjective enhancements of flexibility and novelty of ideas, associations, and contextual understanding, empathic relatedness to people and things, and ability to see solutions to problems. Earlier, Berlin and colleagues (1954, cited in Sessa 2007, erratum 2008) found that a panel of experts rated the paintings of four artists completed during an LSD experience of higher aesthetic value than their typical work.

Alcohol

In addition to disinhibition, creative people may attribute creative inspiration to alcohol, and there appears to be an association between alcohol dependence and writing prose professionally (Post, 1996). However, there is little objective evidence to support the creative connection. When pharmacological and expected effects of alcohol were experimentally dissociated using a balanced placebo design, Lapp and colleagues (1994) demonstrated that the creative inspiration attributed to alcohol is probably due to expectation rather than direct drug effects.

Stimulants

As a class, stimulants might increase components of creativity through dopamine, which is purported to reduce latent inhibition (enables fixing into sensations), and is correlated with novelty-seeking (Swerdlow *et al.*, 2003; Savitz & Ramesar, 2004). In a double-blind placebo-controlled study, Farah *et al.* (2008) tested the effects of mixed amphetamine salts (Adderall) on creativity in 16 healthy young adults and demonstrated no effect on divergent tasks, but those with a higher range of normal creativity were unaffected or impaired on convergent tasks, whereas those with convergent task impairments had enhanced functioning. Amphetamines promote CNS plasticity and accelerate motor learning in post-stroke patients (Walker-Batson *et al.*, 2001; Grade *et al.*, 1998). Perhaps there could be a role in the creative arts such as enhancing skills acquisition in learning to play a musical instrument and the disciplined practice it entails (Chatterjee, 2004).

Conclusion

The use of medications for performance improvement is an ill-defined, but certainly increasing, phenomenon in our society. As the chapter above demonstrates, the definition of "cosmetic" psychopharmacology is clearly in the eye of the beholder – a cosmetic weight reduction for one might be deemed as medically necessary for another. Improving function by relieving a person of depression is one thing, but removing bothersome personality traits with the exact same medication is perceived as quite another.

Given the demonstrated fluidity of conceptual and diagnostic paradigms, the clinician should carefully weigh the potential benefits to a patient against potential risks, while respecting both patient autonomy and professional obligations. It is in this "no-man's land" of conflicting needs and desires that the modern clinician must make recommendations, suggestions, and prescriptions.

Acknowledgments

The section on anabolic androgenic steroids is adapted from Westreich (2008).

References

Åkerstedt, T. & Ficca, G. (1997). Alertness-enhancing drugs as a countermeasure to fatigue in irregular work hours. *Chronobiology International*, **14**, 145–58.

Amiri, S., Mohammadi, M. R., Mohammadi, M. *et al.* (2008). Modafinil as a treatment for attention-deficit/hyperactivity disorder in children and adolescents: a double blind, randomized clinical trial. *Progress in Neuro-Psychopharmacology and Biological Psychiatry*, **32**(1), 145–9. Epub August 8, 2007.

Arrington, M. (2008). How many silicon valley startup executives are hopped up on provigil? *TechCrunch.com*, July 15, 2008. http://www.techcrunch.com/2008/07/15/how-many-of-our-startup-executives-are-hopped-up-on-provigil/Downloaded November 23, 2008.

Avois, L., Robinson, N., Saudan, C. *et al.* (2006). Central nervous system stimulants and sport practice. *British Journal of Sports Medicine*, **40**(Suppl. 1), 116–20.

Babcock, Q. & Byrne, T. (2000). Student perceptions of methylphenidate abuse at a public liberal arts college. *Journal of American College Health*, **49**, 143–5.

Ballon, J. S. & Feifel, D. (2006). A systematic review of modafinil: potential clinical uses and mechanisms of action. *Journal of Clinical Psychiatry*, **67**(4), 554–66.

Baranski, J. V., Pigeau, R., Dinich, P. & Jacobs, I. (2004). Effects of modafinil on cognitive and meta-cognitive performance. *Human Psychopharmacology*, **19**, 323–32.

Biederman, J., Swanson, J. M., Wigal, S. B. *et al.* (2005). Efficacy and safety of modafinil film-coated tablets in children and adolescents with attention-deficit/hyperactivity disorder: results of a randomized, double-blind, placebo-controlled, flexible-dose study. *Pediatrics*, **116**(6), e777–84.

Bramstedt, K. A. (2007). Caffeine use by children: the quest for enhancement. *Substance Use & Misuse*, **42**(8), 1237–51.

Brantigan, C. O., Brantigan, T. A. & Joseph, N. (1982). Effect of beta blockade and beta stimulation on stage fright. *American Journal of Medicine*, **72**(1), 88–94.

Broderick, P. & Benjamin, A. B. (2004). Caffeine and psychiatric symptoms: a review. *Journal of the Oklahoma State Medical Association*, **97**(12), 538–42.

Brower, K. J., Blow, F. C., Beresford, T. P. & Fuelling, C. (1989). Anabolic-androgenic steroid dependence. *Journal of Clinical Psychiatry*, **50**(1), 31–2.

Brower, K. J., Eliopulos, G. A. *et al.* (1990). Evidence of physical and psychological dependence on anabolic androgenic steroids in weight lifters. *American Journal of Psychiatry*, **147**(4), 510–12.

Brower, K. J., Blow, F. C., Young, J. P. & Hill, E. M. (1991). Symptoms and correlates of anabolic-androgenic steroid dependence. *British Journal of Addiction*, **86**, 759–68.

Bryant, H. (2005). *Juicing the Game*. New York: Viking.

Caldwell, J. A. Jr, Caldwell, J. L., Smythe, N. K. 3rd & Hall, K. K. (2000). A double-blind, placebo-controlled investigation of the efficacy of modafinil for sustaining the alertness and performance of aviators: a helicopter simulator study. *Psychopharmacology (Berlin)*, **150**(3), 272–82.

Canceso, J. (2005). *Juiced*. New York: Harper Collins.

Carneiro, J. R., Nader, A. C., Oliveira, J. E., da Silveira, V. G. & Barroso, F. L. (2006). Past use of amphetamines in candidates for gastric bypass surgery in a university hospital. *Obesity Surgery*, **16**(1), 31–4.

Carter, O. L., Burr, D. C., Pettigrew, J. D. *et al.* (2005). Using psilocybin to investigate the relationship between attention, working memory, and the serotonin 1A and 2A receptors. *Journal of Cognitive Neuroscience*, **17**(10), 1497–508.

Cassidy, J. (2008). Birdies in a bottle. *Men's Vogue*, April 2008, p.72.

CDC (2002). Annual smoking-attributable mortality, years of potential life lost, and economic costs – United States, 1995–1999. *Morbidity and Mortality Weekly Report*, **51**, 300–3.

Chatterjee, A. (2004). Cosmetic neurology: the controversy over enhancing movement, mentation, and mood. *Neurology*, **63**, 968–74.

Colman, E. (2005). Anorectics on trial: a half century of federal regulation of prescription appetite suppressants. *Annals of Internal Medicine*, **143**(5), 380–5.

Csordas, T. J., Storck, M. J. & Strauss, M. (2008). Diagnosis and distress in Navajo healing. *Journal of Nervous and Mental Disease*, **196**(8), 585–96.

Dahlsgaard, K., Peterson, C. & Seligman, M. E. P. (2005). Shared virtue: the convergence of valued human strengths across culture and history. *Review of General Psychology*, **9**, 203–13.

De Silva, D. A., Wong, M. C., Lee, M. P., Chen, C. L. & Chang, H. M. (2007). Amphetamine-associated ischemic stroke: clinical presentation and proposed pathogenesis. *Journal of Stroke & Cerebrovascular Diseases*, **16**(4), 185–6.

Drug and Alcohol Services Information System (DASIS) Report, 9/12/04, accessed at oas.samsha.gov, February 15, 2006.

Dupont, R. L., Coleman, J. J., Bucher, R. H. & Wilford, B. B. (2008). Characteristics and motives of college students who engage in nonmedical use of methylphenidate. *American Journal of Addiction*, **17**(3), 167–71.

Elliott, R., Sahakian, B. J., Matthews, K. *et al.* (1997). Effects of methylphenidate on spatial working memory and planning in healthy young adults. *Psychopharmacology*, **131**, 196–206.

Escher, M., Desmeules, J., Giostra, E. *et al.* (2001). Hepatitis associated with kava, a herbal remedy for anxiety. *British Medical Journal*, **322**, 139.

Farah, M. J., Illes, J., Cook-Deegan, R. *et al.* (2004). Neurocognitive enhancement: what can we do and what should we do? *Nature Reviews Neuroscience*, **5**(5), 421–5.

Farah, M. J., Haimm, C., Sankoorikal, G. & Chatterjee, A. (2008). When we enhance cognition with Adderall, do we sacrifice creativity? A preliminary study. *Psychopharmacology (Berlin)*, November 15 [Epub ahead of print].

Ferreira, S. E., de Mello, M.T., Pompeia, S. & de Souza-Formigoni, M. L. (2006). Effects of energy drink ingestion on alcohol intoxication. *Alcoholism: Clinical and Experimental Research*, **30**, 598–605.

Frias, C. (2006). Baseball and amphetamines. *Palm Beach Post*, Sunday, April 2.

Gable, R. S. (2007). Risk assessment of ritual use of oral dimethyltryptamine (DMT) and harmala alkaloids. *Addiction*, **102**(1), 24–34.

Galanter, M. & Kleber, H. D. (2004). *Textbook of Substance Abuse Treatment*, 3rd edn. Washington: American Psychiatric Publishing.

Gill, M., Haerich, P., Westcott, K., Godenick, K. L. & Tucker, J. A. (2006). Cognitive performance following modafinil versus placebo in sleep-deprived emergency physicians: a double-blind randomized crossover study. *Academic Emergency Medicine*, **13**(2), 158–65. Epub January 25, 2006. Erratum in: Academic Emergency Medicine, **13**(4), 477.

Grade, C., Redford, B., Chrostowski, J., Toussaint, L. & Blackwell, B. (1998). Methylphenidate in early poststroke recovery: a double-blind, placebo controlled study. *Archives of Physical Medicine and Rehabilitation*, **79**, 1047–50.

Griffiths, R. R., Richards, W. A., McCann, U. & Jesse, R. (2006). Psilocybin can occasion mystical-type experiences having substantial and sustained personal meaning and spiritual significance. *Psychopharmacology (Berlin)*, **187**(3), 268–83; discussion 284–92. Epub July 7, 2006.

Griffiths, R. R., Richards, W. A., Johnson, M. W., McCann, U. D. & Jesse, R. (2008). Mystical-type experiences occasioned by psilocybin mediate the attribution of personal meaning and spiritual significance 14 months later. *Journal of Psychopharmacology*, **22**(6), 621–32. Epub July 1, 2008.

Grob, C. S., McKenna, D. J., Callaway, J. C. *et al.* (1996). Human psychopharmacology of hoasca, a plant hallucinogen used in ritual context in Brazil. *Journal of Nervous and Mental Disease*, **184**, 86–94.

Halpern, J. H., Shuster, T. D., Siegel, A. J. & Naidoo, U. (2008). MDMA-assisted therapy in people with anxiety related to advanced stage cancer. http://www.clinicaltrials.gov/ct2/show/NCT00252174, accessed November 27, 2008.

Harman, W. W., McKim, R. H., Mogar, R. E., Fadiman, J. & Stolaroff, M. J. (1966). Psychedelic agents in creative problem-solving: a pilot study. *Psychedelic Reports*, **19**, 211–27.

Horne, J. A. & Reyner, L. A. (2001). Beneficial effects of an "energy drink" given to sleepy drivers. *Amino Acids*, **20**(1), 83–9.

Huxley, A. (1954). *The Doors of Perception*. London: Chatto and Windus.

Ivy, J. L., Costill, D. L., Fink, W. J. & Lower, R. W. (1979). Influence of caffeine and carbohydrate feedings on endurance performance. *Medicine & Science in Sports & Exercise*, **11**(1), 6–11.

Janiger, O. & Dobkin de Rios, M. (1989). LSD and creativity. *Journal of Psychoactive Drugs*, **21**(1), 129–34.

Jarvis, M. J. (1993). Does caffeine intake enhance absolute levels of cognitive performance? *Psychopharmacology*, **110**, 45–52.

Johnson, M. W., Richards, W. A. & Griffiths, R. R. (2008). Human hallucinogen research: guidelines for safety. *Psychopharmacology*, **22**, 603, originally published online July 1, 2008.

Jones, M. T. (2007). The creativity of Crumb: research on the effects of psychedelic drugs on the comic art of Robert Crumb. *Journal of Psychoactive Drugs*, **39**(3), 283–91.

Keepnews, O. (1988). *The View from Within: Jazz Writings 1948–1987*. New York: Oxford University Press, p. 91.

Kerr, B., Shafer, J., Chambers, C. & Hallowell, K. (1991). Substance use of creatively talented adults. *Journal of Creative Behavior*, **25**(2), 145–53.

Kleber, H. D. (1967). Prolonged adverse reactions from unsupervised use of hallucinogenic drugs. *Journal of Nervous and Mental Disease*, **144**(4), 308–19.

Kramer, P. D. (1993). *Listening to Prozac, a Psychiatrist Explores Antidepressant Drugs and the Remaking of the Self*. New York: Viking Books.

Kumar, R. (2008). Approved and investigational uses of modafinil: an evidence-based review. *Drugs*, **68**(13), 1803–39.

Lagarde, D., Batejat, D., Van Beers, P., Sarafian, D. & Pradella, S. (1995). Interest of modafinil, a new psychostimulant, during a sixty-hour sleep deprivation experiment. *Fundamental and Clinical Pharmacology*, **9**, 1–9.

Lane, J. R. & Connor, J. D. (1994). The influence of endogenous and exogenous sex hormones in adolescents with attention to oral contraceptives and anabolic steroids. *Journal of Adolescent Health*, **15**(8), 630–4.

Lanni, C., Lenzken, S. C., Pascale, A. *et al.* (2008). Cognition enhancers between treating and doping the mind. *Pharmacology Research* **57**(3), 196–213. Epub February 15, 2008. Review.

Lapp, W. M., Collins, R. L. & Izzo, C. V. (1994). On the enhancement of creativity by alcohol: pharmacology or expectation? *American Journal of Psychology*, **107**(2), 173–206.

Laseter, J. T. & Russell, J. A. (1991). Anabolic steroid-induced tendon pathology: a review of the literature. *Medicine & Science in Sports & Exercise*, **23**(1), 1–3.

Leake, J. (2004). Downtime is over as pill offers 24-hour living. *Timesonline*. July 4, 2004. http://www.timesonline.co.uk/tol/news/uk/health/article453615.ece, accessed November 23, 2008.

Lukas, S. E. (2009).The pharmacology of anabolic androgenic steroids. In *Principles of Addiction Medicine*, 4th edn, ed. R. K. Ries. Philadelphia PA: Lippincott Williams & Wilkins, Inc, pp. 251–63.

McCabe, S. E., Knight, J. R., Teter, C. J. & Wechsler, H. (2005). Non-medical use of prescription stimulants among US college students: prevalence and correlates from a national survey. *Addiction*, **100**, 96–106.

McCusker, R. R., Goldberger, B. A. & Cone, E. J. (2003). Caffeine content of specialty coffees. *Journal of Analytical Toxicology*, **27**(7), 520–2.

McCusker, R. R., Goldberger, B. A. & Cone, E. J. (2006). Caffeine content of energy drinks, carbonated sodas, and other beverages. *Journal of Analytical Toxicology*, **30**(2), 112–14.

McEvoy, A. W., Kitchen, N. D. & Thomas, D. G. (2000). Intracerebral hemorrhage and drug abuse in young adults. *British Journal of Neurosurgery*, **14**(5), 449–54.

Maher, B. (2008). Poll results: look who's doping. *Nature*, **452**(7188), 674–5.

Malinauskas, B. M., Aeby, V. G., Overton, R. F., Carpenter-Aeby, T. & Barber-Heidal, K. (2007). A survey of energy drink consumption patterns among college students. *Nutrition Journal*, **6**, 35.

Martinez, M., Devenport, L., Saussy, J. & Martinez, J. (2002). Drug-associated heat stroke. *Southern Medical Journal*, **95**(8), 799–802.

Mehta, M. A., Owen, A. M., Sahakian, B. J. *et al.* (2000). Methylphenidate enhances working memory by modulating discrete frontal and parietal lobe regions in the human brain. *Journal of Neuroscience*, **20**, RC65.

Metzner, R. (1998). Hallucinogenic drugs and plants in psychotherapy and shamanism. *Journal of Psychoactive Drugs*, **30**(4), 333–41.

Miskowiak, K., Inkster, B., Selvaraj, S. *et al.* (2008). Erythropoietin improves mood and modulates the cognitive and neural processing of emotion 3 days post administration. *Neuropsychopharmacology*, **33**(3), 611–18. Epub May 2, 2007.

Mithoefer, M. (2008). A test of MDMA-assisted psychotherapy in people with posttraumatic stress disorder NCT00090064. http://www.clinicaltrials.gov/ct2/show/NCT00090064, accessed November 27, 2008.

Monitoring the Future (MFT), University of Michigan, December 2005.

Morein-Zamir, S., Turner, D. C. & Sahakian, B. J. (2007). A review of the effects of modafinil on cognition in schizophrenia. *Schizophrenia Bulletin*, **33**(6), 1298–306. Epub July 18, 2007.

Mottram, D. R. (2005). *Drugs in Sport.* New York: Taylor & Francis, p. 283.

Nawrot, P., Jordan, S., Eastwood, J. *et al.* (2003). Effects of caffeine on human health. *Food Additives and Contaminants*, **20**(1), 1–30.

O'Brien, M. C., McCoy, T., Rhodes, S. D., Wagoner, A. & Wolfson, M. (2008). Caffeinated cocktails: energy drink consumption, high-risk drinking, and alcohol-related consequences among college students. *Academic Emergency Medicine*, **15**, 453–60.

Pary, R., Lewis, S., Matuschka, P. *et al.* (2002). Attention deficit disorder in adults. *Annals of Clinical Psychiatry*, **14**, 105–11.

Perry, P. J., Andersen, K. H. & Yates, W. R. (1990). Illicit anabolic steroid use in athletes, a case series analysis. *American Journal of Sports Medicine*, **18**(4), 422–8.

Pope, H. G. & Katz, D. L. (1988). Affective and psychotic symptoms associated with anabolic steroid use. *American Journal of Psychiatry*, **145**(4), 487–90.

Pope, H. G., Phillips, K. A. & Olivardia, R. (2000). *The Adonis Complex, The Secret Crisis of Male Body Obsession.* New York: The Free Press.

President's Council on Bioethics. (2003). *Beyond Therapy: Biotechnology and the Pursuit of Human Improvement.* Washington DC: Dana Press.

Post, F. (1996). Verbal creativity, depression and alcoholism: an investigation of one hundred American and British writers. *British Journal of Psychiatry*, **168**, 545–55.

Rao, A., Hu, H. & Nobre, A. C. (2005). The effects of combined caffeine and glucose drinks on attention in the human brain. *Nutritional Neuroscience*, **8**(3), 141–53.

Reissig, C. J., Strain, E. C. & Griffiths, R. R. (2009). Caffeinated energy drinks – a growing problem. *Drug and Alcohol Dependence*, **99**(1–3), 1–10.

Rosenthal, R. N. & Solkhah, R. (2005). Psychopharmacology of club drugs. In *Clinical Manual of Addiction Psychopharmacology*, eds. H. R. Kranzler & D. A. Ciraulo. Washington DC: American Psychiatric Publishing, Inc, pp. 243–67.

Savitz, J. B. & Ramesar, R. S. (2004). Genetic variants implicated in personality: a review of the more promising candidates. *American Journal of Medical Genetics B Neuropsychiatric Genetics*, **131B**(1), 20–32.

Sessa, B. (2005). Can psychedelics have a role in psychiatry once again? *British Journal of Psychiatry*, **186**, 457–8.

Sessa, B. (2007). Is there a case for MDMA-assisted psychotherapy in the UK? *Journal of Psychopharmacology*, **21**(2), 220–4. Erratum in *Journal of Psychopharmacology*, **22**(6), 699, 2008.

Silverberg, D. S., Iaina, A., Wexler, D. & Blum, M. (2001). The pathological consequences of anaemia. *Clinical & Laboratory Haematology*, **23**(1), 1–6. UI: 11422223.

Smith, A. P. (2005). Caffeine at work. *Human Psychopharmacology*, **20**, 441–5.

Spencer, T., Biederman, J., Wilens, T. *et al.* (2001). Efficacy of a mixed amphetamine salts compound in adults with attention-deficit/hyperactivity disorder. *Archives of General Psychiatry*, **58**(8), 784–5.

Sunram-Lea, S. I., Foster, J. K., Durlach, P. & Perez, C. (2002). The effect of retrograde and anterograde glucose administration on memory performance in healthy young adults. *Behavioural Brain Research*, **134**, 505–16.

Swerdlow, N. R., Stephany, N., Wasserman, L. C. *et al.* (2003). Dopamine agonists disrupt visual latent inhibition in normal males using a within-subject paradigm. *Psychopharmacology (Berlin)*, **169**(3–4), 314–20. Epub February 28, 2003.

Teitelman, E. (2001). Off-label uses of modafinil. *American Journal of Psychiatry*, **158**, 1341.

Tinklenberg, J. R., Darley, C. F., Roth, W. T., Pfefferbaum, A. & Kopell, B. S. (1978). Marijuana effects on associations to novel stimuli. *Journal of Nervous and Mental Disease*, **166**(5), 362–4.

Trenton, A. J. & Currier, G. W. (2006). Behavioural manifestations of anabolic steroid use. *CNS Drugs*, **19**(7), 571–95.

Trice, I. & Haymes, E. M. (1995). Effects of caffeine ingestion on exercise-induced changes during high-intensity, intermittent exercise. *International Journal of Sport Nutrition*, **5**(1), 37–44.

Turner, D. C., Clark, L., Dowson, J., Robbins, T. W. & Sahakian, B. J. (2004). Modafinil improves cognition and response inhibition in adult attention deficit/hyperactivity disorder. *Biological Psychiatry*, **55**(10), 1031–40.

van der Watt, G., Laugharne, J. & Janca, A. (2008). Complementary and alternative medicine in the treatment of anxiety and depression. *Current Opinion in Psychiatry*, **21**, 37–42.

Volkow, N. D. & Swanson, J. M. (2008). The action of enhancers can lead to addiction. *Nature*, **451**, 31.

Walker-Batson, D., Curtis, S., Natarajan, R. *et al.* (2001). A double-blind, placebo controlled study of the use of amphetamine in the treatment of aphasia. *Stroke*, **32**, 2093–8.

Wasson, R. G. (1980). *The Wondrous Mushroom: Mycolatry in Mesoamerica*. New York: McGraw-Hill.

Westover, A. N., Nakonezny, P. A. & Haley, R. W. (2008). Acute myocardial infarction in young adults who abuse amphetamines. *Drug & Alcohol Dependence*, **96**(1–2), 49–56.

Westreich, L. M. (2008). Anabolic androgenic steroid use pharmacology, prevalence, and psychiatric aspects. *Psychiatric Times*, **25**(1).

Wilens, T. E. (2008). Effects of methylphenidate on the catecholaminergic system in attention-deficit/hyperactivity disorder. *Journal of Clinical Psychopharmacology*, **28** (3Suppl. 2), S46–53.

Williams, S. J., Seale, C., Boden, S., Lowe, P. & Steinberg, D. L. (2008). Waking up to sleepiness: modafinil, the media and the pharmaceuticalisation of everyday/night life. *Sociology of Health & Illness*, **30**(6), 839–55. Epub April 25, 2008.

Yesavage, J. A., Mumenthaler, M. S., Taylor, J. L. *et al.* (2002). Donepezil and flight simulator performance: effects on retention of complex skills. *Neurology*, **59**(1), 123–5.

Zegans, L. S., Pollard, J. C. & Brown, D. (1967). The effects of LSD-25 on creativity and tolerance to regression. *Archives of General Psychiatry*, **16**(6), 740–9.

Psychotherapeutic paradigms and the prescription pad: treating drug addiction with drugs

Ed Paul

Prescribing medication is fraught with psychological sequelae, especially in addiction psychiatry. Patients are told to be wary of medications, that meds are just a crutch, or, worse still, that they invite continued abuse. Our patients are told, and often feel, that they are not "really sober" if they rely on modern medicines. They echo the sentiments of an earlier time, the era of Bill W., when allopathic physicians had little to offer in the way of addiction treatment, one result being that our patients' families, friends, and sponsors take an unusual and often critical interest in what the doctor is up to.

It is important to be aware of what we are up to, because prescribing is a hydra-headed beast. Writing a prescription involves much more than mere awareness of the statistics, efficacy data, side-effects, and potential interactions with other drugs. It is always a psychodynamically loaded event as well.

How a medication is prescribed is just as important as why it is prescribed.

What follows is a description of therapies organized under three main rubrics, and a discussion of how these impact our behavior whenever we write a 'scrip.'

Psychotherapeutic interventions in addiction psychiatry can be categorized as *theurgic*, *contractual*, or *experiential*.

Theurgic therapy is therapy by fiat: the doctor tells the patient what to do, arguing by authority (a kind of suasion frequently favored in therapeutic communities, by "hard-core" AA sponsors, drug counselors, and "control freak" psychiatrists). Manipulative threats run in tandem. Clearly, there is a world of difference between telling someone that "millions of people have stayed sober using AA," and telling someone "you will die if you don't go to meetings." Since none of us possesses a crystal ball (outcome data apply to groups, not to individuals) – and addicts are already far beneath the wheel when it comes to feeling controlled – this approach is not ideal.

Often, I fall into the trap of telling a reluctant patient who wants to try one more time to stay off heroin by attending NA, or going to their 15th detox, that scientific evidence shows that detox doesn't work, that they need to go on buprenorphine, methadone, or commit to a lengthy (i.e. 2-year) stint in a therapeutic community. This rarely works. Occasionally, pointing out the parallel between their treatment of choice and the definition of insanity ("trying the same thing over and over and expecting different results") broadens such a patient's perspective.

The family members, much less dependent on the doctor, are even less likely accept the doctor's recommendations. The theurgic approach is on very shaky ground. It often sounds like the harping of unliked relatives.

Contractual therapy has much more to offer. It is the set of therapies that broker interactions between the patient and significant others, or the community at large. It is based on operant conditioning, i.e. rewarding patients for approaching goals such as sobriety. This is a particularly powerful way of thinking about prescribing Antabuse. It is one thing to say "you have to take this or you'll keep drinking," yet quite another to say "if you take this we may be able to get your spouse to calm down and stop nagging." This is the basis for the Antabuse contract (Onken *et al.*, 1995). A patient takes Antabuse in full view of his spouse, then says, "I am taking this in front of you so that you don't have to worry about my drinking today." The spouse says, "Thank you," and then adds, "Because I know it is difficult for you if I predict relapse, or tell you all my worries about your drinking, I will refrain for today." The patient says, "Thank you." This has the effect of both lowering expressed emotion and quelling anxiety among the concerned, a benefit beyond that typically attributed to disulfiram alone.

Contractual therapies include contingency contracting (a form of negative reinforcement, in which a dreaded outcome is avoided by consistent daily sobriety. A typical contingency contract is a letter, drawn up by the identified patient, in which he documents in painful detail the severity and dreadful consequences of his addiction; what is specifically contractual about any of this is that the writer agrees that this letter will be mailed to his employer the next time he picks up his addiction of choice. A variant of this is seen in community reinforcement programs, in which teens are given vouchers for sports supplies, etc. in return for negative urines. This procedure was studied in teenage cocaine abuse, but could likely be used in conjunction with buprenorphine during the current pharmaceutical opioid epidemic, especially rampant among teens (McCance-Katz & Clark, 2004).

CRAFT is a form of family intervention which helps families get their addicted loved ones into treatment by a detailed behavioral analysis of the identified patient's drug use, appropriate positive reinforcement of sobriety, and helping the significant others to improve their own social networks (Smith & Meyers, 2004). Examples range from encouraging a husband to see friends instead of staying home waiting up for an alcoholic spouse, or going to the movies with the spouse before he gets the phone call that inevitably leads to cocaine. This approach has promising results, with better outcomes than the isolated recommendation to families to attend Al-Anon.

A closely related treatment for alcoholism is behavioral marital therapy, which aims to abrogate typical vicious cycles, including intoxication and recrimination, or distance and withdrawal by either partner. Behavioral marital therapy utilizes operant conditioning principles, i.e. the partners have fun together without talking about drinking if the alcoholic partner is sober (Fals–Stewart *et al.*, 2000).

Experiential therapies are essentially learning experiences. Disulfiram (Antabuse) can play a very interesting role here. The patient – rather than feeling monitored, feeling constantly watched – uses the disulfiram to learn.

To learn? Consider: patients who are sober and in relapse-prevention mode can begin to use disulfiram more judiciously (it is, after all, moderately toxic), and learn for themselves what constitutes a high-risk occasion. Should they take an Antabuse right after an argument, before a wedding, on a cruise, etc.? This sensitization to drinking cues increases self-awareness and promotes autonomy and self-regard. Heightened self-awareness/self-confidence can actually complement AA's emphasis on surrender, on giving up one's

will; heightened autonomy helps to place some of the AA philosophy ("keep it simple, stupid" or "your best thinking got you here") in proper context. Ultimately, true healing – recovery – involves self-reliance (even if it means emulating a sponsor, or acting in a way deemed consistent with a higher power's wishes).

A particularly dramatic and frequently effective way of prescribing Antabuse is during an initial intake. By elucidating a patient's central emotional conflicts (psychodynamic life narrative, described by Veiderman in 1980) and explaining how drinking has become a desperate attempt to handle these, a therapist can promote change.

For instance, someone who grew up in an authoritarian home (to be loved they had to squelch their own individuality, feelings, conscience) may feel as an adult that she can only be loved if she submits. Otherwise, she fears, she will be bereft, alone.

This developmental scenario makes fertile ground for substance abuse later on in life. Drinking and/or drugging have been the patient's habitual response to conflict. Often they are reliving earlier unresolved conflicts in the current relationship ("Oh, maybe that's why I can't ever commit?"). Sure, change is tough – but if the patient really wants to stop this way of relating *now*…he can! He can achieve these goals by becoming sober, and by taking the Antabuse you place in his hand.

Patients in this situation become wide-eyed. They stare at the pill in your hand. The tension is palpable. Often they gulp and say "okay." You get a glass of water, they down it, heaving a sigh of giddy relief. The prognosis is good.

Akin to the psychodynamic method is the motivational interviewing technique (Miller & Rollnick, 2004). This technique involves non-judgmental exploration of motive, encouraging the patient to speak for him or herself – to speak aloud or write on paper their reasons for drinking or drugging, what drinking achieves, and what drinking destroys. By not telling the patient what to do (theurgic or exhortative), they find out for themselves.

A note on the psychodynamic approach: telling an active alcoholic that he is unconsciously satirizing his need for the breast by sucking (alcohol) from a poison tit is not helpful. Two years later, perhaps, the same strategy could be an effective component of relapse prevention.

Wurmser used free association with early recovery alcoholics; his patients took the Antabuse daily, right before lying on the couch! Wurmser noted that his patients lived with double binds and with contradictory superego demands (Wurmser, 2001).

My patient, likewise unable to satisfy all his superego demands, became a fervent devotee of AA. He said (referring to his peers), "We're all either sociopaths or anti-sociopaths."

Patients and family members frequently have emotional reactions to medication and to doctors in general. Some patients love pills; they want medication without psychotherapy or self-help (and may be abusing their meds). Other patients have a hostile relationship toward medication, compounded at times by the attitudes of sponsors and significant others. A history of adverse reactions or of a medication-abusing relative may explain a given patient's resistance to potentially life-changing medication. Some AA sponsors are kind, well informed, and provide a steady and stable resource. At times, it is appropriate to consider inviting the sponsor to a session to discuss the pros and cons of medication.

I have focused on Antabuse and Suboxone because of their efficacy and because of the emotional issues attendant on prescribing them. Pharmacotherapy such as naltrexone to diminish alcohol craving and use, off-label use of Topiramate, Baclofen, ondansetron, or over-the-counter drugs like glutamate, SAMe, or melatonin – these drugs are usually more acceptable to patients.

The patient's style quite often augurs the response to your suggestion of pharmacotherapy. Some patients become panicky when confronted with lots of data and risks regarding a prescription; others take umbrage at being reassured soothingly, and, to their minds, dismissively. Assess whether the patient wants lots of data (obsessive style) or reassurance (dependent style). For the dependent patient, a leaflet may be more appropriate than a recitation of warnings. Of course, all patients should be encouraged to call if they notice side-effects.

Addicts and alcoholics do tend to displace their fears about their own "self-medication" (Khantzian, 2008) onto prescription medication. Patients often fear that "methadone will rot (my) bones." That myth derives at least in part from the frequent observation that heroin addicts' teeth are rotted, sometimes beyond repair, by poor dental hygiene and chronic suppression of (dental) pain via opiate dependence.

Resistance to pharmacotherapy may be wholly psychological in origin. One patient with attention deficit disorder (ADD) and cocaine dependency was started on Concerta. Stimulant treatment of ADD tends to mitigate cocaine use. This patient had a family history of Tourette's syndrome, and she began writing angry letters to me about the risk involved in prescribing stimulants to anyone with such a family history. The strident complaints and fears somehow did not extend to her own cocaine use!

The following example of displacement involves a non-clinical situation. An architect I know positively glowed while describing his 100% organic cigars: they had "nothing bad in them." Really?!

Most patients have fears, all kinds of fears, about their addiction. Experiential therapy? There is nothing like Suboxone to convince a patient that opiate addiction is a biological process, not a moral deficit or soul sickness. Opioid/opiate dependence involves (demonstrable by brain imaging) structural and functional physical disease. This becomes immediately apparent when the patient in opiate withdrawal experiences the immediate, dramatic relief of the very first dose of buprenorphine. Patients often say that they "immediately feel normal." I had a patient who described it as "hitting the reset button" (the elimination of the misery of protracted abstinence symptomatology).

Patients typically feel a dissipation of all craving, an experience that is hard to convey to others – others who might accuse them of being "legally" high. Psychological support for the patient's own experience becomes crucial at this point; merely telling him that he must stay on it will make him feel more trapped, more controlled, and conflicted.

Families, in particular, may not appreciate the subtle, multiple benefits of buprenorphine, and are often insistent that a patient come off it and go to rehab. Multifamily psychoeducational groups could be quite helpful. An experiential point of view would also help to clarify the large multicenter study of disulfiram (Schuckit, 1985). This study found that disulfiram was no better than placebo, unless the patient relapsed. After publication of this finding, many practitioners stopped prescribing Antabuse.

References

Fals-Stewart, W., O' Farell, T.J. *et al.* (2000). Behavioral couples therapy versus individual-based treatment for male substance-abusing patients. An evaluation of significant individual change and comparison of improvement rates. *Journal of Substance Abuse and Treatment*, **18**(3), 249–54.

Khantzian, E.J. (2008). Supportive psychotherapy: the nature of the connection to patients. *American Journal of Psychiatry*, **165**(10), 1355.

McCance-Katz, E. F. & Clark, H. W. (2004). *Psychosocial Treatments*. New York: Brunner-Routledge.

Miller, W. R. & Rollnick, S. (2002). *Motivational Interviewing: Preparing People for Change*, 2nd edn. New York: Guilford Press.

Onken, L. S., Blaine, J. D. *et al.* (1995). *Integrating Behavioral Therapies with Medications in the Treatment of Drug Dependence*. Rockville, MD: U.S. Department of Health and Human Services, Public Health Service, National Institutes of Health Support of Doctors.

Schuckit, M. A. (1985). A one-year follow-up of men alcoholics given disulfiram. *Journal of Studies on Alcohol and Drugs*, **46**, 191–5.

Smith, J. E. & Meyers, R. J. (2004). *Motivating Substance Abusers to Enter Treatment*. New York: Guilford Press.

Viederman, M. (1980). Management of emotional reactions to acute medical illness. *General Hospital Psychiatry*, **2**(3), 177–85.

Wurmser, L. (2001). *Flight from Conscience: Psychodynamic Treatment of Character Perversion, Obsessive-compulsive Disorder, and Addiction*. Northvale, NJ: J. Aronson.

Six key areas when working with addicts

Kathleen Tracy

Clinicians and addicts in recovery agree that addiction treatment works. But how exactly are we defining success? And what do clinicians do that contributes to treatment success, and what do they do that has no effect on treatment success or, even worse, actually slows down recovery? The answers to these questions are vitally important to clinicians and administrators who must design effective treatment programs to help their suffering patients. The second section of this book will lay out the answers as they stand now, in hopes of guiding clinicians toward the most effective strategies for their individual patients.

Of course, the treatment of addiction is in many ways an art rather than a science, and the data-based studies mentioned in this section only approximate the kind of information necessary for treating the individual addict. However, by insisting upon a clear-eyed and comprehensive understanding of the scientific data available, the clinician can make the best possible choices in treatment planning. This introductory chapter will describe just those sorts of treatment success measures that the clinician can use in judging the treatment methods suggested in this book and elsewhere.

First, this chapter will look at how exactly success is defined in addiction, with an emphasis on what clinicians need to know. Then, an examination of the traditional therapies and the newer, data-based treatment will allow the reader to consider these two modalities side by side. The anti-addiction medications which are increasingly touted by both addicts and clinicians will be discussed, with an emphasis on the treatment success data available. After reviewing the data and some clinical lore on the use of inpatient versus outpatient treatment, the chapter will conclude with a discussion on the philosophical issues involved in recommending abstinence and the need for a holistic addiction treatment model.

When working with individuals with addiction there are six key areas that one should address to provide treatment effectively. These are not the only items to consider in treatment; however, these are universal and typically emerge when addressing the needs of someone who is using substances and interacting with treatment systems in attempts to obtain or sustain abstinence. These include issues for the person with the substance use disorder to address and also include issues for the treatment system to address.

1. Readiness for treatment

In the past it was characteristic to say that individuals were not ready for treatment if they dropped out or were resistant when in fact those who are struggling may need treatment the most. It is useful to make treatment continuously available to those in need and to adapt the treatment to permit focus on the immediate needs of the patients such as food and shelter and other immediate crises.

Ask the patient the following: is your current approach working to the point where you feel good about yourself and your world?

Most patients will acknowledge that their approach has not been working for quite some time. Provide them with the opportunity to try something new with the option that if it does not work they can always return to their previous approach; their willingness to try a new approach is the only way they can find out what treatment might offer.

It is amazing how therapeutic dialog such as this can help shift the direction of someone who is ambivalent about treatment. The safety of knowing that the individual can return to his or her previous (dysfunctional) approach if they do not like what treatment has to offer is often the impetus that allows them to change.

2. Treatment-resistant patients or treatment-resistant treatment?

Is the patient resistant to treatment or is the treatment itself really creating the resistance? It has not been easy in the addiction field to develop treatment strategies with demonstrable effectiveness. Further, the dissemination of such treatment strategies has been slowed by the resistance shown by established treatment programs. None the less, whenever a patient does not engage, clinicians tend to (almost automatically) remark that "the patient is treatment-resistant" – the patient is the problem, not the treatment. Clinicians need to regularly re-assess the effectiveness of their treatment methods, always with a view toward improving their practice. In addition, we should, whenever possible, consider whether the patient–treatment match is optimal – perhaps a misguided triage or other treatment decision has contributed to a therapeutic stand-off or failure.

3. Reconnecting with strengths

Individuals who are dependent on substances have often lost their interpersonal roles in the family and community. Treatments are often focused on the "here and now" and may not address personal and interpersonal strengths and resources that the patient actually possesses. Ask patients to remember what goals they had before substance use became a regular part of their lives. This can be difficult for the person in early recovery; persevere, ask them to try! An alternate, somewhat less direct, approach involves asking the patient to describe the first thing that comes to mind when he or she thinks about their pre-addiction goals and aspirations. The main point? The main point is to introduce your patient to his premorbid self, who had goals, ambitions, and hope for the future. If the individual had an abusive or otherwise troubled past, early childhood or fleeting memories may be where the patient will find his or her life-embracing self. Help them to know that they can reconnect to their dreams; people do it all the time (!), or some aspect of their dreams again.

Setting specific, concrete goals necessitates invoking and then using personal strength. Short-term goals, admittedly the necessary precursors of longer term goals, should be goals that are *achievable*, that work toward long-term goals. For example, money may be a trigger to use. An excellent short-term goal is the patient's decision to put aside a certain amount of money each day or week. Patients may literally have to be reminded of some of the other pleasures (aside from drugs) that money can buy. Help your patient to frame short-term goals that are both healthful and provide immediate or short-term gratification (i.e. "See a movie, or go to a spa to get massaged"). Longer term goals might include saving for a short vacation or for a return to school.

Some may question the wisdom of encouraging further spending on anything but the chronic and large and recurrent bills that patients almost without exception have. The counterargument is that if the new activities promote abstinence, then the patient will be saving a great deal of money as a result of his new lifestyle.

When addicts decide to stop using and to move forward, they are often unprepared for setbacks; the first reversal or barrier the patient encounters may be a trigger to immediate relapse. (Things may get worse before they get better.)

4. Rebuilding relationships

Individuals who abuse substances have often severed or significantly damaged their relationships with friends, family members, and co-workers who do not take. The substance abuser's modus operandi – which often includes hiding drug use, challenges related to honesty, inability to fulfil obligations, and financial strain associated with continuing use is extremely toxic to relationships with significant others. The addict's "intact" relationships are often those he or she has with drug dealers and/or other drug users. This is quite challenging for the individual who is attempting to stop using drugs and sustain abstinence. Significant others who are actively using alcohol or drugs may react negatively to the individual in early recovery and may sabotage his or her efforts to abstain. The individual's attempts to reconnect with those who are not drug users or abusers may be frustrated; former friends and family may no longer trust him or her and may either summarily or covertly reject him or her. It is important to provide opportunities for relationships that are based on abstinence for the person in recovery. This can be accomplished through self-help groups, treatment groups, or various forms of mentorship groups. It is important for the patient to experience the possibility of healthy relationships; this can occur in the aforementioned settings. The individual then views himself as someone who has something to offer.

5. Trauma and negative life events

The prevalence of trauma is higher in those with substance use disorders than in the general population. Individuals may have had traumatic events in their past that influence how they interact with others in the present. Some patients will have co-occurring post-traumatic stress disorder (PTSD). It is important to address these issues while treating the substance use disorder, because "undigested" trauma can go on provoking recidivism and relapse. Addicts have often experienced negative life events related to their substance use and these too should be addressed.

There are effective behavioral treatments that facilitate the psychological processing of trauma and negative life events; these include seeking safety; mentorship for substance abuse and trauma (MSAT); and response exposure techniques. The best place to start is first to discuss the patient's negative life events and experiences of trauma.

6. Perspectives on success

It is important not to become frustrated with expectations of large gains in short periods of time. When working with individuals who are struggling with substance use disorders, one should appreciate small gains and reinforce that progress with praise. These small gains eventually lead to larger changes. It takes time to undo what was previously done.

During early recovery the patient is at high risk for relapse. Many clinicians do not practise therapeutic "harm reduction." It is critically important for the therapist to continue "accentuating the positive," and to reframe current events – if and when appropriate – so the patient does not feel that all is lost. "Catastrophizing" is another common relapse trigger. Perhaps the patient succeeded at lengthening the interval between the previous relapse and this one.

Closing remarks

Treating substance abuse can be challenging; however, there are essential items to address across all treatments. When these issues are addressed, better treatment outcomes are obtained and there is a higher likelihood that the individual will achieve and sustain abstinence. The six areas discussed – readiness for treatment, ownership of resistance to treatment, reconnecting with strengths, rebuilding relationships, trauma and negative life events, and perspectives on success – can provide a solid foundation for the treatment of individuals with substance use disorders.

Part 2 Real World

The twelve-step approach

Marc Galanter

Every day, people who want to overcome their problems with addiction walk into one of the 200 000 Alcoholics Anonymous (AA) meetings held worldwide. If you look in on any of these meetings, you will find a tone of earnestness and mutual concern among members who have been successful, and you will also find others who still struggle with the demons within them. If you speak English, you will understand what people are saying in most of these meetings, but in others, you would hear their tales told in French or German, Mandarin, Russian or – in Aboriginal Australia – in Pidgin English. From this medley of voices emerges the redemptive experiences of AA's two million members worldwide, each struggling with the "baffling and cunning" disease of addiction, each playing a role in this "spiritual fellowship," as AA has called itself.

Outcome evaluations on AA are hard to implement because of the program's requirement of anonymity among its members. None the less, a large sample of (AA) people entering alcoholism treatment clinics for the first time from referral or detoxification centers were evaluated at intervals up through 16 years. It was found that longer participation in AA made a positive contribution to both alcohol and social function outcomes independent of the quantity of treatment these patients experienced (Moos & Moos, 2006). It seems clear, as well, that attendance at AA meetings is effective in achieving a positive effect, and does not just reflect greater motivation for recovery before attending. In one large-scale study of alcoholics discharged from the hospital, the level of AA attendance in the first year after admission was found to predict lower alcohol-related problems at follow-up, independent of their previously measured motivation for change (McKellar *et al.*, 2003).

AA and the experience of spiritual redemption

To appreciate the essence of this movement of personal renewal, we can begin with a key moment in the life of

Bill Wilson, its co-founder. Bill W.'s seminal experience led to his lifelong commitment to promoting AA's mission. He had been a successful stockbroker in his day, but by the age of 40 he had suffered many failed hospitalizations in attempts to dry out from his drinking, and had been pronounced "a hopeless alcoholic" by the physician who had earnestly tried to move him toward recovery. During what would be his final hospitalization in December, 1934, Bill had a revelation that became a turning point in his life: he later described it in the book, *Alcoholics Anonymous Comes of Age* (1957). As he lay despairing in his room in the Towne Hospital on the Upper West Side of Manhattan:

> I found myself crying out, "If there is a God, let him show himself! I am ready to do anything, anything!"

> Suddenly, the room lit up with a great white light. I was caught up on an ecstasy which there are no words to describe. It seemed to me in my mind's eye, that I was on a mountain and that a wind not of air but of spirit was blowing. And then it burst upon me and I was a free man. . . . Things are "alright with God and His world."

The next day, Bill was given a copy of William James' classic, *The Varieties of Religious Experience* (1929), that helped him to understand what happened from the perspective of spiritual rebirth. From there he moved on, abstinent from alcohol, a missionary committed to saving others who chose to struggle with their compulsions as he did.

Some AA members experience sudden, spiritual revelations. Others are relieved of their remorse as they achieve a gradual realization of the benefits of not drinking. Bill W.'s experience parallels that of the many millions of AA members who have reached a state of despair because of alcohol and other drugs.

Over the 4 years following his spiritual experience, Bill W. worked with other alcoholics, the first among them a physician, Dr. Bob, who went on to co-found AA with him. In time, Bill decided to lay out the Twelve Steps toward recovery which have become so central to the many "Anonymous" groups that exist today.

AA's place in American society

In a sense there are two kinds of redemptive experiences. In one, a remorseful person remains a tainted sinner who may be forgiven, but he or she carries out ritual because of a lingering sense of guilt. The confessional, whether to a religious or a political body, can leave the person retaining this taint.

Other redemptive experiences, when they are achieved in an accepting context with mutuality and a sense of optimism, leave the person with a differing feeling. This is more like the AA experience, and a positive tone like this is evident in certain elements in contemporary American culture. We see it not only in the tone of AA meetings, but also in the positivity and optimism of many of America's evangelical movements; collectively these movements led to the optimistic culture shared by many of the large interdenominational churches which have gained popularity in recent years.

Ironically, an openness to new religious views apparently allowed Americans to become more religiously oriented than western Europeans. Whereas little more than 15% of the American population claimed church membership in 1790, over succeeding years, religious affiliation came to be increasingly common in the US (Melton, 1996). Survey data today show that 84% of Americans self-identify with some religious denomination (The Pew Forum on Religion and Public Life; http://religions.pewforum.org, accessed February 20, 2010); 95% say they believe in God or a higher power; and 87% report that they go to church regularly (Gallup, 2002). This stands in marked contrast to many western European countries. In Sweden, for example, only 10% believe that religion is important and only 5% are church attendees (DeMarinis, 2003). The emergence of AA as a spiritual fellowship was not surprising in light of this religiosity, but a degree of restlessness caused old traditions to be cast aside and new ones to emerge, as people struggled to develop a sense of community, and as traditional European roots were weakened.

Bill W. underwent a transformation with his religious renewal which came to be associated with the religiously oriented Oxford Group that he joined. The Oxford Group was not a religious organization, but was characterized by a belief in surrendering one's life to God and carrying that message to others. Along with his co-founder, Bill brought an initially small group of committed believers together. Importantly, though, Bill's emerging philosophy and his expectation of people's acceptance of behavioral change was in line with the values of the general society, and the group he founded moved into the American mainstream, rather than isolating itself in a remote geographic locale.

A psychological perspective on the disease

We are increasingly coming to "medicalize" many aspects of human behavior, reifying physiologic and psychological explanations of the struggles that addicts confront. American society makes a tremendous investment – in the hundreds of millions of dollars each year – in the National Institutes of Health in the hope of finding a genetic locus that leaves people vulnerable to compulsive alcohol and drug use, and of developing a medication that will make it easier for the addicted person to turn down the offer of a drink or a habit-forming drug. This approach has great merit, and may indeed have a profound impact on future treatment for the problems of compulsivity and addiction, but many of its advocates are disinclined to be hospitable to AA as a redemptive community. Understandably, they think in terms of physiology and laboratory experimentation when framing their research and advocating the way we should approach the problem of addiction.

On the other hand, people sympathetic to the twelve-step approach, and those who have become abstinent by turning to twelve-step programs, are more inclined to look at self-examination and emotional rejuvenation as roads to helping the addicted person. "Twelfth-step work" (following the injunction of the last of AA's twelve steps) emphasizes the importance of this latter approach: "Having had a spiritual awakening as a result of these Steps, we tried to carry this message to alcoholics, and to practice these principles in all our affairs." This is a process of personal and communal rejuvenation, and almost every AA meeting is characterized by it. It is a testimony that sounds religious in nature, and has an intensity of support and engagement that is certainly more reminiscent of a revival meeting than a research laboratory. But the two approaches, research-grounded and spiritual, are not incompatible. Bill W. was certainly respectful of the work that Vincent Dole did in developing methadone, a medication for heroin addiction that emerged from the laboratory and clinic. Bill W. expressed the hope that some day there would be a methadone-like agent for treating alcoholism.

One problem that the medical research community encounters in understanding AA as complementary to its armamentarium is that the movement did not derive from experimental research, but rather from a grounds-up process from lay members. AA is therefore suspect to those who rely on empirical proof before accepting a treatment option. AA's effectiveness, often very difficult to study and evaluate, can be approached from the perspective of systematic scientific research. In actuality, one of the principal ways that AA achieves its results is similar to the technique of cognitive behavioral therapy, a research-based approach that is increasingly popular within the psychological and psychiatric communities. In the case of AA, however, the approach is embedded in a structure of advice and exhortation.

The cognitive behavioral therapist systematically queries the patient on the kind of thoughts and circumstances that precipitate the problem being treated (Kadden et al., 1992). In the case of depression, for example, these relate to situations that are incorrectly construed in a negative light. These are then reinterpreted by the therapist with the patient in a more benign and realistic way. In the treatment of alcoholism, this approach involves questioning the patient about "triggers," such as the sight of a liquor bottle, or circumstances, like becoming anxious, associated with the pressure to turn to drinking. The patient is then taught how to anticipate the impact of such triggers for picking up a drink, and is taught to pre-empt them with considered reflection, or by adopting a pre-emptive behavior (i.e. calling another recovering addict for help).

There are numerous aphorisms in AA to help deal with triggers to drink, but they do so in a context of exhortation. An AA sponsor will admonish a sponsee to be careful about "H-A-L-T," or situations when one is hungry, angry, lonely, or tired. Each of these is a well understood trigger for relapse, as recognized in AA lore.

In addition, there are numerous exchanges among members, including examples given by speakers in AA meetings, that reinforce such caution, and enlarge the lexicon of situations to avoid, all of which fits well with a cognitive behavioral approach.

Positive psychology

The concept of "positive psychology" (Seligman et al., 2005) has recently gained currency in academic psychological circles. Advocates of this approach focus on enhancing a person's positive, gratifying experiences rather than offering heuristic relief through psychopathological explanations of etiology. Their goal is to increase the potential for enjoyment of life, and to promote resiliency in the face of problems a person may confront. This perspective may be useful in understanding AA's ethos of life improvement; the way a concept is framed can help to anchor an approach to research and clinical intervention.

There are some interesting examples of studies associated with positive psychology, suggesting how it can be related to improved health. While these do not suggest specific mechanisms of its therapeutic impact, they do offer a useful way of categorizing certain health outcomes. A positive outlook has been shown to be associated with improved outcome in relation to better pulmonary function (Kubzansky et al., 2002), decreased incidence of stroke among the elderly, and increased longevity among both older community-dwelling individuals (Duckworth et al., 2005) and monastic nuns (Danner et al., 2001). Conversely, an association between depression and poor outcome following myocardial infarction has been reported (Frasure-Smith et al., 1995). Depressed patients have also been found to be less likely to comply with medical treatment (Chwastiak et al., 2002), with attendant ill consequences.

Attributing meaning

To understand how engagement into spiritually oriented movements takes place, we can turn to a body of social psychology that has informed research on group influence. This will shed light on both the affective and affiliative aspects of AA, and how they can lead to recovery oriented attitudes. One issue is the way people attribute meaning to their experiences. Research on attribution theory suggests that people are most likely to adopt a new or unusual explanation for their situation when they have lost confidence in themselves and encounter a quandary they cannot solve, and then experience a social context that promotes the new perspective that is different from their own (Kelley, 1967). They may then adopt this new perspective and reorder how they attribute meaning to subsequent experiences. They will explain new observations by using the new perspective they have adopted, so that their circumstances make more sense to them. This is evident in the transformation one sees in despairing addicted people who encounter the new perspective on their plight offered by AA in the supportive atmosphere of its group meetings.

Spiritual recovery movements

How does the intense phenomenon of self-transformation relate to recovery from addiction by means of spiritual and social support? There is a parallel between the way attitudes are transformed in intensely zealous groups and the way that the denial of illness and the self-defeating behaviors of alcoholics and drug addicts may be reversed through induction into a twelve-step group like AA.

AA can be considered a highly successful example of a social phenomenon which may be termed a "spiritual recovery movement" (Galanter, 1997). Such movements have three primary characteristics. First, they claim to provide relief from disease; second, they operate outside the modalities of established empirical medicine; and, third, they ascribe their effectiveness to higher metaphysical powers. The current appeal of such movements is due in part to the fact that physicians often overlook the spiritual or emotional concerns of their patients (Galanter, 2005).

Clearly, the attitudes and behavioral norms that AA espouses conform much more with the values of the larger culture than those of zealous religious sects. The expectation of avoiding drunkenness in AA, normative in our culture, illustrates this. Additionally, adherence to a spiritual recovery movement like AA and its health-related philosophy does not involve every area of the inductee's life; for example, there are limited, if any, constraints on personal property, family ties, or residence. As a spiritual recovery movement, however, AA does engage its followers in behavioral expectations related to the health issues it addresses.

People who are highly distressed over the consequences of their addiction are therefore candidates for response to the strong ideologic recovery orientation of AA. AA members are operantly reinforced by the relief produced by affiliation with the group's ideology and behavioral norms, all related to abstinence and a spiritually grounded lifestyle. Significantly, AA generates distress in its members by pressing them to give up their addictive behaviors, but the distress associated with this conflict is relieved if they sustain affiliation and cleave to the group.

Defining recovery on the basis of spirituality

In the clinical context, recovery is based on a person's behavioral and physiologic status, which can be assessed by recourse to criteria employed in the DSM. Some of these criteria are also embodied in the Addiction Severity Index (McLellan et al., 1992), which is employed widely in addiction outcome research. These items can be assessed relatively easily, since they rate observable behavior.

A spiritually grounded definition of recovery, however, can be useful too. Spirituality, a non-demographic subject factor, originally proposed as a "quality of life" issue (Campbell et al., 1976), is critically important to recovery. In this context, a series of suitable criteria for "diagnosing" addiction ("addiction" is more apt a term than "substance dependence") could be developed. They could then be used to assess the spiritual aspect of recovery associated with the twelve-step experience. Resolution of these issues could be considered to be related to the spiritual aspect of recovery from addiction. A series of criteria could include items such as:

1. Loss of sense of purpose due to excessive substance use.
2. A feeling of inadequate social support because of one's addiction.
3. Continued use of a substance while experiencing moral qualms over its consumption.
4. Loss of the will to resist temptation when the substance is available.

Conclusion

We have considered a number of approaches to understanding the ongoing impact of AA: spiritual redemption; the social context of religion in the US; medical and psychological perspectives; positive psychology; and social movements. This multi-faceted approach illustrates the complexity of the AA phenomenon, and reinforces the need for a multidisciplinary approach to understanding how a self-help movement like AA "works." The clinician should be mindful of each patient's potential response to an encounter with AA, and should be sensitive to the many ways a patient may react to its use.

References

Alcoholics Anonymous. (1957). *Alcoholics Anonymous Comes of Age*. New York: Alcoholics Anonymous Publishing.

Campbell, A., Converse, P. E. & Rogers, W. L. (1976). *The Quality of American Life*. New York: Russell Sage Foundation.

Chwastiak, L., Ehde, D. M., Gibbons, L. E. *et al.* (2002). Depressive symptoms and severity of illness in multiple sclerosis: epidemiologic study of a large community sample. *American Journal of Psychiatry*, **159**, 1862–8.

Danner, D. D., Snowdon, D. A. & Friesen, W. V. (2001). Positive emotions in early life and longevity: findings from the nun study. *Journal of Personality and Social Psychology*, **80**, 804–13.

DeMarinis, V. (2003). *Pastoral Care, Existential Health, and Existential Epidemiology: A Swedish Postmodern Case Study*. Stockholm: Verbum.

Duckworth, A. L., Steen, T. A. & Seligman, M. E. P. (2005). Positive psychology in clinical practice. *Annual Review of Clinical Psychology*, **1**, 629–51.

Frasure-Smith, N., Lesperance, F. & Talajic, M. (1995). Depression following myocardial infarction: impact on 6-month survival. *Journal of the American Medical Association*, **270**, 1819–25.

Galanter, M. (1997). Spiritual recovery movements and contemporary medical care. *Psychiatry*, **60**, 211–23.

Galanter, M. (2005). *Spirituality and the Healthy Mind: Science, Therapy and the Need for Personal Meaning*. New York: Oxford University Press.

Gallup, G. H. (2002). *Religion in America 2002*. Princeton, NJ: Princeton Religious Research Center.

James, W. (1929). *The Varieties of Religious Experience*. New York: Modern Library.

Kadden, R., Carroll, K., Donovan, D. *et al.* (eds.) (1992). *Cognitive-Behavioral Coping Skills Therapy Manual*. Rockville MD: US Department of Health and Human Services.

Kelley, H. H. (1967). Attribution theory in social psychology. In *Nebraska Symposium on Motivation*, Vol. *XV*, ed. D. Levine. Lincoln: University of Nebraska Press.

Kubzansky, L. D., Wright, R. J., Cohen, S. *et al.* (2002). Breathing easy: a prospective study of optimism and pulmonary function in normative aging study. *Annals of Behavioral Medicine*, **24**, 345–53.

McKellar, J., Stewart, E. & Humphreys, K. (2003). Alcoholics Anonymous involvement and positive alcohol-related outcomes. *Journal of Consulting and Clinical Psychology*, **71**, 302–8.

McLellan, A. T., Kushner, H., Metzger, D. *et al.* (1992). The fifth edition of the Addiction Severity Index. *Journal of Substance Abuse Treatment*, **9**, 199–213.

Melton, J. G. (1996). *Encyclopedia of American Religions*. Detroit, MI: Gale Publishing.

Moos, R. H. & Moos, B. S. (2006). Participation in treatment and Alcoholics Anonymous: a 16-year follow-up of initially untreated individuals. *Journal of Clinical Psychology*, **62**, 735–50.

Seligman, M. E. P., Steen, T. A., Park, N. & Peterson, C. (2005). Positive psychology progress. Empirical validation of interventions. *American Psychologist*, **60**, 410–21.

Alcoholism

Jerome Levin

Alcoholism: an equal opportunity destroyer

Alcoholism: "cunning, baffling and insidious," in Alcoholics Anonymous' words, is an equal opportunity destroyer. Although science has rendered it somewhat less baffling, and advances in clinical technique have made it more treatable, the folk wisdom inherent in AA's characterization continues to resonate. A disease whose essence is prolonged, persistent, and self-poisoning (and that is the essence of alcoholism) is indeed baffling. Ask anyone who has struggled to recover from it and he or she will tell you that alcoholism is indeed cunning and insidious.

Although prevalence figures are notoriously unreliable, alcoholism is known to be a widespread disorder. It affects the young and the old; college students and late-onset residents of retirement communities; men and women; straights and gays; the disabled and the bodily intact; whites, Asians, Native Americans, and blacks; all social classes, economic levels, occupations, and religious groups – even those that forbid alcohol consumption. There is a vast literature discussing the differential prevalence rates across groups and the possible reasons (cultural and/or genetic) for these differentials; discussion of that literature is beyond the scope of this chapter. Suffice it to say that some cultures and subcultures sanction extremely heavy drinking; some gene pools predispose. Both heredity and environment are powerful risk factors. A professor at Cornell used to say, "Give me a man of Irish ethnicity who attended Princeton in the fifties or sixties, who now works on Madison Avenue in advertising – and I'll diagnose him as alcoholic before I see him." Not the best medical practice perhaps, yet allowing for polemical overstatement, the formulation was not entirely unreasonable. It makes the point, dramatically, that both genetic predisposition and culture are powerful predictors of alcoholism and that some populations are more susceptible than others.

Why are reliable and accurate prevalence rates so hard to come by? They elude us for two reasons: we lack universally accepted, operational definitions useful in epidemiological studies; and most such research is survey research, depending on self-report by alcoholics. As a group, alcoholics are not terribly reliable as historians. (Denial of the problem, of course, is pathognomonic of the syndrome.) In some sense, alcoholism, at least in its milder manifestations, is a "soft disease," difficult to pin down. Up to a point it exists in the eye of the beholder. There is the story of the fire and brimstone preacher who, in his intensely emotional peroration, thunders, "Is there anyone in this congregation in favor of sin?" A little old lady in the back of the church sticks up her hand. The incredulous preacher bellows, "What? You're in favor of sin?" To which the old lady replies, "Oh, I thought you said gin." To the preacher, gin consumption, let alone heavy drinking, *was* sin; in contemporary terms, an illness. Not so to the old lady, for whom drinking, even heavy drinking, was a sustaining and reliable source of pleasure. Similar discrepancies in the evaluation of drinking behavior and the definition of alcoholism plague epidemiologists.

Prevalence data

With these caveats in mind, let me share some statistics (National Institute on Alcohol Abuse and Alcoholism [NIAAA], 1990; Nephew *et al.*, 2003; 2004).

These studies report that one-third of the adult population abstain, one-third are light drinkers, and one-third are moderate or heavy drinkers. They also found that *10% of the population drank half of the total alcohol consumed.* Men are more likely to drink than women at all ages; young and early middle-aged men more often than the late middle-aged and the old; the unattached more often than the attached; the better educated more often than the less educated; the economically better off more often than the poor; and the urban more often than the rural. The one group that has shown a consistent increase in the percentage of heavy drinkers is young women. Ethnicity also matters, with Jews reporting the least problem drinking, the Irish reporting the most. In general, the strongly religious report low rates of problem drinking.

Although the poor are less likely to drink, if they do they are more likely to be problem drinkers. The same is true of the less educated. African Americans of both sexes are less likely to drink; if they do, they are more likely to be problem drinkers. Problem drinking is most prevalent among men in their twenties, but frank alcoholism is more prevalent among men in their forties. The percentage of drinkers who manifest problem drinking has remained remarkably consistent, being reported at 7–10% by all researchers. The distinction between problem drinking and alcoholism is fuzzy, and the diffuseness of this differential bedevils all of the survey literature (Fingarette, 1988). Nevertheless, in 1990 (NIAAA, 1990) *one million* Americans described themselves as alcoholic and there is little reason to think that this has changed. And if that is the self-identified, then the actual number of alcoholics must be much higher.

For the most part prevalence figures have reported a 2:1 male:female ratio (Brady *et al.*, 1993), but there's reason to think that this is changing as the social sanctions against women drinking have weakened. AA "old-timers" will tell you that when they first came into the program they saw few women – but that is no longer the case. The "old-timers" are not necessarily pleased by this gender shift. The phenomenon could be the result of female alcoholism coming out of the closet rather than an actual increase in pathological drinking in women.

The notion that alcoholism is an equal opportunity destroyer has important clinical implications. It is easy to miss the diagnosis in fluently articulate high achievers, whose very success sustains their denial. People with drinking problems play both sides of the fence. Those from cultures or subcultures where heavy drinking is the norm will strenuously maintain that they drink like everyone else they know, even as they are admitted to the hospital for the third or fourth time for delirium tremens (DTs). Others will use their membership in a low prevalence group to insist that they couldn't possibly have a problem. Don't be fooled! I once treated an elderly, Orthodox Jewish woman who lived in a rural community in the deep South and who was passionately devout. Her presenting problem was anxiety. In spite of membership in not one, but many low incidence groups – she was old, female, Jewish, religious, and rural – she was none the less alcoholic. Further, she used all this in the service of her resistance. "People my age don't have drinking problems . . . Jews aren't drunks . . . people in my town don't drink." Her claim had statistical validity, but unfortunately it didn't apply to her. Another patient was a professor in a top medical school who of course maintained that a man of his distinction couldn't possibly have a drinking problem.

Alcoholism: a biopsychosocial disorder

There are four factors involved in the etiology and maintenance of any addiction, including alcoholism: heredity; environment (including the cultural attitudes of both the larger societal surround and the family toward use and abuse); personality (including emotional and dynamic forces); and the pharmacology of the drug. Both the etiology and the consequences of alcoholism are truly biopsychosocial. Alcoholism's sources are multidimensional and its effects are all-pervasive to mind, body, and human surround. Let us start with the biological.

Heredity

There is strong evidence of several sorts for genetic predisposition to alcoholism. First, alcoholism has long been known to run in families. Casual observation has been validated by countless studies and the phenomenon is not in doubt, but its meaning is (Bleuler, 1955; Pitts & Winokur, 1966). Family attitudes toward drinking, modeling, maladaptive efforts to cope with the pain and trauma of growing up in an alcoholic family, identification with the aggressor, and social learning have all been implicated. All of these factors play a role, but current thinking leans toward genetic transmission of vulnerability as a primary causal element in this running in families. Nevertheless, in themselves family studies cannot determine the relative influence of the various factors. Twin studies (see below) offer much stronger evidence for the role of heredity in the etiology of alcoholism.

That evidence for the heritability of alcoholism is of several sorts: family studies, studies of twins, studies of adoptees (also called population genetic studies), animal studies, and comparison of family history-positive and family history-negative students' response to alcohol.

Studies of twins

Studies of twins have contributed evidence for a genetic factor in alcoholism. Such studies are conducted by calculating the concordance between identical (monozygotic) and fraternal (dizygotic) twins for alcoholism; the concordance rate is the percentage of twins sharing a given trait or condition. In this case, the percentage of alcoholic twins with an alcoholic twin is calculated for populations of identical and fraternal twins. The concordance rates are then compared. Since identical twins are the product of the same fertilized egg, or zygote, and fraternal twins are the product of different fertilized eggs, a higher concordance between identical than fraternal twins is taken as evidence of a genetic factor in the transmission of the trait or condition. The results consistently show that identical twins of alcoholics have a statistically significantly higher incidence of alcoholism than do fraternal twins of alcoholics. In a typical study, Kaij (1960), using male twins, found a concordance of 53.5% in identical twins and a concordance of 28.3% in fraternal twins. These findings have been replicated many times.

Studies of adoptees

A promising research design is to study the children of alcoholics who were adopted very early in life by non-alcoholic adoptive parents, following them into adulthood and determining their rates of alcoholism and comparing those rates to their generational peers. The first, and one of the most important, of these adoption studies was conducted by Goodwin, Schulsinger, Hermansen, Guze, and Winokur (1973[a]) in Denmark. Goodwin *et al.* followed children of alcoholics who were adopted at or shortly after birth and raised by non-alcoholic parents. An early study (Roe, 1945) found almost no alcoholism in children of alcoholics who were raised by non-alcoholic adoptive parents. This result may be confounded by the disproportionate number of girls in the study. Goodwin *et al.*'s results were the opposite. In their study, chronic alcoholism was four times more common in 55 adopted-out sons of alcoholic fathers than among 78 adopted-out sons of non-alcoholics. The sons of alcoholics had a 25% rate of alcoholism – higher than the 17% rate Goodwin *et al.* found for male children of alcoholics raised by those alcoholics. This, of course, means that 75% of the sons of alcoholics raised by non-alcoholic adoptive parents did not become

alcoholic; therefore, simple Mendelian inheritance of alcoholism is not the case. Moreover, alcoholism was not found to be significantly more prevalent in adopted-out daughters of alcoholics raised by non-alcoholics. It is of considerable interest that Goodwin *et al.*'s adopted-out male children of alcoholics had significantly higher rates of hyperactivity, shyness, sensitivity, and aggression than adopted-out male children of non-alcoholics. Adoptees whose biological parents were not alcoholics but who were raised by alcoholic parents did not have significantly higher rates of alcoholism. In contrast to their findings on alcoholism, Goodwin *et al.* found no correlation between "problem drinking" and alcoholism in biological parents. They concluded that alcoholism in children of alcoholics is not transmitted by learning, modeling, or unconscious identification, let alone by the maladaptive use of alcohol to ameliorate the pain of being raised in an alcoholic home, although environmental provocation is necessary for "milieu-limited" alcoholism to occur (see below). However, there may be a confounding variable here. It is known that many children of alcoholics become teetotalers, and it may be that the environmental, emotional, and interpersonal, as opposed to the genetic, influences of parental alcoholism may be to increase the likelihood of *either* alcoholism or total abstinence, while decreasing the likelihood of becoming a social drinker. This hypothesis was not tested in either the Danish or the Swedish studies. The Swedish study reported by Cloninger (1983) confirms Goodwin *et al.*'s results although it made a distinction between "male limited" (severe, early onset, highly hereditable) alcoholism and "milieu limited" (late onset, less hereditable) alcoholism. A more recent American study (Cadoret *et al.*, 1984; 1986; 1995) using the same design found that adopted-out sons of alcoholics were three times as likely to develop alcoholism as adopted sons of non-alcoholics. An important additional finding was that these Iowa children of alcoholics had a significantly higher rate of conduct disorder than their peers, a finding congruent with the high rates of hyperactivity in the Danish study and with retrospective evidence (Tartar, 1981; Tarter & Alterman, 1989) of childhood hyperactivity in clinical alcoholic populations.

Animal studies

Because people are among the few animals that naturally drink ethanol, finding animal models for alcoholism is difficult. Elephants are apparently an exception, getting smashed on fermented palms and going on rampages, but it is not clear that it is the alcohol rather than the palms that attract them, nor are we certain whether alcoholic elephants see pink elephants. Alcohol is not strongly reinforcing for most animals. This is strikingly different from the animal response to cocaine. If a rodent is given a choice of pushing a lever that delivers cocaine and one that delivers food, he or she will choose the cocaine, continuing to do so until collapse. Nevertheless, animal subjects are used to study drinking behavior and alcoholism.

Appetite for alcohol and preference for alcohol are traits that occur in some but not all rodent individuals and strains, and strains of mice and rats have been bred not only to drink alcohol but to prefer it to water (Goodwin & Warnock, 1991). There are even rodents that will voluntarily drink enough alcohol to have withdrawal symptoms when they stop. The way these anomalies are created is by breeding with each other those animals that show some appetite for alcohol and in turn selecting those of their offspring with the greatest appetite for alcohol to mate with others similarly inclined. This process of selective breeding is continued over the generations until a strain of rodents with a distinct appetite for alcohol emerges. Surprisingly, Martini Mickey can be bred in as little as 10 generations. With some strains, continued selective breeding results in animals that prefer alcohol and even animals that show a physical dependence. These results argue strongly for the existence of a genetically transmitted appetite for alcohol in rodents. Although extrapolating from animal models to humans is inferential, and it is not certain that similar propensities are inherited by humans, the heritability of an appetite for alcohol in rodents is a striking finding that strongly suggests that similar mechanisms exist in humans. Additionally, the heritability of a tolerance for alcohol, as measured by the righting response (the ability to remain on or regain one's paws after a heavy dose of ethanol), has been demonstrated in rodents.

Response to alcohol by family-positive students

There are numerous studies (Newlin & Thomson, 1990; Volavka et al., 1990) comparing family history-positive (FHP) to family history-negative college students to "challenge doses" (i.e. three to five drinks) on a variety of responses. The results consistently show that alcohol has more positive effects on FHP students and fewer negative effects, which suggests that genetic

predisposition may make alcohol highly reinforcing for these, perhaps pre-alcoholic students, predisposing them to the disorder. The relative absence of negative effects in the FHP group removes a deterrent to heavy drinking that may protect others against developing alcoholism. Pollock et al. (1983), using the electroencephalograph (EEG), showed that drinking was reinforcing, albeit in different ways, for both Cloninger type 1 (milieu limited) and type 2 (male limited) FHP students, reducing anxiety by slowing and synchronizing alpha waves in the first group and by reducing evoke potentials in the second. Again, these are differential responses that would predispose to alcohol addiction. Further, attention deficit disorder (ADD), shown by many researchers (Biederman et al., 1998; Hallowell & Ratey, 1995) to be comorbid with and frequently antecedent to alcoholism, correlates with these evoke potential irregularities.

What conclusion can be drawn from all this? The best evidence that we have shows that a predisposition to some forms of alcoholism is inherited. Alcoholisms can probably be arranged in a continuum, ranging from those in which constitutional factors play little or no role to those in which constitutional factors play a determining role. One-third of alcoholics report no family history of alcoholism. From a clinical standpoint, the most important finding of these studies is that children of alcoholics are at extremely high risk for alcoholism, even if this predisposition is not necessarily exclusively genetic. That brings up the question of what is inherited that predisposes to the development of alcoholism. An appetite for alcohol? Enjoyment of alcohol? Relief of some dysfunction or dysphoria by alcohol? More than normal reinforcement by alcohol? A high tolerance for alcohol (hollow leg)? A deviant response to alcohol by the nervous system or the liver? Some combination of the above? We don't know, but most probably each of these mechanisms plays a greater role in some of the predisposed than in others.

Pharmacology

The effects of alcohol on the body are delineated elsewhere in this volume, but let me say that ethanol is a small molecule, as organic molecules go, that is easily soluble in both water and fat, giving it easy access to every cell in the body. That easy access, combined with high toxicity and the absence of any one receptor site, means that the somatic consequences of very heavy drinking can be catastrophic. Any part of the body can be affected, but by far the most frequent pathologies are of the liver and nervous system. It has been said that alcohol is a miracle drug – evidence its popularity across cultures and eras – with horrendous side-effects, at least from prolonged heavy use. Not all of these side-effects are physical, but the physical ones can indeed be serious and indeed life-threatening. As a result of alcohol's effect on the nervous system and other parts of the body, full-blown alcoholics aren't playing with a full deck, and that makes treating them all the more difficult. Cognitive impairment, combined with emotional lability, renders "getting through" problematic. In terms of therapeutic technique, this means simplicity, clarity, and a high degree of redundancy. The therapist's interventions should carry emotional valence without being overwhelming. AA refers to the mental state of those in early recovery as "mokus," an onomatopoeic word meaning mentally confused. I have even speculated that part of alcoholic denial may be the result of brain damage resulting in a form of anosognosia, in which the potential for the awareness of the disease is radically diminished consequent upon neurological deficit.

It is important for the treating person to keep in mind that alcohol is a central nervous system (CNS) depressant (its pharmacology, including the withdrawal syndrome, is discussed more fully in Chapter 3), and abrupt withdrawal can be dangerous. Withdrawal symptoms, often not recognized as such, also serve to maintain the addiction, as the alcoholic takes "the hair of the dog" to "calm" his or her nerves. A "subacute withdrawal syndrome" manifesting itself in ill-defined dysphoria and emotional lability, may lead to self-medication of these symptoms, thereby sustaining the addiction.

Role of culture and the environment

Social cultural factors are powerful determinants of drinking behavior and alcoholism and of drug use and addiction in general. Witness the sharp decline in American middle-class cigarette smoking in recent years. There has been no change in the gene pool or in the pharmacology of nicotine. But there has been a radical change in the cultural evaluation of smoking. Conversely, in male subcultures where heavy drinking, even drunkenness, is proof of "machismo," the rates of alcoholism are high. Youth subcultures may put a premium on getting high and that too boosts the prevalence rates.

American attitudes toward heavy drinking, indeed toward drinking in general, have changed, and Americans are drinking less (Substance Abuse and Mental Health Services Administration, 2006) particularly of the hard stuff. Our attitudes towards drunkenness have also changed. It is much less tolerated. The campaign against drunken driving or even driving while impaired has played a major role in this shift. How much this will impact on the occurrence of alcoholism remains to be seen. During American prohibition, the rates of cirrhosis of the liver fell, but not that strikingly. Socialization into moderation in general and moderate alcohol use in particular are believed to "inoculate" against alcoholism. (Heard at an AA meeting: "I'm getting used to moderation, I've passed through it so many times going between the extremes.")

The strength of social–cultural factors is vividly illustrated by the expectancy literature (MacAndrew & Edgerton, 1969). That literature demonstrates that cognitive factors, which are internalized from the culture, determine, at least in part, how a drug, or in our case alcohol, is experienced and how it influences behavior. For example, there are heavy drinking cultures (Rooney, 1991) in which alcohol consumption has no correlation with violence. This is strongly at variance with the strong association between drinking and violence in western culture. The resurgence of religion and participation in religious ritual and ceremony may also be having a moderating effect on American drinking.

Sociologists have traditionally contrasted two sets of cultures in terms of their attitudes toward drinking and rates of alcoholism. They are French–Italian and Irish–Jewish (Pittman & White, 1991). In France, it is an insult to refuse a drink; drinking is both familial, usually with meals, and non-familial, with peers at all hours of the day and night. Perhaps most significantly, there is little sanction against drunkenness. By contrast, Italian drinking tends to be intergenerational, with meals, in the family, and what is consumed is low-proof wine. This stands in contrast to France, where consumption is of both wine and liquor. Drinking is less central to Italian social life, and, most importantly, drunkenness is strongly disapproved of. Not surprisingly, France (with the highest rate in the world) has strikingly more alcoholism per capita than Italy.

Ireland, where excessive drinking was regarded as "a good man's vice," and where a socially and politically oppressed culture with a high level of sexual repression gave its men a social remission in the pub where high-proof whiskey went down, has had a high incidence of alcoholism. By contrast, in Jewish society, which believed "shikker is a goy" (i.e. the drunk is a gentile) and in which drinking was highly ritualized and associated with the family and with sacred observance, there was a low incidence of alcoholism. Certainly the Irish rate was substantially higher. In contrast to the "safety" of the Irish pub, being drunk was dangerous for the Jews as a small, persecuted minority in Eastern Europe. In the sociologists' typography of drinking behavior, Irish drinking was "instrumental" (i.e. in the service of getting drunk), whereas Jewish drinking was "convivial" and/or "sacred" and highly ritualized in both cases. As both the Jews and the Irish have assimilated into the American mainstream, these distinctions blur and become less etiological, but the point of these studies, namely, that the culture and values are strikingly determinative of drinking behavior and rates of alcoholism, remains valid, and indeed, the efficacy of one of the most successful of treatments, participation in Alcoholics Anonymous (AA), can be conceptualized as a change in culture. As anyone who has worked with alcohol- and drug-abusing youth can tell you, if they don't change their social surround their chance of remaining in recovery is nil. Sociologists have also pointed to drinking as a passive–aggressive act of rebellion by marginalized groups against the perceived oppressors. In this context, Native American drinking has been described as the oldest extant protest movement in the world.

Personality: emotional–psychological factors

Personality factors are the third etiological factor in the development of alcohol addiction. People who use externalization, projection, and denial as primary defense mechanisms/coping strategies are at heightened risk of alcoholism, as are those who suffer from lack of affect tolerance and/or impulsivity (Ciarrocchi et al., 1991). An angry, rebellious, acting-out configuration of personality traits sharply predisposes to alcoholism, and plays a central role in maintaining the addiction. So do depression, anxiety, low self-esteem, and poor interpersonal skills. It seems that high-rolling, devil-may-care types and withdrawn, isolated, emotionally tormented types are especially prone to substance abuse, including alcohol abuse, albeit for

different reasons. And each of these sets of personality traits mitigates against recovery.

For many problem drinkers, self-medication of neurotic conflict is both etiological and intrinsic to the alcoholism itself. Larry had a prolonged neurotic conflict with his Orthodox Jewish family. He hated what he experienced as their judgmental rigidity and he particularly hated his father, who would weep, his tears falling on Larry's head, as he pronounced the New Year's blessing on his apostate, unbelieving son. But Larry also loved and admired the hated father. He was torn between rage and guilt. Then Larry, who had long been a heavy "social" drinker, discovered that by the third or fourth drink, he could feel both his love and his hate of his father without conflict and without guilt. From there, the pharmacology of ethanol took over and within a few years Larry was a full-blown alcoholic. His was an alcoholism in which genetic predisposition played little or no role, environmental factors a modest one, and emotional conflict a major one.

There is general agreement that a clinical or "post-alcoholic" personality characterized by negative affect, low self-esteem, lack of affect tolerance, and other characteristics adumbrated below exists (Barnes, 1983). There is a great deal of empirical evidence to support this (Barnes, 1979). The existence of a "pre-alcoholic" personality is much more doubtful, and the empirical evidence for one is weak or non-existent. However, we do know that conduct disorder and ADHD are clear predispositional factors.

One of the oldest theories of the psychological substrate of alcoholism is the dependency conflict theory first articulated by McCord and McCord (McCord and McCord with Gudeman, 1960; McCord and McCord, 1960). Derived from a longitudinal empirical study, it postulates that men whose dependency needs are not reliably met in childhood develop a counterdependent defense against forbidden, overwhelming need and then use alcohol to meet that need covertly: the hard-drinking, two-fisted "Lone Ranger" style cowboy being the stereotypic embodiment of the syndrome. As the drinking becomes alcoholic, the defense collapses and the infantile dependency re-emerges. If such a dependence is ego-alien, more alcohol is used to obliviate the painful self-perception and a vicious cycle is set up. A syndrome of counter-dependence, alternating with open, primitive dependence without interdependence anywhere in sight, is the end result. There is anthropological evidence that societies that frustrate the meeting of dependency needs are heavy drinking societies. In the 1972 classic, *The Drinking Man*, David McClelland *et al.* offer evidence based on Thematic Apperception Tests (TAT) research of male drinkers, that they drink to feel "powerful." McClelland looks at this as disproving the dependency conflict theory, though his data can be seen as supporting it. The counterdependent power-seeking comes from a profound sense of powerlessness. McClelland's theory was derived from an empirical study that followed Boston working class youth from adolescence into maturity.

In 1983 (revised edition 1995), George Vaillant published another longitudinal study entitled *The Natural History of Alcoholism*. Vaillant reported on two relatively large research samples. One consisted of Harvard University students chosen for their mental health who were followed from their sophomore years into their 50s, and the other consisted of normal core-city working-class subjects who were followed from their childhoods into their 40s. Vaillant found that childhood and adolescent emotional problems and overtly disturbed childhoods did not predict adult alcoholism in either sample, although such disturbed childhoods did predict adult mental illness. He found that ethnicity (Irish or northern European ancestry) and parental alcoholism did predict adult alcoholism. He argued that the clinical alcoholic personality is the result of drinking, not of premorbid personality factors. Vaillant also argued that adult alcoholics retrospectively falsify the degree of pathology in their childhood environments to rationalize their drinking. I have found that retrospective idealization of their childhoods is at least as characteristic of adult alcoholic patients as retrospective devaluation or denial of whatever may have been positive in their childhoods; this, however, is a clinical and not a research finding. Vaillant's data cannot be dismissed, but his interpretation of them is not entirely persuasive.

Zucker and Gomberg (1986) argue that methodological artifacts are responsible for Vaillant's conclusion that childhood experience and antecedent psychopathology play no role in adult alcoholism. They also suggest that he was looking for the wrong stuff, pathological dependency and negative affect, whereas if he had looked for non-conformity, impulsivity, and reward seeking at high enough levels to constitute an antisocial trend, he would have found it. In fact, they re-analyzed Vaillant's data (by changing the order of regression of his variable) and did find

childhood antecedents, including disturbed homes and psychopathology, of alcoholism.

Interestingly, although Vaillant didn't find a correlation between disruptive childhood environment and alcoholism, he did find a correlation between disruptive childhood environment and early onset and severity of alcoholism. Vaillant basically argues that culture and parental alcoholism are far more powerful determinants of (male) alcoholism than psychological factors.

Be this as it may, cause or consequence or both, emotional–psychological factors are a huge proportion of what we must address and can treat in the biopsychosocial mix that is alcoholism.

A psychological intervention derived from Vaillant's work that often resonates with alcoholics and indeed may be mutative is the following confrontation: "You think that you drink because you're crazy. Did it ever occur to you that you're crazy because you drink?" Even if the patient is comorbid, stopping his or her drinking is a *sine qua non* of recovery and, if this intervention arrests the drinking, the therapist can deal with any other psychopathology that may be there, whether it be cause or consequence.

I would like to single out one emotion, alcoholic rage, because it is so central to the dynamics of relapse. I believe that most "slips" are rage reactions and that the clinician who understands this phenomenon can intervene to circumvent some of these slips. Alcoholic rage is multifactorial, being: 1) consequent on the pharmacology of alcohol and the prolonged withdrawal syndrome; 2) self-hatred projected outward; 3) in the service of justifying the next drink; 4) the result of narcissistic vulnerability – that is, the liability of being easily hurt that low self-esteem and ego weakness make inevitable – leads to reactive or prophylactic rage at the perceived hurt or threat; and 5) a defense against experiencing overwhelmingly painful guilt and shame. All this can be discussed/interpreted in a treatment. A useful intervention at the beginning of treatment: "It is vital that we discuss it when you are angry, frustrated, anxious or down. It is especially important that we talk about your anger and rage. Sometimes we will be able to understand why you feel the way you do at that particular time; that is, we will be able to point to something going on within you that is emotional or something going on in your world that is interpersonal that is making you so angry. However, sometimes we won't be able to understand what your emotional reaction is about and it will be important for us to realize that these feelings are part of the recovery process. That is, ups and downs are just part of healing. You've done a lot of damage to your nervous system, assaulting it with a powerful poison for a long period of time. It will heal, but it will take time for it to do so. And during that time neurochemical events are going on which you will experience as rage and anger and other forms of emotional discomfort that are not really psychologically meaningful." The therapist should probe for underlying rage, which may be minimized, denied, or not even overtly experienced. Be suspicious of your patient saying, "I'm annoyed." "I'm annoyed" almost certainly means "I want to kill somebody."

Types of alcoholism

There are many typographies of alcoholism, and, like any other abstraction, they are imperfect fits with reality. Further, there are classification systems that have come and gone. Nevertheless, the following conceptualizations are both theoretically illuminating and clinically useful.

Jellinek and gamma alcoholism

Emil Jellinek (1960) not only has a classificatory scheme, he was one of the first to elaborate and defend the disease concept of alcoholism. Jellinek had predecessors, going back to Benjamin Rush (1785), surgeon-general of the American revolutionary army, and British naval physician Thomas Trotter (1820, in Levin & Weiss, 1994), who believed "inebriety" was a disease caused by premature weaning and heredity, and, more proximally, AA's notion that "alcoholism is an obsession of the mind and an allergy of the body," which its co-founder, Bill Wilson, learned from William Silkworth, the physician in charge of Towns Hospital where Wilson finally got sober. But it was Jellinek who made the notion scientifically respectable. He also affected social policy, resulting in the American Medical Association, both the American Psychiatric and American Psychological Associations and, more ambivalently and conflictively, the legal system subscribing to the disease concept.

In *The Disease Concept of Alcoholism* (1960) Jellinek took a very careful and painstaking look at each of the possible ways of understanding alcoholism as a disease. In doing so he evaluated available empirical evidence and the conceptual strength of each approach. Two major findings emerged. One was the concept of alcoholism as a progressive disease culminating in loss

of control (that is, the inability to stop drinking after having begun). He called this *gamma alcoholism*. Jellinek derived this conceptualization largely from responses to a questionnaire on drinking histories that he submitted to a sample of AA members. Few pieces of survey research have had such influence. Every alcohol rehabilitation program has a chart of Jellinek's stages of progression, which it uses to teach the disease concept of alcoholism to patients. According to this scheme (Jellinek, 1952), alcoholism progresses from "occasional relief drinking" to "obsessive drinking continuing in vicious cycles," having passed through such stages as "onset of blackouts," "grandiose and aggressive behavior," "family and friends avoided," and "indefinable fears." The order of progression is seen as invariant. This concept of alcoholism as a progressive, fatal disease is canonical in AA. Later research (Park, 1973; Vaillant, 1983) has shown that neither progression per se nor Jellinek's invariant order is necessarily the case. Nevertheless, for most problem drinkers, things do not get better; if they continue to drink, they get worse, and their problems get worse in pretty much the way the respondents to Jellinek's questionnaire said they do.

Although Jellinek's conceptualization of at least one form of alcoholism as a disease is based on a nuanced, subtle analysis that recognizes that not all problem drinking is best understood as a disease (see below), his ideas have come under increasing attack. Critics point to the fact that the progression is not inevitable or invariant, and to experiments that show that alcoholics do not always drink themselves to oblivion when they have the opportunity.

Herbert Fingarette (1988), one of the most thoughtful of the critics, cites survey research (Clark & Cahalan, 1976; Polich *et al.*, 1981) that purports to show that symptoms of problem drinking come and go but do not progress, and Vaillant's (1983) longitudinal study showed that youthful problem drinking is a poor predictor of middle age alcoholism, and that the rate of "spontaneous recovery" from alcoholism is substantial. Fingarette attacks the notion of loss of control by citing Mello and Mendelson's (1972) study that showed that hospitalized alcoholics who had open access to alcohol did not drink themselves into oblivion and that they drank less when they had to "work" for their drinks. Fingarette also attacks the disease concept from a clinical standpoint, maintaining that teaching alcoholics that they have an uncontrollable disease becomes a self-fulfilling prophecy.

Marlatt and Gordon (1985) speak of the abstinence violation effect (AVE) in which alcoholics who believe that if they take one drink they will be unable to stop, will in fact not be able to stop, not because of a "disease" but because of a cognitive expectancy. As for the loss-of-control issue, Jellinek's original formulation of it is clearly untenable. What loss of control does mean is that "alcoholics" cannot predict what will happen when they pick up a drink. The social drinker may decide to get drunk, say as a way of dealing with frustration. That may be foolish or immature from somebody else's standpoint, but that is not evidence of loss of control. Alcoholics, on the other hand, decide to have one beer and sometimes do, but if they continue to experiment, they find that sooner or later the desire to have one drink will not prevent them from winding up completely smashed. This is extremely important clinically and must be explained to patients, especially to those who have been able to stop after one or two, and use this to justify continued drinking.

Critics of the unpredictability notion of loss of control maintain that the alcoholic has simply decided to get drunk. This contradicts many alcoholics' subjective experience and they report: "I found myself drinking in spite of not wanting to," and just about everybody's clinical experience. I have not found that alcoholics who subscribe to the disease concept continue to drink; on the contrary, the disease concept makes sense of a bewildering experience, reduces anxiety and guilt, and facilitates taking responsibility for one's recovery.

The therapist can usefully reflect that alcoholism entails progressive impoverishment, with the alcoholic winding up with an empty bottle, empty world, and empty self, and that recovery is a process of progressive enrichment.

Jellinek's second major contribution is his taxonomic system. At any given time all alcoholics will fall into one of his categories, but the alcoholic may move across categories with the passage of time. Jellinek's categories are as follows: alpha, beta, gamma, delta, and epsilon.

Alpha alcoholism is characterized by the presence of such symptoms as hangovers or blackouts and by psychological, not physical, dependence. The alpha alcoholic is the person who needs alcohol on a regular basis and who becomes anxious if it is not available. However, he or she will not experience withdrawal symptoms upon cessation of drinking. The person who "requires" alcohol to do a particular thing, such as make love, can also be considered an alpha since this is a psychological dependency on alcohol. Alpha alcoholism is not necessarily progressive. Some drinkers remain psychologically dependent on alcohol for life without deteriorating physically or mentally.

Beta alcoholism is characterized by physical symptoms such as ulcers or liver disease but not by physical dependence. The typical beta alcoholic is a heavy drinker, usually of beer, who continues to function socially and economically in a fairly adequate way as he or she continues to inflict somatic injury on himself or herself. The beta alcoholic's drinking pattern remains stable in terms of quantity consumed and the relative absence of psychological and social symptomatology. Although beta alcoholism is not a progressive disease, it, too, is a form of pathological drinking. There is something manifestly crazy about continuing to inflict bodily damage on oneself in this way. Beta alcoholism is strongly associated with male, blue collar, culturally syntonic heavy drinking.

According to Jellinek, gamma alcoholism is the most prevalent form of alcoholism in the US. Gamma alcoholics are both symptomatic and physically dependent (at least in the late stages). That is, they suffer emotional and psychological impairment, their social and economic functioning is compromised, and they develop a tolerance to alcohol and experience withdrawal symptoms if they stop drinking. Jellinek thought that gamma alcoholism was characterized by *progression* and *loss of control.*

Delta alcoholism is characterized by physical dependence but few or no symptoms. Jellinek believes that alcoholism in heavy wine-drinking countries such as France is largely delta alcoholism. The delta drinker does not lose control or get drunk, violent, or pass out, but cannot stop drinking without experiencing withdrawal symptoms. High rates of liver disease are associated with delta alcoholism.

Jellinek's final category is epsilon alcoholism. Epsilon alcoholism is binge drinking, which the old psychiatric literature called dipsomania. Epsilon drinkers go on binges, for no apparent reason, of indeterminate length, usually lasting until they collapse. They then do not drink again until the next binge. The interval between binges may be weeks, months, or even years.

Knight: essential versus reactive alcoholism

Psychoanalyst Robert Knight (1937) made a clinically vital distinction between essential and reactive alcoholism. Essential alcoholics are those who never really established themselves in life. They had trouble from adolescence onward. They are often financially and emotionally dependent on their families; they have spotty educational and work histories with very little evidence of accomplishment or achievement. Their object relations are at the need-gratifying level. Knight, who was the first to describe the syndrome, noted that many essential alcoholics have borderline personality structures.

The reactive alcoholics are those who have managed some life successes. They have achieved economic independence and have vocational attainments. They have generally succeeded in marrying and establishing families. The quality of their object relations had once been fairly adequate, even if now they are gravely impaired by their drinking. Most had had a period of social drinking before crossing the "invisible line" into alcoholism. Knight saw their addiction as a reaction to life stresses or losses. From his description of his reactives, they seem to be a mix of "normals" with drinking problems and narcissistic personality disorders (NPD). Essentials require *habilitation*, while reactives require *rehabilitation*. The biphasic nature of the alcoholic population has been noted by many observers who give the two groups differing labels. What matters is recognition that the two groups require different treatment approaches.

Winokur, Rimmer, and Reich's primary versus secondary alcoholism

Winokur, Rimmer, and Reich (1971) drew a distinction between primary alcoholism and secondary alcoholism. Actually, their typology is trichotomous: primary alcoholism, depressive alcoholism, and sociopathic alcoholism. Primary alcoholics are those whose alcoholism is not preceded by a major psychiatric illness. Secondary alcoholics are those whose alcoholism follows a major psychiatric illness. By major psychiatric illness, Winokur primarily meant a major affective disorder. Clinically, Winokur's distinction is of great importance. Both primary and secondary alcoholics may be seriously depressed. However, the depression associated with primary alcoholism will remit with treatment consisting of abstinence and appropriate psychotherapeutic intervention, whereas that associated with secondary alcoholism will not. Participation in AA helps to alleviate depression associated with primary alcoholism. This is not the case

with patients suffering from secondary alcoholism. Their affective disorders are not a consequence of their alcoholism, which is an attempt at self-medication of that depression, and treatment of the alcoholism will not cure it. This is not to say that the alcoholism need not be arrested for the depression to remit. As the old cowboy song would have it, "Cigarettes and *whiskey,* and wild, wild women will drive you crazy, drive you insane." Secondary alcoholism is more common in women. Winokur also drew attention to another important differential – that between primary alcoholism and alcoholism that is secondary to sociopathy. Primary alcoholics may display sociopathic behavior, but they are not sociopaths; sociopaths, however, are often heavy drinkers without necessarily being alcoholic. Alcoholism secondary to sociopathy is generally found in men and is extremely difficult to treat.

Cloninger's male-limited and milieu-limited alcoholisms

We have already met Cloninger in our discussion of the heritability of alcoholism. We return to his theory to highlight his distinction between male-limited and milieu-limited alcoholism. The alcoholics in his 1983 study (Cloninger, 1983; Coloninger, Bohman and Sigvardsson, 1981) who manifested early-onset severe alcoholism characterized by inability to abstain, fighting, arrests, and little or no guilt about their drinking, had a type of alcoholism that is heavily influenced by heredity and is limited to men. He called this male-limited or type 2 alcoholism. The other group of alcoholics in his study showed late-onset, progression, psychological dependence, and guilt about that dependence. This type of alcoholism occurs in men and women, and, although Cloninger believes that genetic factors are involved here too, they do not manifest themselves without environmental provocation. He called this milieu-limited or type 1 alcoholism.

Cloninger's male-limited alcoholism overlaps with Winokur's alcoholism secondary to sociopathy. It is vital to distinguish clinically those alcohol addicts who may have done really dreadful things in the course of their addiction, but who feel intense shame and guilt from those who do not. That guilt can be so painful that it leads to what Leon Wurmser (1978) calls "flight from conscience," through relapse.

Diagnosis

Alcoholism is a disease that tells you that *you* don't have it. Paradoxically it is also a disease that must be in some sense self-diagnosed if recovery is to occur. The primary goal in treatment is facilitating that self-diagnosis.

There are, of course, formal diagnostic criteria, the most widely applied being those of the APA's DSM-IV-R (1994). A less structured diagnostic tool is simply to ask, "Does the drinking persist in spite of serious consequences to one or more vital areas of functioning" – health, personal relations, relationship with self, work, school, or family.

In the DSM-III-R and DSM-IV, alcoholism is treated as a subspecies of psychoactive substance dependence. Such dependence is diagnosed by the presence of three or more of the following: 1) substance taken in larger amounts than wished; 2) persistent desire or failure to cut down; 3) frequent intoxication (or withdrawal symptoms that interfere with functioning); 4) significant time spent obtaining supplies or dealing with consequences of use; 5) activities given up to use; 6) persistent use despite adverse consequences; 7) marked tolerance; 8) withdrawal symptoms; and 9) use of the substance to treat withdrawal. The symptoms must be of at least 1 month's duration.

The DSM series made a distinction between abuse and dependence. In the earlier editions, dependence meant physical dependence, so psychological dependence was diagnosed as abuse. This changed with DSM-IV. Now psychological dependence without withdrawal symptoms can be diagnosed as psychoactive dependency, with alcohol specified as the drug of abuse. Although they are the required diagnostic standards in most treatment settings, to me the DSM criteria do not add much to a more intuitive approach. As AA says, "It's not how much you drink, but what it does to you." AA has a series of twelve questions (Alcoholics Anonymous World Services, 1952) intended for self-diagnosis that are helpful.

Another useful diagnostic tool is the Michigan alcoholism screening test (Selzer, 1971). It too is easy to administer and quite helpful clinically.

Today it is hard to find a "pure" alcoholic. Almost everyone you treat has at least dabbled in other drugs and more than a few will be cross-addicted. For example, many cocaine users drink to come down, and some alcoholics use "uppers," including cocaine, so they can drink more. The potential for cross-addiction in either scenario is obvious. Being a "garbage head" used to be pathognomonic of severe psychopathology, but as the culture has changed, that is less true. Nevertheless, polysubstance abuse is a serious matter and is usually more treatment-resistant than plain old alcoholism.

Investigation of drinking and drugging behavior is intrinsic to any competent mental status exam or intake protocol. But even with judicious probing, the diagnosis can easily be missed, alcoholics being canny minimizers as well as self-deceivers. Tom was referred by the employee assistance program (EAP) of a research lab for a work problem. He just couldn't get his reports in on time. Since he was a safety engineer at a nuclear reactor, this was not a trivial problem. Neither in the referral nor the intake nor in several months of weekly therapy did any indication of a drinking problem surface. Then Tom started a session by relating a dream in which he was wearing shit-stained underpants on backwards and inside out. Since Tom suffered all sorts of anal conflicts, not unrelated to his presenting problem, we worked hard on the dream, but the work was unproductive. The session turned in a different direction until at the very last moment, Tom sat bolt upright and said, "I know why I had that dream. I got shitfaced last night." So Tom, or at least his unconscious, diagnosed and communicated his quite serious alcohol involvement and in subsequent sessions we were able to move him away from the brink of disaster as he stood on the border between (in DSM-IV terms) abuse and dependence.

Psychological theories of causality and dynamics

Learning theory

There are three primary ways in which human beings learn – classical conditioning, operant conditioning, and modeling. Learning theory helps make sense of addiction. We know that rewards and punishments need to be closely associated with actions for them to increase or decrease the frequencies of those actions. That is, reinforcement needs to be closely paired with an event. Alcohol's first effects: tension reduction, anxiety modulation, disinhibition, and euphoria are positively reinforcing. Its regressive, negative effects (punishments), for example, cirrhosis, job loss, and self-hatred, are long delayed. Therefore the connection between the negative consequences and excessive drinking is not established in the mind.

Table 12.1 Michigan alcoholism screening test (MAST)

Points		
	0. Do you enjoy a drink now and then?	Yes _____ No _____
(2)	1. Do you feel you are a normal drinker? (By normal we mean you drink less than or as much as most people)	Yes _____ No _____
(2)	2. Have you ever awakened the morning after some drinking the night before and found that you could not remember a part of the evening?	Yes _____ No _____
(1)	3. Does your wife, husband, a parent or other relative ever worry or complain about your drinking?	Yes _____ No _____
(2)	4. Can you stop drinking without a struggle after one or two drinks?[a]	Yes _____ No _____
(1)	5. Do you feel guilty about your drinking?	Yes _____ No _____
(2)	6. Do friends or relatives think you are a normal drinker?	Yes _____ No _____
(2)	7. Are you able to stop drinking when you want to?	Yes _____ No _____
(5)	8. Have you ever attended a meeting of Alcoholics Anonymous (AA)?	Yes _____ No _____
(1)	9. Have you gotten into physical fights while drinking?	Yes _____ No _____
(2)	10. Has drinking ever created problems between you and your wife, husband, a parent, or other relative?	Yes _____ No _____
(2)	11. Has your wife, husband (or other family members) ever gone to anyone for help about your drinking?	Yes _____ No _____
(2)	12. Have you ever lost friends because of your drinking?	Yes _____ No _____
(2)	13. Have you ever gotten into trouble at work because of drinking?	Yes _____ No _____
(2)	14. Have you ever lost a job because of drinking?	Yes _____ No _____
(2)	15. Have you ever neglected your obligations, your family, or your work for 2 or more days in a row because you were drinking?	Yes _____ No _____
(1)	16. Do you drink before noon fairly often?	Yes _____ No _____
(2)	17. Have you ever been told you have liver trouble? Cirrhosis?	Yes _____ No _____
(2)	18. After heavy drinking, have you ever had delirium tremens (DTs) or severe shaking, or heard voices, or seen things that really weren't there?[b]	Yes _____ No _____
(5)	19. Have you ever gone to anyone for help about your drinking?	Yes _____ No _____
(5)	20. Have you ever been in a hospital because of drinking?	Yes_____No_____
(2)	21. Have you ever been a patient in a psychiatric hospital or a psychiatric ward of a general hospital where drinking was part of the problem that resulted in hospitalization?	Yes_____No_____
(2)	22. Have you ever been seen at a psychiatric or mental health clinic or gone to any doctor, social worker, or clergyman for help with any emotional problem, where drinking was part of the problem?	Yes _____ No _____
(2)	23. Have you ever been arrested for drunk driving, driving while intoxicated, or driving under the influence of an alcoholic beverage?	Yes _____ No _____
(2)	24. Have you ever been arrested, or taken into custody, even for a few hours because of other drunk behavior? [c]	Yes _____No_____
	If YES, how many times?	

Scoring: [a]alcoholic response is negative; [b]5 points for the DTs; [c]2 points for each arrest. 5 points or more, alcoholism; 4 points, suggestive of alcoholism; 3 points or less, subject is not alcoholic.

The second learning theory principle, which is highly relevant to the dynamics and treatment of alcoholism, is the resistance to extinction of random patterns of reinforcement. If the pigeon pecking at the bar is reinforced with a food pellet the third time, the fortieth time, the forty-second time, the ninety-ninth time, and then not at all, the pigeon will go on pecking almost forever. Something very similar happens with alcoholics. Once their drinking was highly and fairly reliably reinforcing; this has long ceased to be the case. However, every once in a while the old magic is there, and the drinking is reinforced. Given this random pattern of reinforcement, it is perfectly rational to go on pecking the bar, or drinking *at* the bar, indefinitely, in the hope that there will be another reward. Participants in twelve-step meetings speak over and over about the euphoria of their first high. Twenty years later, they may still be searching for that euphoria, long since unavailable in a glass or bottle. This seems to be totally irrational and self-destructive behavior, but given the power of random (or, as it is technically called, "variable interval") intermittent reinforcement and its resistance to extinction, the behavior makes perfect sense. Escape behavior is also highly resistant to extinction. Alcohol provides cessation of pain, or escape from anxiety. This is indeed escape behavior and it is highly resistant to extinction. Even if drinking has long ceased to provide escape, the drinker goes on looking for it for a very long time. Both classical and operative conditioning play a role in the creation of "triggers" or "drink signals." Social learning theory teaches us the importance of cognitive elements in alcoholism. Beliefs, expectations, and attitudes profoundly affect the way in which people use alcohol. Modeling influences are highly potent. Perhaps that is one of the reasons that self-help groups work so well. They provide models of sustained, happy sobriety – models with which the members readily identify.

Empirical findings

There are a few consistent, well replicated findings about the clinical (male) alcoholic. Because alcoholism is a regressive process, it is not surprising that there is a high degree of commonality in psychological test scores of people in detox or rehab. This commonality consists of elevated psychopathic deviance score on the Minnesota multiphasic personality inventory (MMPI), field dependency on a variety of measures, low self-esteem and impoverished self-concepts, ego weakness, and stimulus augmentation (Ciarrocchi *et al.*, 1991).

The MMPI is a 550-item self-report. Subjects respond to each item by indicating if it is true of them. Subjects' responses to the items are reported as scores on 11 scales. The most consistent and frequently replicated MMPI finding with alcoholic populations is significant elevation of the psychopathic deviate (Pd) scale score. This finding goes back to Hewitt's (1943) study of an early AA group in Minneapolis. Subsequent MMPI studies (Morganstern *et al.*, 1997) of a wide variety of alcoholic populations have also reported elevated Pd. What does this mean? An examination of the Pd items reveals that a number of them refer to excessive drinking and others to situations likely to be associated with heavy drinking. Then are the elevated Pd findings trivial? Not necessarily. Later investigators (MacAndrew, 1965; MacAndrew & Geertsma, 1963) modified the Pd scale to eliminate these items, and the findings of elevated Pd held. The most reasonable interpretation of the elevated PD scores is that alcoholics tend to have a "devil-may-care" attitude. Interestingly, Pd scores fall, but not to the average range, with sobriety. It is the abnormal personality measure most resistant to change with continuing sobriety, psychotherapeutic treatment, and participation in AA. Furthermore, it is known that at least some pre-alcoholics show elevated Pd scores on the MMPI. The University of Minnesota once required entering freshmen to take the MMPI, and Loper *et al.*, (1973) back-checked the MMPIs of the University of Minnesota graduates admitted to the university hospital for treatment of alcoholism. These alcoholics showed significantly elevated Pd scores 13 years earlier when they were college freshmen. Thus, there is something extremely persistent and characteristic of (male) alcoholics that is measured by this scale. It is not known how much the presence of type 2 alcoholism accounts for the elevation of Pd scores. The Pd scores of female alcoholics are also elevated relative to non-alcoholic females, but neither their absolute scores nor the differential is as high as that of males. The Pd scale has been called the "anger" scale.

The other consistent MMPI finding is elevation in the depression (D) scale in alcoholics. Unlike elevated Pd, elevated depression does remit with sobriety. The pre-alcoholic University of Minnesota students scored high on the hypomanic (Ma), but not the depression scale; however, they had elevated scores on the depression scale when they were admitted to the hospital for treatment. This suggests that an acting-out hypomanic lifestyle may serve as a manic defense against an underlying depression.

Clinical alcoholics also manifest elevated scores on scale 7, psychasthenia (Pt), of the MMPI. The Pt scale is a measure of neuroticism indicative of high levels of anxiety, irrational fears, ruminative self-doubt, and self-devaluation. This finding is corroborated by the consistently high scores of alcoholics on the neuroticism scale of the Eysenck personality inventory (Cox, 1985). Alcoholics also score high on Zuckerman's (1979) sensation seeking scale, a finding that corroborates elevation on the Pd scale.

MacAndrew (1965) developed a scale that distinguishes alcoholics by determining to which MMPI items they responded differently. The MacAndrew alcoholism scale (MAC) accurately identifies 85% of male alcoholics. The MAC alcoholics are reward-seeking, bold, aggressive, impulsive, and hedonistic, sharing traits with high Pd scorers. The scale still works 40 years later.

MacAndrew also developed a scale that identifies the 15% of male alcoholics not identified by the MAC. He called them secondary alcoholics. They are tense, fearful, depressed punishment-avoiders. MacAndrew concluded that there are two types of male alcoholics: high-rolling, devil-take-the-hindmost, hell raisers, and depressed neurotics. This is consistent with other research.

The second important and consistent empirical psychological finding is that alcoholics tend to be field-dependent. Field dependence refers to the way a person organizes his or her perceptive field. The field-dependent person relies on the environment and on external cues, rather than on introceptive, internal cues, in orienting himself or herself in space. The field-dependent person experiences events globally and diffusely, with the surrounding field determining the way those events are organized. Since field dependency is associated with organic brain damage, this finding may be a consequence of prolonged heavy drinking rather than etiological.

Alcoholics have impoverished self-concepts. The self-concept is a person's conscious image of himself or herself. It is usually measured by some form of self-report.

One of the most illuminating self-concept studies is that of Conner (1962). His form of self-report was an adjective checklist. Active alcoholics studied early in treatment checked very few adjectives. Their self-concepts were impoverished and the adjectives they did check were neurotic traits such as "anxious." Their self-concepts were impoverished, depressed, and diffuse. When Conner tested a group of recovering alcoholics who had been sober for 3 years in AA, he found that their self-concepts were radically different. They checked many adjectives, demonstrating an enriched self-concept, and the reported neurotic traits radically diminished in recovery.

Many personality studies have found evidence of ego weakness in clinical alcoholics. Ego weakness is manifested by impulsivity, inability to delay gratification, low-affect tolerance, confused sense of identity, and lack of clear boundaries.

Another dimension of personality first elucidated and measured by Rotter (1966) is locus of control.

A self-report is used to determine if a subject sees himself or herself as controlling or being controlled by a situation. Those who see themselves as in control of themselves and their actions are said to have an internal locus of control. Active alcoholics tend toward an external locus of control.

The last consistent finding in alcoholic populations is stimulus augmentation. The concept of stimulus augmentation–stimulus attenuation was developed by Asenath Petrie (1978). She studied the way that subjects responded to the pressure of a wooden block pressed against their hands but out of their sight. It was found that the perception of the size of the block and the intensity of the pressure was an individual difference that ranged along a continuum from those who perceived the block as greatly magnified and the pressure as highly intense (stimulus augmenters) to those who perceived the block as smaller and the pressure as less than it was (stimulus attenuators). Alcoholics are stimulus augmenters. Petrie's findings have been confirmed (Volavka *et al.*, 1996) by recent EEG studies of evoke potentials. Because stimulus augmentation–stimulus attenuation is a relatively stable personal characteristic, there may be something constitutional in alcoholics that leads them to experience stimuli in a particularly intense way. This may help explain their lack of affect tolerance and their attraction to a "down" drug.

From a clinical perspective, what all this adds up to is that alcoholics far progressed in their disease and those in early recovery suffer from far more than hangnails and require strong therapeutic interventions sensitive to the issues, conflicts, and deficits spotlighted by these research findings.

Psychodynamic theories

Psychoanalysts have contributed a host of insights into the dynamics and treatment of alcoholism. There follows a highlight of those contributions.

Freud

In *Civilization and its Discontents*, Freud (1930) stated:

> The service rendered by intoxicating media in the struggle for happiness and in keeping misery at a distance is so highly prized as a benefit that individuals and peoples alike have given it an established place in the economics of the libido. We owe to such media not merely the immediate yield to pleasure, but also a greatly desired degree of independence from the external world. For one

knows that, with the help of this "drowner of cares," one can at any time withdraw from the pressure of reality and find refuge in a world of one's own with better conditions of sensibility [p. 78].

Freud (1985) also postulated that all later addictions are displacements of and re-enactments of the original addiction to masturbation. This is a dynamic that highlights the dead-end nature of addiction, its compulsive repetition, the guilt and shame that accompany the failure to follow through on the resolve, originally not to masturbate, later not to use, a failure that is driven by withdrawal into a world of fantasy and narcissistic pleasure. Many alcoholics describe themselves as "doing nothing but jerking off," and this can be put to use clinically. In his essay on *Dostoevsky and Parricide,* Freud (1928) analyzes Dostoevsky's compulsive gambling as a displacement of his conflict about masturbation. He points out that Dostoevsky's violent, alcoholic father was murdered by his peasants, enacting Dostoevsky's unconscious wish to kill that father, and that the enactment in reality of the fantasy inculcated guilt – overwhelming guilt – in Dostoevsky. This analysis allows Freud to focus on the pay-off in Dostoevsky's compulsive gambling, namely losing. The pleasure is in the pain. Addictions, including alcoholism, offer one a rare opportunity to express aggression and be punished for it simultaneously. This is an extraordinarily powerful hook.

In *Beyond the Pleasure Principle,* Freud (1920) speaks of the repetition compulsion as a manifestation of the death instinct. He uses addiction as one of his examples of the repetition compulsion. The centrality of guilt and the use of substance abuse for self-punishment is highly salient, and its interpretation is often mutative in treating substance abusers, including alcoholics.

Glover

Edward Glover (1928) emphasized not the pleasure of self-punishment, but the aggression inherent in some alcohol abuse. This is drinking *at* someone – the "fuck you martini" as an infantile expression of rage.

Rado

Sandor Rado (1933) captured the tragic trap of alcoholism. He spoke of a state of tense depression, a sort of agitated depression that is felt to be intolerable, and its concomitant feelings of worthlessness and low self-esteem. The alcohol is then taken for its euphoric properties. The drinker goes from tense depression to manic joy. In that manic joy, the constraints of reality are obliterated. So far, so good. Unfortunately, it cannot be sustained and there is the crash, returning the nascent alcoholic to an even tenser and deeper depression. The claims of reality come back in spades, necessitating another round of drinking. But it is less effective this time, and the manic or euphoric state is briefer and more tenuous, necessitating yet more drinking until there is almost no euphoria and almost continuous bleak and black depression. In his elucidation of this cycle, Rado noted the similarity between alcohol addiction and manic depression. Rado also underlines the highly salient centrality of self-esteem in the entire process.

Fenichel

Otto Fenichel (1945) noted the narcissistic regression concomitant with addictive drinking, and AA, with no debt to Fenichel, makes the amelioration of that regression central to its "treatment strategy." As Bill Wilson, co-founder, said, "Alcoholism is self-will run riot" (Alcoholics Anonymous World Services, 1952, p. 37).

Menninger

There is no question but that alcoholic drinking eventuates in self-destruction. The question is, "Is that self-destruction motivated or is it an unintended consequence of the addictive process?" In a no-longer fashionable formulation, Karl Menninger (1938) described alcoholism as "chronic suicide." Edward Khantzian (1981; 1999) is the counterpoint to this darker side of psychoanalytic formulations.

Khantzian

Edward Khantzian is the author of the self-medication hypothesis, the notion that people use alcohol to remediate ego deficits and developmental arrest. In his view, the taking of the substance is an initially adaptive attempt to cope with a deficit state. He sees these deficits as involving both ego and self. Although these deficits encompass many areas of functioning and self-regulation, they are primarily deficits in the area of self-care, affect regulation, self-esteem, and a subjective sense of wellbeing. The self-medication hypothesis has also been called the prosthetic theory of alcohol use and abuse. Khantzian is very clear that the motivation, conscious or unconscious, driving substance abuse is the attempt to relieve suffering, not to destroy the self.

Khantzian's view is of the utmost clinical saliency. If the therapist does not recognize, as one of the most central dynamics of addiction, the adaptive nature of alcohol use and the attempt at self-cure through that use, there is no way in which the alcoholic or drug addict will feel understood. Nevertheless, my clinical experience is that self-punishment, especially self-punishment for the addictive behavior itself, is not infrequent.

AA's twelve steps of recovery provide mechanisms to attenuate guilt and prevent self-hatred and the need for self-punishment, leading to relapse. Freud's insight (1926) that the hardest resistance to overcome is the resistance from the superego that tells the patient that he or she doesn't deserve to be well comes to mind. Although Khantzian's self-medication hypothesis is enormously useful, both as explanation and as guiding clinical intervention, Menninger was onto something too. At any rate, whether the guilt and self-hatred were antecedent to the alcoholism which served as a self-punisher from the beginning or is consequential to it, the clinician must still deal with it.

Krystal and Raskin

Krystal and Raskin (1970), building on their theory of affect development from a preverbal, somatized, undifferentiated stage to an articulated, de-somatized, verbal stage, postulated that in the course of addiction, affect regression occurs and that treatment needs to reverse the process. Developmentally, we have to be taught to recognize and label feelings. Many alcoholics have grown up in highly dysfunctional alcoholic homes where such learning was less than optimal, making affect regression, often to a state of virtual alexithymia, all too likely as the addictive drinking progresses. Clinically, this means that the therapist needs to identify and label feelings. This is one of the most helpful interventions of early recovery.

Hans Kohut

Hans Kohut (1977) has an elaborate developmental scheme, discussion of which is beyond the scope of this chapter. However, his insight that addiction, including alcoholism, is driven by a futile attempt to remediate self and ego deficits, a process he compares to trying to cure a gastric fistula by eating, is right on the money. In his terms, this is a consequence of regression/fixation to the state of the archaic self. Kohut also points out that alcoholics form idealizing and mirror transferences to alcohol. That is, their magical expectation is that alcohol is a powerful parent that will fulfil their every wish and affirm the splendor of the self. Of course, alcohol cannot do this and a vicious cycle ensues. The empirical psychological findings discussed above are characteristics of Kohut's stage of the archaic self and lend support to the saliency of his conceptualization of the psychic concomitant of alcohol addiction. I have developed (Levin, 1987; 1995; 1999) a set of suggested interventions based on both clinical experience and Kohut's model. They are the following.

1. This intervention addresses the narcissistic wound inflicted by not being able to drink "like other people." The admission that one is powerless over alcohol, as twelve-step programs put it, or that one cannot use without the possibility of losing control, as I would put it, is extremely painful. It is experienced as a defect in the self, which is intolerable. The self must not be so damaged. The therapist must recognize and articulate the conflict between the patient's wish to stop using and the patient's feeling that to do so entails admitting that he or she is flawed in a fundamental way: "You don't so much want to use, as not want not to be able to use," is a formulation that can be "heard" by the alcoholic patient.

2. Alcoholism is one long experience in narcissistic injury. Failure stalks the alcoholic like a shadow. As one of my patients put it, "When I drink everything turns to shit." Even if the outward blows have not yet come, the inner blows – self-hatred and low self-regard – are there. The therapist must empathize with the suffering. "Your disease has cost you so much," "You've lost so much," and "Your self-respect is gone" are some ways to make contact with the alcoholic's pain and facilitate experiencing it instead of denying, acting out, or anesthetizing it.

3. Alcoholics feel empty. Either they never had much good stuff inside or they have long ago flushed out the good stuff with alcohol. "You drink so much because you feel empty" makes the connection and brings into awareness the horrible feelings of an inner void.

4. Alcoholics lack a firm sense of identity. How can you know who you are if your experience of self is tenuous and lacks consistent cohesion? The therapist can comment on this and point out that

being an alcoholic is at least something definite. When AA members say, "My name is _____, and I am an alcoholic," they are affirming that they exist and have at least that one attribute. The manifest purpose of such identification is to deal with denial. But the latent meaning is existential. Not being sure of their very existence, alcoholics need to assert it. One way of conveying this to the patient is to say, "You're confused, and not quite sure who you are. That is partly because of your drinking. Acknowledging your alcoholism will lessen your confusion as to who you are, and give you a base on which to build a firm and positive identity."

5. Many people use alcohol because they cannot stand to be alone. This should be interpreted: "You drink so much because you can't bear to be alone, and getting high gives you the illusion of having company, of being with a friend."

6. Alcoholics form transferences to alcohol. The image of the archaic, idealized parent is projected onto the drink and it is regarded as an all-powerful, all-good object with which the drinker merges in order to participate in this omnipotence. "Martinis will deliver the goods and give me love, power, and whatever else I desire" is the drinker's unconscious fantasy. The therapist should interpret this: "Alcohol feels like a good, wise, and powerful parent who protects you and makes you feel wonderful, and that is why you love it so much. In reality, it is a depressant drug, not all the things you thought it was."

7. One of the reasons that drinkers are devoted to drinking is that it confirms their grandiosity. The therapist should make this conscious: "When you drink, you feel you can do anything, be anything, achieve anything, and that feels wonderful. No wonder you don't want to give it up."

8. Alcoholics have low self-esteem no matter how well covered over by bravado. At some point the therapist needs to say: "You feel like shit, and think that you are shit, and all your claims to greatness are ways to avoid knowing that you feel that way." The reasons, both antecedent and consequent to the addiction, that the patient values himself or herself so little need to be elucidated and worked through.

9. Many drinkers have a pathological need for omnipotent control. The drink is simultaneously experienced as an object they believe they can totally control and coerce into doing their will, and an object they believe gives them total control of their subjective states and of the environment. Alcoholics frequently treat people, including the therapist, as extensions of themselves. The twelve-step slogans, "Get out of the driver's seat" and "Let go and let God," are cognitive behavioral ways of loosening the need to control. Therapists should interpret this need to control in the patient's relationship to the alcohol, to other people, and to the therapist. For example, "You think that when you drink you can feel any way you wish." "You go into a rage and get high whenever your wife doesn't do what you want." "You thought of drinking because you were upset with me when I didn't respond as you thought I should."

10. Alcoholics suffer greatly from shame experiences. They are ashamed of having been shamed, and often drink to obliviate feelings of shame. Therapists need to help these patients experience, rather than repress, their feelings of shame now that they no longer anesthetize them, by saying, for example, "You felt so much shame when you realized you were an alcoholic that you kept on drinking so you wouldn't feel the shame."

Carl Jung

Carl Jung (1973) famously opined that alcoholism is a case of *spiritus contra spiritum*, spirits against the spiritual, and that the cure was necessarily spiritual in nature. Jung thought that "hitting bottom," a state of deep despair, akin to the mystic's dark night of the soul, was a required prolegomena to recovery. AA made Jung's formulation central to its teaching, and the psychoanalyst rabbi, Abe Twersky (1998), teaches that "addiction is a spiritual deficiency disease." They are onto something. Among the things lost in alcoholic regression are values, beliefs, and sustainable ideals, and their rediscovery or reformulation does seem to be of the essence of recovery.

Existential factors

These existential factors are a vital part of the alcoholic dynamic. At the end of the addictive process life is indeed "a tale told by an idiot, full of sound and fury, signifying nothing." And this loss of meaning, however unconscious, is intolerably painful. It needs to be introduced into the therapy, if not by the patient, then by the therapist. Erik Erikson tells us that "final integrity" (1968, p. 139) entails "the acceptance of the one and only life that has been possible." A developmental task imperfectly achieved by most, but seemingly completely out of reach for those, like many alcoholic patients, whose life has been importantly characterized by destroyed opportunity and by injury to self and others. This too must be addressed. As must mortality.

Alcoholics enact an unconscious drama of death and resurrection when they drink themselves into oblivion only to wake, however hungover, alive. This enactment provides an illusion of immortality. Ironically, this very same enactment of reassurance does the opposite of conveying immortality as it slowly, but inexorably, kills. The flight from death hastens it. Given that all patients in sustained psychotherapy harbor the unconscious belief/fantasy that the therapist will make them immortal, and I believe they do, there is a particularly rich matrix for psychotherapeutic work around existential issues including one's mortality in work with alcoholics. They have been swimmers at the deep end of the pool for a long time and the therapist needs to be willing to go there too.

Treatment

Alcoholism is a complex disorder affecting body, mind, and spirit, as well as relationships, family, and the workplace (if any). That argues for a multimodal approach and, indeed, that is usually the most efficacious form of treatment. It is helpful to think in terms of a treatment decision tree. Does the patient need detoxification? Inpatient rehabilitation? Individual therapy? Group therapy? Family therapy? Is the patient a good candidate for participation in AA or another twelve-step program? Most often the patient will require, or at least can profitably make use of, more than one of these modalities. How to sequence these interventions is another question that needs to be answered. And what is the treatment goal: abstinence or least harm? Is the patient likely to do better with a cognitive approach? A dynamic one? Or would DBT (dialectical behavior therapy) be helpful? What about medical and psychiatric issues? Are they being addressed? To come up with an optimal treatment plan, a first step is an in-depth assessment. Then, depending on the patient's needs and the physician's treatment philosophy, a plan can be actualized. If at all possible, the alcoholic should participate in that planning.

Alcoholics Anonymous

Alcoholics Anonymous participation is part of most treatments. The therapist can and should learn more about "The Program" by reading AA literature and attending "open" meetings. The more concurrent psychopathology present, the less likely that AA will "work." AA is not for every alcoholic and should not be mindlessly insisted upon. Professional help and self-help are not antithetical, and if the therapist is feeling competitive with the "program," there is a countertransference problem that needs to be worked through.

Change theory

Stages of change theory can be helpful in treatment planning. It was developed by Prochaska et al. (1992). They conceptualize change as taking place in five stages: precontemplation, contemplation, preparation, action, and maintenance. In the first stage, the pleasurable effects of drinking predominate and the drinker isn't even entertaining the thought of quitting. After all, he is without pain. Expectancies play a role here. Thus, if hangovers are accepted as "part of the game," their onset will not lead to change.

In the next stage, contemplation, the aversive consequences have become too insistent to be completely ignored and the thought of stopping is now allowed to enter into consciousness. No action is yet actually contemplated, but it is at least a possibility. In the contemplative stage, the pleasure:pain ratio has changed and there is intense ambivalence. The therapist needs to acknowledge and reflect back the patient's ambivalence and minimize countertransferential frustration by understanding where the patient is at.

In the preparation stage, the patient actually considers a concrete plan of action. Then, finally, the action stage is reached and change occurs. Unlike the AA model, which tends to envision "hitting bottom" and "surrender" as sudden moments of illumination, the stage of change model sees a long developmental process preceding eventual action. Prochaska et al. stressed that the action stage involves more than stopping drinking and that action must include changes that help maintain sobriety such as a change in peer group, attitude, and expectancies. The change process ends in the maintenance stage, where the emphasis is on relapse prevention.

Table 12.2 Alcoholics Anonymous twelve questions

1. Have you ever decided to stop drinking for a week or so, but only lasted for a couple of days? Yes _____ No _____

2. Do you wish people would mind their own business about your drinking – stop telling you what to do? Yes _____ No _____

3. Have you ever switched from one kind of drink to another in the hope that this would keep you from getting drunk? Yes _____ No _____

4. Have you ever had an eye-opener upon awakening during the past year? Yes _____ No _____

5. Do you envy people who can drink without getting into trouble? Yes _____ No _____

6. Have you had problems connected with your drinking during the past year? Yes _____ No _____

7. Has your drinking caused trouble at home? Yes _____ No _____

8. Do you ever try to get "extra" drinks at a party because you do not get enough? Yes _____ No _____

9. Do you tell yourself you can stop drinking any time you want to even though you keep getting drunk when you don't mean to? Yes _____ No _____

10. Have you missed days of work or school because of drinking? Yes _____ No _____

11. Do you have "blackouts"? Yes _____ No _____

12. Have you ever felt that your life would be better if you did not drink? Yes _____ No _____

If you answered YES to four or more questions, you are probably in trouble with alcohol.

The questions, from *Is AA for you?*, are reprinted with permission from Alcoholics Anonymous World Services, Inc.. Use of this material does not imply affiliation with AA.

A therapeutic model

My own model envisions treatment as a three-stage process: confrontation; teaching coping skills and recognition of drink signals; and, finally, working through underlying conflicts and remediating underlying deficits.

Of course, diagnosis precedes confrontation. In that confrontation the therapist needs to be on the side of reality, not on the side of the punitive superego that alcoholics too easily project onto therapists. Confrontation needs to be firm, persistent, and non-judgmental. This stage of treatment is didactic and directive and may involve explaining alcoholism and the disease model. The more evidence the therapist can muster and present non-threateningly, the better. It is important to avoid being drawn into a debate or a discussion with the patient, who may be all too ready to turn the session in that direction.

The next stage is a cognitive behavioral one. The alcoholic patient has long forgotten whatever coping skills he or she possessed before using alcohol as a ubiquitous coper. A strenuous process of (re)education is indicated. A vital part of the work is making drink signals conscious before they are acted out and helping the patient find alternatives to drinking in response to them. For example, if the therapy has revealed that Friday night is a powerful trigger, alternative modes of celebration and relaxation can be suggested. Avocational activities are lost along with everything else during the progression of alcoholism. Internal triggers like fear and sadness must also be identified. Here the therapy itself may be the alternative coping strategy.

The final stage of treatment is a dynamic one aimed at working through underlying conflicts and remediating deficits long self-medicated. Not all recovering alcoholics choose to participate in third stage treatment; however, termination during the "pink cloud" period of early recovery is not uncommonly followed by a return for more dynamic work. In my experience, this most frequently occurs somewhere around 2 years into recovery.

A case example

George, who came for therapy because he was depressed, casually mentioned that he sometimes drank too much, then angrily closed off discussion of the topic when I tried to explore it. He had plenty to be depressed about. A once-successful composer, he hadn't had a commission for years, his marriage was lifeless, and his often abrasive, sometimes explosive, style of interpersonal relating had left him isolated. It turned out that his "explosions" were invariably associated with drinking, but it took a long time to uncover this as George tenaciously protected his most important remaining "friendship," that with alcohol.

His childhood had many bizarre elements, with a highly seductive, radically inappropriate, mother who enlisted George's assistance in her frequent douching, and a withdrawn, ineffectual father who managed not to see the many prolonged affairs his wife openly engaged in, not to mention being blind to her aberrant relationship with her son. Their economic situation was marginal. George was deeply resentful and contemptuous of his highly conventional, "upright," yet ultimately successful brother, who in turn denigrated George's bohemian life as he extolled his own corporate lifestyle. George's talent, early recognized, provided a ladder that took him out of the family morass. There was a series of scholarships, awards, and eventually a splash in the classical music scene. George's career seemed assured. His family, for all its neurotic tensions, encouraged and supported his talent. He had been traditionally trained and had real ability as a tonal composer. In fact, he had even made a few bucks orchestrating movie scores, but he considered this beneath him. His "real" work was 12-tone serialism. He later conceded that he turned away from the tonal because he couldn't come close to producing work of the quality of the Romantic masters he so deeply admired, even revered. His grandiosity was destroying him by not allowing him to do work that he could market. But the most profound reason he turned away from the tonal was that he unconsciously feared depicting and evoking the emotional horrors of his childhood. Further, his style was so tightly geometrical that, however brilliantly executed, it allowed for virtually no emotional force or content to manifest itself. George railed against the philistine imbeciles who did the programming and gave out the recording contracts, as he quoted Dorothy Parker (who died of alcoholism) to the effect that, "Euclid alone looked on beauty bare." No John Cage-style spontaneity for him. He feared the "explosion," not so unconsciously associated with the discharge of his mother's erotic douches he overheard as a child, not to mention the explosiveness of his own rage. George's brother wasn't the only "uptight" sibling.

George's style had once been fashionable and he had a certain cachet, but the wheel turned and his work had long been "out." But the "real" reason that his career had collapsed was his drinking. He had fought with virtually everyone of significance in the music world, alienating conductors, critics, and patrons. And always when drunk. His personal life was as chaotic as his work was rigid. As talented as he was and as capable, technically anyway, of modifying his compositional approach, few were now willing to put up with his demeaning, insulting, drunken tirades.

Like all alcoholics, George defended his drinking, rationalizing it as intrinsic to his creativity. After all, hadn't Beethoven and Moussorgsky drunk heavily? I countered with, "Yes, but Moussorgsky died in the DTs." Fortunately, George, for all his defensiveness, was as honest as he was able to be, and within a few months of therapy I had more than ample material for a confrontation. He gave me an opening when he related being "eighty-sixed," (i.e. thrown out of his favorite bar and told not to come back) and I took advantage of it. I used all the evidence I had and, surprisingly, it worked. With the exception of a few brief slips, George hasn't drunk since. Denial is never absolute and somewhere George had long known that he had to stop. Rejection by his sole remaining social support, the crowd at his "favorite place," was George's bottom.

George's depression was both cause and consequence of his drinking, as was his rage. His narcissistic regression and reactive grandiosity were right there on the surface and could not have been more apparent. I gently confronted him with this. As tempting for a therapist as all of the rich material he presented was, nothing useful could be accomplished until his alcoholism was arrested. Over and over again I connected his misery with his drinking, empathizing with his futile attempt at self-medication, and suggesting that repair of ruptured relationships was not impossible. After all, he operated in the world where difficult people were often tolerated and this did not seem an unrealistic hope.

The second stage, teaching alternative coping strategies, was vital, as George had few of these. One of the most helpful turned out to be physical. This pathetically tense, tight-as-a-drum, man got into jogging and mountain climbing and it was enormously helpful. I told him, "Whenever you feel uptight, just run," and he did. As he remained sober his love for literature re-entered his life and that helped too. Booze was replaced by Bellow and Beckett. As time went on, George became more attuned to internal signals of anger, despair, and sorrow, and became able to mourn them rather than anesthetize or act them out. The dynamic stage had begun and the work continues.

References

Alcoholics Anonymous World Services (1952). *Twelve Steps and Twelve Traditions.* New York: American Psychiatric Association.

Barnes, G. E. (1979). The alcoholic personality: a reanalysis of the literature. *Journal of Studies on Alcohol*, **40**, 571–634.

Barnes, G. E. (1983). Clinical and prealcoholic personality characteristics. In *The Biology of Alcoholism*: Vol. **6**. *The Pathogenesis of Alcoholism: Psychosocial Factors*, eds. B. Kissin & H. Begleiter. New York: Plenum, pp. 113–96.

Biederman, J., Wilens, T., Mick, E., Faraone, S. V. & Spencer, T. (1998). Does attention-deficit hyperactivity disorder impact the developmental course of drug and alcohol abuse and dependence? *Biological Psychiatry*, **44**(4), 269–73.

Blane, H. T. & Leonard, K. E. (eds.) (1987). *Psychological Theories of Drinking and Alcoholism.* New York: Guilford.

Bleuler, M. (1955). Familial and personal background of chronic alcoholics. In *Etiology of Chronic Alcoholism*, ed. O. Drethem. Springfield, IL: Charles C. Thomas, pp. 110–66.

Brady, K. T., Grice, D. E., Dustan, L. & Randall, C. (1993). Gender differences in substance use disorders. *American Journal of Psychiatry*, **150**, 1707–11.

Cadoret, R. J., O'Gorman, T. W., Troughton, E. & Heywood, L. (1984). Alcoholism and anti-social personality: interrelationships, genetic and environmental factors. *Archives of General Psychiatry*, **42**, 161–7.

Cadoret, R. J., Troughton, E., O'Gorman, T. W. & Heywood, E. (1986). An adoption study of genetic and environmental factors in drug abuse. *Archives of General Psychiatry*, **43**, 1131–6.

Cadoret, R. J., Yates, W. R., Troughton, E., Woodworth, G. & Stewart, M. A. (1995). Adoption study demonstrating two genetic pathways to drug abuse. *Archives of General Psychiatry*, **52**, 42–52.

Ciarrocchi, J. W., Kirschner, N. M. & Falik, F. (1991). Personality dimensions of male pathological gamblers, alcoholics, and dually addicted gamblers. *Journal of Gambling Studies*, **7**, 133–44.

Clark, W. B. & Cahalan, D. (1976). Changes in problem drinking over a four-year span. *Addictive Behaviors*, **1**, 251–9.

Cloninger, C. R. (1983). Genetic and environmental factors in the development of alcoholism. *Journal of Psychiatric Treatment and Evaluation*, **5**, 487–96.

Cloninger, C. R., Bohman, M. & Sigvardsson, S. (1981). Cross-fostering analysis of adopted men. *Archives of General Psychiatry*, **36**, 861–8.

Conner, R. (1962). The self-concepts of alcoholics. In *Society, Culture and Drinking Patterns*, eds. D. Pittman & C. Snyder. Carbondale: Southern Illinois University Press, pp. 455–67.

Cox, W. M. (1985). Personality correlatives of substance abuse. In *Determinants of Substance Abuse: Biological, Psychological, and Environmental Factors*, eds. M. Galizio & S. A. Mausto. New York: Plenum, pp. 209–46.

Erikson, E. (1968). *Identity, Youth and Crisis.* New York: Norton.

Fenichel, O. (1945). *The Psychoanalytic Theory of Neurosis.* New York: Norton.

Fingarette, H. (1988). *Heavy Drinking: The Myth of Alcoholism as a Disease.* Berkeley: University of California Press.

Freud, S. (1920). Beyond the pleasure principle. *Standard Edition*, **18**, 1–64.

Freud, S. (1926). Inhibitions, symptoms, and anxiety. *Standard Edition*, **20**, 87–175.

Freud, S. (1928). Dostoevsky and parricide. *Standard Edition*, **21**, 173–94.

Freud, S. (1930). Civilization and its discontents. *Standard Edition*, **21**, 64–148.

Freud, S. (1985). *The Complete Letters of Sigmund Freud to Wilhelm Fliess.* J. M. Mason, ed. and translator). Cambridge, MA: Harvard University Press, 1897.

Glover, E. (1928). The etiology of alcoholism. *Proceedings of the Royal Society of Medicine*, **21**, 1351–5.

Goodwin, D. W. & Warnock, J. K. (1991). Alcoholism: a family disease. In *Clinical Textbook of Addictive Disorders*, eds. R. J. Frances & S. I. Miller. New York: Guilford, pp. 486–500.

Goodwin, D. W., Schulsinger, F., Hermansen, L., Guze, S. B. & Winokur, G. (1973). Alcohol problems in adoptees raised apart from alcoholic biological parents. *Archives of General Psychiatry*, **28**, 283–343.

Hallowell, E. & Ratey, J. J. (1995). *Understanding Attention Deficit Disorder and Addiction: Workbook.* Center City, MN: Hazelden.

Hewitt, C. C. (1943). A personality study of alcohol addiction. *Quarterly Journal of Studies on Alcohol*, **4**, 368–86.

Jellinek, E. M. (1952). Phases of alcohol addiction. *Quarterly Journal of Studies on Alcohol*, **13**, 673–84.

Jellinek, E. M. (1960). *The Disease Concept of Alcoholism.* New Haven, CT: College and University Press.

Jung, C. G. (1973). In *C.G. Jung: Letters, Vol. II, 1951–1961*, ed. G. Adler. Princeton, NJ: Princeton University Press, pp. 623–5.

Kaij, L. (1960). *Alcoholism in Twins: Studies on the Etiology and Sequels of Abuse of Alcohol*. Stockholm: Almquist & Wiksell.

Khantzian, E. J. (1981). Some treatment implications of ego and self-disturbances in alcoholism. In *Dynamic Approaches to the Understanding and Treatment of Alcoholism*, eds. M. H. Bean & N. E. Zinberg. New York: Free Press, pp. 163–88.

Khantzian, E. J. (1999). *Addiction as a Human Process*. Northvale, NJ: Jason Aronson.

Knight, R. P. (1937). The dynamics and treatment of chronic alcohol addiction. *Bulletin of the Menninger Clinic*, **1**, 233–50.

Kohut, H. (1977). *Psychodynamics of Drug Dependence (National Institute on Drug Abuse Monograph 12, pp. vii–ix)*. Washington, DC: US Government Printing Office.

Krystal, H. & Raskin, H. (1970). *Drug Dependence: Aspects of Ego Function*. Detroit: Wayne State University Press.

Levin, J. D. (1987). *Treatment of Alcoholism and Other Addictions: A Self-psychology Approach*. Northvale, NJ: Jason Aronson.

Levin, J. D. (1995). *Introduction to Alcoholism Counseling: A Biopsychosocial Approach*, 2nd edn. Washington, DC: Taylor & Francis.

Levin, J. D. (1999). *Therapeutic Strategies for Treating Addiction*. Northvale, NJ: Jason Aronson.

Levin, J. D. & Weiss, R. H. (eds.) (1994). *The Dynamics and Treatment of Alcoholism: Essential Papers*. Northvale, NJ: Jason Aronson.

Loper, R. G., Kammeier, M. L. & Hofmann, H. (1973). MMPI characteristics of college freshmen males who later became alcoholics. *Journal of Abnormal Psychology*, **82**, 159–62.

MacAndrew, C. (1965). The differentiation of male alcoholic outpatients from non-alcoholic outpatients by means of the MMPI. *Quarterly Journal of Studies on Alcohol*, **26**, 238–46.

MacAndrew, C. & Edgerton, R. B. (1969). *Drunken Comportment*. Chicago: Aldine.

MacAndrew, C. & Geertsma, R. H. (1963). Analysis of responses of alcoholics to Scale 4 of the MMPI. *Quarterly Journal of Studies on Alcohol*, **26**, 23–38.

Marlatt, G. A. & Gordon, J. R. (1985). *Relapse Prevention: Maintenance Strategies in the Treatment of Addictive Behaviors*. New York: Guilford.

McClelland, D. C., Davis, W., Kalin, R. & Wanner, E. (1972). *The Drinking Man: Alcohol and Human Motivation*. New York: Free Press.

McCord, W. & McCord, J., with Gudeman, J.(1960). *Origins of Alcoholism*. Stanford, CA: Stanford University Press.

McCord, W. & McCord, J. (1960). A longitudinal study of the personality of alcoholics. In *Society, Culture and Drinking Patterns*, eds. D. J. Pittman & C. R. Snyder. Carbondale: Southern Illinois University Press, pp. 413–30.

Mello, N. K. & Mendelson, J. H. (1972). Experimentally induced intoxication in alcoholics: a comparison between programmed and spontaneous drinking. *Journal of Pharmacology and Experimental Therapeutics*, **173**, 101–16.

Menninger, K. (1938). *Man Against Himself*. New York: Harcourt Brace.

Morganstern, J., Langenbucher, J., Labouvie, E. & Miller, K. J. (1997). The comorbidity of alcoholism and personality disorders in a clinical population: prevalence rates and relation to alcohol typology variables. *Journal of Abnormal Psychology*, **106**, 74–84.

National Institute on Alcohol Abuse and Alcoholism. (1990). *Seventh special report to the U.S. Congress on alcohol and health from the Secretary of Health and Human Services* (DHHS Publication No. 90–16556). Rockville, MD: Washington DC, US Government.

Nephew, T. M., Williams, G. D., Yi, H. *et al.* (2003, September). *Surveillance report #59: Apparent per capita alcohol consumption: National, state, and regional trends, 1977–2000*. Rockville, MD: NIAAA Division of Biometry and Epidemiology, Alcohol Epidemiologic Data System.

Nephew, T. M., Yi, H., Williams, G. D., Stinson, F. S. & Dufour, M. C. (2004, June). *Alcohol epidemiological data reference manual, Vol. 1, 4th edn, US apparent consumption of alcoholic beverages based on state sales, taxation, or receipt data*. (NIH Publication No. 04–5563). Bethesda, MD: National Institutes of Health, National Institute on Alcohol Abuse and Alcoholism, Alcohol Epidemiologic Data System.

Newlin, D. B. & Thomson, J. B. (1990). Alcohol challenge with sons of alcoholics: a critical review and analysis. *Psychological Bulletin*, **108**, 383–402.

Park, P. (1973). Developmental ordering of experiences in alcoholism. *Quarterly Journal of Studies on Alcohol*, **34**, 473–88.

Petrie, A. (1978). *Individuality in Pain and Suffering*, 2nd edn. Chicago: University of Chicago Press.

Pittman, D. & White, R. H. (eds.) (1991). *Society, Culture and Drinking Patterns Reexamined*. New Brunswick, NJ: Rutgers Center for Alcohol Studies.

Pitts, F. N. Jr. & Winokur, G. (1966). Affective disorder – VII: alcoholism and affective disorder. *Journal of Psychiatric Research*, **4**, 37–50.

Polich, J., Armor, D. & Brainer, H. (1981). *The Course of Alcoholism*. New York: Wiley.

Pollock, V. E., Volavka, J., Goodwin, D. W. *et al.* (1983). The EEG after alcohol administration in men at risk of alcoholism. *Archives of General Psychiatry*, **40**, 857–61.

Prochaska, J. V., DiClemente, C. C. & Norcross, J. C. (1992). In search of how people change: applications to addictive behaviors. *American Psychologist*, **47**, 1102–14.

Rado, S. (1933). The psychoanalysis of pharmacothymia. *Psychoanalytic Quarterly*, **2**, 2–3.

Roe, A. (1945). The adult adjustment of children of alcoholic parents raised in foster homes. *Quarterly Journal of Studies on Alcoholism*, **5**, 378–93.

Rooney, J. F. (1991). Patterns of alcohol use in Spanish society. In *Society, Culture, and Drinking Patterns Reexamined*, eds. D. Pittman & H. R. White. New Brunswick, NJ: Rutgers Center of Alcohol Studies, pp. 78–86.

Rotter, J. B. (1966). Generalized expectancies for internal versus external control of reinforcement. *Psychological Monographs*, **80**(1), 1–28.

Rush, B. (1994). An inquiry into the effects of ardent spirits upon the human body and mind. In *The Dynamics and Treatment of Alcoholism: Essential Papers*, eds. J. Levin & R. Weiss. Northvale, NJ: Jason Aronson, pp. 11–27.

Selzer, M. (1971). The Michigan alcoholism screening test: the quest for a new diagnostic instrument. *American Journal of Psychiatry*, **127**, 1653–8.

Substance Abuse and Mental Health Administration Services. (2006). *National Survey on Drug Use and Health.* Washington, DC: US Government.

Tarter, R. E. (1981). Minimal brain dysfunction as an etiological disposition to alcoholism. In *Evaluation of the Alcoholic: Implications for Research, Theory and Treatment (NIAAA Monograph Series)*, ed. R. E. Meyer. Washington, DC: National Institute on Alcohol Abuse and Alcoholism.

Tarter, R. E. & Alterman, A. I. (1989). Neurobehavioral theory of alcoholism etiology. In *Theories of Alcoholism*, eds. C. D. Choudron & D. A. Wilkinson. Toronto: Addiction Research Foundation.

Twersky, A. (1998). *Talk on Spirituality and Addiction.* New York: New School for Social Research.

Vaillant, G. E. (1983). *The Natural History of Alcoholism: Causes, Patterns and Paths to Recovery.* Cambridge, MA: Harvard University Press.

Volavka, J., Czobor, P., Goodwin, D. W. *et al.* (1990). The electroencephalogram after alcohol administration in high-risk men and the development of alcohol use disorders 10 years later: preliminary findings. *Archives of General Psychiatry*, **53**, 258–63.

Winokur, G., Rimmer, J. & Reich, T. (1971). Alcoholism IV: is there more than one type of alcoholism? *British Journal of Psychiatry*, **18**, 525–31.

Wurmser, L. (1978). *The Hidden Dimension: Psychodynamics in Compulsive Drug Use.* New York: Jason Aronson.

Zucker, R. A. & Gomberg, E. S. L. (1986). Etiology of alcoholism reconsidered: the case for a biopsychosocial process. *American Psychologist*, **41**, 783–93.

Zuckerman, M. (1979). *Sensation Seeking: Beyond the Optimal Level of Arousal.* New York: Wiley.

Real World

Alcoholism in primary care

Mack Lipkin, Andrea Truncali & Joshua D. Lee

PORTER: Faith, sir, we were carousing till the second cock, and drink, sir, is a great provoker of three things.

MACDUFF: What three things does drink especially provoke?

PORTER: Marry, sir, nose-painting, sleep and urine. Lechery, sir, it provokes and unprovokes: it provokes the desire but it takes away the performance. *Therefore much drink may be said to be an equivocator with lechery: it makes him and it mars him; it sets him on and it takes him off.* –

Macbeth (Act 2 Scene 3): William Shakespeare

Shakespeare said what needs saying. *Equivocal* is the central reality about alcoholism in primary care. Consider these primary care truisms and attitudes we hear stated often in teaching about this subject:

Alcohol is protective; there is a J shaped curve, so you live longer if you have a drink a day and shorter if you have none or three. Alcohol is a major cause of deteriorating disease, of the liver, the blood system, the nerves, the brain, social function, and psychological well-being. It is a man's disorder – women worry, men drink. As a co-morbidity, it makes everything worse. Don't treat the other stuff until the alcoholism is controlled or you are spitting in the wind. If their hypertension, diabetes, anemia . . . is not getting better despite proper care, consider alcoholism.

The typical medical attitudes about detection, assessment, and treatment might be less equivocal but are comparably nihilistic.

People lie about whether or not they drink. Double the quantity they tell you they drink. It is a blue-collar problem. It is an ethnic problem. It is normal, social, and expected. Jews don't drink (it interferes with their suffering). The Irish are all drunks. Arabs don't drink. It is not an Asian problem because they don't tolerate it. It is not worth detecting because it is not treatable. Label a patient alcoholic and they will not come back – better to have them inside the tent. Drugs don't work. Psychotherapy doesn't work. Only AA works, and that not often.

It is frustrating, an exercise in futility, to spend time on an alcoholic.

The end result of such equivocal, ambivalent attitudes and realities is that alcoholism is easier ignored than managed and so it is often overlooked.

The reasons for this are complex, cultural, medical, grounded in the confusing reality, and driven by idiosyncratic experience for most doctors, who have their own and disturbing relationship to drinking in their family, neighbors, patients, and in themselves. In seminars with practising doctors about their most difficult patients, dozens of variants come up. These include:

My father was an abusive alcoholic so I hate to hear about it; my mother was a silent sneaky alcoholic, so I feel betrayed as soon as a patient tells me or hides it; when I was 11, I was attacked at a Seder by these cackling, blue-haired old Jewish women who thought I was cute and got drunk on the wine; so many times I have poured my self into trying to help someone about to wreck his life through drinking, only to have him lie over and over that he is doing what needs to be done to stop.

Importance of alcoholism

Alcoholism is lifetime prevalent in about 15% of the US population (measurements vary, range 12–20%). It is twice as common in men as in women. It is more prevalent in patients. It is associated with family history, about 50% of the risk being genetic (Kendler *et al.*, 1992) and more likely heritable in more severe cases (Partanen *et al.*, 1966). It is more common in persons of lower socioeconomic status, bachelors, the uniformed services, and Native Americans, and in persons with high life stress scores. It is more common in smokers – and most smokers drink – and in patients with psychiatric disorders, especially the depressed female and anxious male. It decreases in war zones.

Thus, in a normal day of primary care practice, seeing between 10 and 30 patients, between one and six will be alcoholic, and several of these would benefit from intervention. Few primary care physicians intervene with an alcoholic each day they practice! In part, this is because the drinking is silent and not detected. In part it is due to a semiconscious belief that to try to intervene would cost a frightening amount of time.

The medical complications of drinking are beyond the scope of this book, but are well known. The most commonly considered is cirrhosis of the liver, which is the leading cause of alcohol-related death and is found in 8% of deaths in the US (National Center for Health Statistics, 2004; Table 13.1). Associated with cirrhosis are portal hypertension, variceal and gastric bleeding, and coagulopathy. Drinking heavily is associated with macrocytosis and anemia, and with cancers of the liver, breast, esophagus and oropharynx. Alcoholics suffer from both peripheral neuropathy and brain disease of the cerebellum and long tracts, although Wernicke–Korsakoff is much less prevalent in the US than in less well nourished places. But the most perplexing primary care problem associated with alcoholism is probably hypertension. For unknown reasons, hypertension in alcoholics is notoriously hard to treat. The experience of the primary care physician is of a hypertensive patient who does not become normotensive, despite escalating treatment. Of course, alcoholics experience accidents and associated trauma, from vehicular- and tool-related crashes and dings to falls and fights. As alcoholism is very common, it is often comorbid with and complicating of other illnesses – hypertension foremost. But alcoholism is associated with increased risk of infection (especially if the spleen is compromised or nutrition lacking), bleeding, poor compliance, and slow healing.

Most alcoholics begin drinking early but become alcoholic in the sense of disordered, sick, and addicted 15–20 years into it (Jellinek, 1952; Vaillant, 1995). There are several overlapping definitions of alcohol-related disorders (from DSM, NIAA, etc.) characterized by the amount of drinking (use, abuse; moderate, heavy, binge), the associated degree of social and psychological impairment, or the duration and intensity (phases). Their utility is not apparent to most primary care physicians, who find it more helpful to characterize the patient according to the individual's various dimensions of impairment such as denial, loss of control in life or mind, dependency and preoccupation, addiction, and toxicities to self and others. The typical medical response to medically or psychiatrically impaired alcoholics is equivocal. The physician knows it is a disease, that it is significantly genetic and rendered more likely by early life disasters and distresses, that the addictive personality is not a choice. Yet the patients are difficult. They lie. They break promises. The normal and treasured premise of the doctor–patient relationship, mutual effort on behalf of the patient's best values, is violated seemingly without limit. The affronted primary care physician feels impotent, frustrated, and helpless. Their puritanical streak may be triggered (why can't you begin to help yourself, unsaid, like a reasonable or a good person would – and sotto voce: and stop tormenting me).

The foundation of the primary care physician's aggravation

The roots of the helplessness and aversion commonly expressed by physicians about alcoholics tap deep into our culture. Drinking, binging, and partying with alcohol are part of high school and college experience, treated as normal, excesses tolerated, and so isolation and denial begin. Families with an alcoholic or three deny their problems, do not talk about them, use avoidance and enabling to manage the disruptive behavior. And physicians learn this early in their lives. Especially those with active alcoholics at home.

The isolation, denial, and avoidance practised at home become further sanitized by the culture. There are bars everywhere; ads glamorizing drinking and drink; TV, movies, and theater showing the comical aspects of the friendly drunk. The most watched video on YouTube at the time of writing (almost a million

Table 13.1 Medical evaluation of drinking

Physical examination
Tachycardia, hypertension, orthostasis
Habitus, grooming, inebriation, breath
Skin (telangiectasias, rhinophyma, spiders, palmar erythema, rubor)
Liver spleen size and texture, tenderness
Peripheral sensation, gait, balance
Folstein
Mental status
Laboratory examination
Liver function
CBC with indices (MCV)
And as indicated

viewings) is of "The most drunk man ever" with comments about how funny he is. Hip hop gives it street cred. Talk radio assumes it. Politicians and athletes model it. So primary care doctors feel they are swimming against the tide of cultural alcohol abuse tolerance when they sit down with a patient about to damage irreversibly his physical, social or psychological health.

Nor is this ameliorated by focused and useful teaching in college, medical school, or residency training. Despite the efforts of groups like the Association for Medical Education and Research in Substance Abuse (AMERSA) and Society of General Internal Medicine (SGIM), the normative graduate emerges as described. This is in part due to the presence in the medical subcultures of drink-tolerant rituals typified by the commonly held "liver" rounds in residencies. It is partly due to the minor curricular standing of substance abuse and alcohol. For example, in new curricula being promulgated now, medical schools are choosing paradigm diseases – what were dubbed in previous eras the grand diseases. Today's versions, e.g. curricular pillars, include diabetes or atherosclerotic coronary artery disease and exclude alcoholism. A second major deficit is the lack of successful role modeling and positive experience with alcoholics. No wonder later they feel it is low yield, so low priority.

In addition, the so-called hidden curriculum is a major contributor to medical alcoholism helplessness. The most formative portion of medical education is what is seen and done on the wards during clinical clerkships and internship. What is seen are end-stage alcoholics, often highly comorbid with majorly impaired mentation, rampant additional mental disorders, socially wrecked, homeless, disengaged, and ejected. These patients are in fact difficult to treat. What is doable is palliation, not cure; rehabilitation is not feasible. Lesson learned and generalized. It is true in general that, of 1000 illness episodes in the community (White *et al.*, 1961, revisited 2001), only one ends up in the university hospital to become the experiential base of the learning clinicians. The comparable figure for alcoholics is doubtless in the same ballpark. Students seldom see first- or second-stage alcoholics, seldom recognize them when they are seen in clinic or their continuity practices, and so develop core attitudes that are difficult to reverse.

Approaches to changing this are generally successful when done diligently with support from above. They include providing comprehensive knowledge, attitudes, and skills training in concentrated doses sufficient to enable students to achieve competence at screening and recognition, sharing the diagnosis and prognosis, and negotiating and implementing an appropriate individualized plan. Some approaches include time for students to discuss and manage their personal idiosyncratic barriers as well. They then need reinforcement and the experience of seeing such processes change lives, more than once or on film. Examples of such programs are the 1-week intensive block we use at NYU in cooperation with Nicholas Pace and a similar block developed at Hazelden-NYC. Model curricula have been published regularly and presented at AMERSA and SGIM. Good overviews abound (see the competencies described in AMERSA's faculty development manual (Abrams, 2003). Good examples are easily assigned (Barnes *et al.*, 1987).

Screening

Prior to assessment comes screening. While most primary care physicians believe they should screen for drinking problems, less than half actually do (Bradley *et al.*, 2007). The United States Preventive Services Task Force (USPSTF) recommends screening all adult patients for alcohol use and dependence using a population-appropriate approach and a standardized questionnaire. Screening begins with query concerning present and prior drinking (do you drink alcohol or have you ever?) and family history (does or did anyone in your family have a drinking problem?) The most widely used and discussed questionnaires are shown in Table 13.2. The CAGE is easily remembered, relatively sensitive, but less useful in early drinkers, heavy drinkers, women, some minorities, and those in the early phases. Nevertheless, doctors can easily remember it and it is not offensive to most patients. The AUDIT is more effective for dependent, heavy, female, and minority drinkers, but it is ten questions and so is seldom adopted in small practices. This may change with computer-based screening availability in practices with Electronic Medical Records (EMRs). A shorter version of three questions, the AUDIT-C, is performing well in early studies. Other contenders for preferred questionnaire are the SMAST (Short Michigan Alcohol Screening Tool); the TWEAK, which is good in women; the T-ACE for pregnant drinkers; and the CRAFFT (Knight *et al.*, 1999) for adolescents. Overall, the number screened to find a treatable case is around 40 (Knight *et al.*, 2003). So, perhaps one every other day.

Table 13.2 Evidence-based alcohol screening tools

1. CAGE

C Have you ever felt you should **Cut down** on your drinking?

A Have people **Annoyed** you by criticizing your drinking?

G Have you ever felt bad or **Guilty** about your drinking?

E Eye opener: Have you ever had a drink first thing in the morning to steady your nerves or to get rid of a hangover?

The CAGE can identify alcohol problems over the lifetime. Two positive responses are considered a positive test and indicate further assessment is warranted

2. AUDIT

1. How often do you have a drink containing alcohol? (0) Never (Skip to Questions 9–10)

(1) Monthly or less

(2) 2 to 4 times a month

(3) 2 to 3 times a week

(4) 4 or more times a week

2. How many drinks containing alcohol do you have on a typical day when you are drinking?

(0) 1 or 2

(1) 3 or 4

(2) 5 or 6

(3) 7, 8, or 9

(4) 10 or more

3. How often do you have six or more drinks on one occasion?

(0) Never

(1) Less than monthly

(2) Monthly

(3) Weekly

(4) Daily or almost daily

4. How often during the last year have you found that you were not able to stop drinking once you had started?

(0) Never

(1) Less than monthly

(2) Monthly

(3) Weekly

(4) Daily or almost daily

5. How often during the last year have you failed to do what was normally expected from you because of drinking?

(0) Never

(1) Less than monthly

(2) Monthly

(3) Weekly

(4) Daily or almost daily

6. How often during the last year have you been unable to remember what happened the night before because you had been drinking?

(0) Never

(1) Less than monthly

(2) Monthly

(3) Weekly

(4) Daily or almost daily

7. How often during the last year have you needed an alcoholic drink first thing in the morning to get yourself going after a night of heavy drinking?

(0) Never

(1) Less than monthly

(2) Monthly

(3) Weekly

(4) Daily or almost daily

8. How often during the last year have you had a feeling of guilt or remorse after drinking?

(0) Never

(1) Less than monthly

(2) Monthly

(3) Weekly

(4) Daily or almost daily

9. Have you or someone else been injured as a result of your drinking?

(0) No

(2) Yes, but not in the last year

(4) Yes, during the last year

10. Has a relative, friend, doctor, or another health professional expressed concern about your drinking or suggested you cut down?

(0) No

(2) Yes, but not in the last year

(4) Yes, during the last year

Add up the points associated with your answers above. A total score of 8 or more indicates harmful drinking behavior (Baber TF, Higgins-Biddle JC, Saunders JB, Monteiro MG, AUDIT: The alcohol use Disorder Identification Test; guidelines for use in Primary Care, 2nd ed. Geneva, World Health Organization, 2001).

Q1: How often did you have a drink containing alcohol in the past year?

Answer	Points
Never	0
Monthly or less	1
Two to four times a month	2
Two to three times a week	3
Four or more times a week	4

(continued)

Table 13.2 (cont.)

Q2: How many drinks did you have on a typical day when you were drinking in the past year?

Answer	Points
None, I do not drink	0
1 or 2	0
3 or 4	1
5 or 6	2
7 to 9	3
10 or more	4

Q3: How often did you have six or more drinks on one occasion in the past year?

Answer	Points
Never	0
Less than monthly	1
Monthly	2
Weekly	3
Daily or almost daily	4

The AUDIT-C is scored on a scale of 0–12 (scores of 0 reflect no alcohol use). In men, a score of 4 or more is considered positive; in women, a score of 3 or more is considered positive. Generally, the higher the AUDIT-C score, the more likely it is that the patient's drinking is affecting his/her health and safety (Bush K, Kiulahum DR, McDonnell MB et al. The audit alcohol consumption questions (AUDIT-C): an effective brief screening test for problem drinking. Arch Internal Med. 1998: 1789-1795).

Table 13.3 Assessment of alcoholics in primary care

Clark's mnemonics for assessment of alcoholics
HALT
Do you drink to get **H**igh?
Do you drink **A**lone?
Do you **L**ook forward to drinking (when your mind should be elsewhere)?
Has your **T**olerance for alcohol increased?
BUMP
Have you had **B**lackouts or noted more recently?
Do you do **U**nplanned drinking (drink in spite of planning not to do so)?
Do you drink **M**edicinally (when you are depressed, angry, sad, etc.)?
Do you **P**rotect your supply of alcohol (so you'll always have enough)?
FATAL DTs
Family history of alcohol problems?
Alcoholics Anonymous attendance, ever?
Thoughts of or attempts at suicide?
Alcoholism, ever thought you might have it?
Legal problems such as driving citations and assault?
Depression, feeling down frequently?
Tranquilizer (or disulfiram) use

Reproduced with permission from Clark (1995).

Assessing

History

The evaluation of the patient screened as potentially alcoholic or a troubled drinker is key to the success of the processes, because the dance of delicacy, frankness, and trust begins before the climax of presenting the diagnosis and negotiating a plan. Clark (1995) recommends using the three mnemonics HALT, BUMP, and FATAL DTs in such assessments (Table 13.3).

Most alcoholic patients need laboratory evaluation of the end organs damaged by ethanol, including liver, blood, nervous system (brain and periphery), and heart. The transaminases are currently used (ALT (SGPT), AST (SGOT), GGT), but are relatively indirect as they measure membrane health rather than hepatocyte function. A new test for small amounts of bile acid in serum, recently FDA-approved, is being widely used in China and may prove more useful for detection and monitoring of liver function. CDT (serum carbohydrate-deficient transferrin) helps with heavy drinkers and to detect relapse but is not widely used. Mean Corpuscular Volume (MCV), high in drinkers due to macrocytosis, is a sensitive marker of hematopoietic deficit and possibly of folate deficiency. No specific laboratory tests are uniformly helpful in diagnosing alcoholism and no specific battery is mandatory.

The same is true of the physical examination; none of it is pathognomonic except unequivocal tolerance. Nevertheless, one should look for frank inebriation, signs of tolerance (if the person drank heavily and does not appear inebriated), skin stigmata of liver disease (spiders, palmar erythema, telangiectasias, rhinophyma; signs of peripheral neuropathy; signs of brain disease, including wide-based gait, past pointing, tremulousness, and abnormal Folstein and mini-mental status examination; and cardiac hydration issues, including tachycardia, orthostatic change, and hypertension.

Presenting the diagnosis

No matter how lax the physician, some alcoholism is undeniable and so all physicians who treat patients will eventually be faced with a patient definitely needing intervention owing to unequivocal evidence of addicted drinking and damage to self or others. Presenting the diagnosis to a patient is a major bottleneck which hangs up many well intentioned physicians. There are personal reasons for this – the patient may deny, get angry, leave the practice, or threaten. The patient will have tough affects, argue, and use all of his or her skills to avoid the feared abstinence. There are the realistic difficulties: for the patient it may feel humiliating, shameful, like an attack, dangerously threatening to something they depend on, as though it may strip their defense against an intolerable life situation. Few guidelines prepare adequately for this complexity. A few are essential. One is to commit the time and space. Second is to believe in it. Third is to keep the discussion empathic, focused on the illness, its effects, and the negotiation of a plan. This requires managing the arguments and affects. Fourth, avoid blaming and scapegoating. Fifth, keep it short, to the point, specific to the patient. Get the patient back soon. Have AA get involved. Clark (1995) offers the mnemonic DR HELPS CD as a menu of things to do and say in these interviews (Table 13.4).

Negotiating a plan

Guiding the patient from the diagnosis to the plan is a second major bottleneck in the course of care. The success of this step is presaged by what has gone before: respectful, non-judgmental elicitation of symptoms, signs, historical markers, and evidence of damage to self and others. By the time all that is accomplished, even an inebriated dull patient knows very keenly where the physician is coming from – if there is censure, judgment, or disapproval, it has been noted.

Bean (1983) clearly delineated the goals of care as: include acceptance of the diagnosis, make the environment safe, learn how to get sober, stay sober, live with it, manage barriers to recovery, and get over the losses of being outside the drinkers' world. If all that goes well, then the person can begin to work to manage their pre-existing problems and remold their recovering self.

Miller and Rollnick (1991; see also Miller *et al.*, 1992) introduced motivational interviewing as a method to achieve mutual agreement concerning goals

Table 13.4 Discussing the diagnosis and plan

1. Commit the time and space
2. Believe in it
3. Keep the discussion empathic
4. Manage argument and affect
5. Focus on the illness and its effects in order to:
6. Negotiate a plan
7. Avoid blaming and scapegoating
8. Keep it short, to the point, specific to the patient
9. Follow up ASAP
10. Initiate AA involvement if feasible

DR HELPS CD

You are **D**ependent on alcohol

Come for a **R**eturn visit on…

Help is necessary and available and useful

The **E**vidence that tells us you are in trouble is…

Leave alcohol behind: abstain (and other mood-altering drugs)

Your **P**erspective is limited; you can't see reality, this is part of the disease

This predicament **S**neaked up on you; no one asks for it

I'm **C**oncerned and worried because you are ill

Your **D**epression and despair result from not living according to your own values, hurting people you love, and not living up to your potential

(DR HELPS CD reproduced with permission from Clark (1995)).

and reasons to get better and barriers to doing that. They are sometimes summarized as the simplistic and yet powerful "OARS:" 1) open-ended questions; 2) affirmations; 3) reflective listening; and 4) summaries. The core concepts are comparable to consensus notions of proper communications, with the additional strategy that whatever iota of motivation exists, it can be used to initiate change. Concepts such as the readiness ruler reify this approach and it has become a world view for its proponents (Carroll *et al.*, 2004).

Intervention

Obviously intervention needs to be appropriate to the stage and severity of the disease. It needs to assess for withdrawal symptom potential, and may require brief or prolonged inpatient treatment. However, most drinkers will require some variant of the NIAA's AAAA approach: ask (about drinking), assess, advise and assist. A fifth "A," plan to do it **a**gain soon, might be appropriately added. Results from such simple efforts are better than most physicians imagine but are still low – a 10–20 response is what the literature promises.

A second level of intervention involves use of one of several well studied methods. It seems within the scope of primary care training to teach one such method. The principle methods are motivational interview and enhancement therapy, cognitive behavioral therapy or a variant such as the combined behavioral treatment used in COMBINE (Anton *et al.*, 2006) or twelve-step intervention facilitation. The latter is simply ensuring referral to an in-practice or both local and culturally appropriate AA group. The three approaches are roughly equally successful.

The reasons to hospitalize boil down to the presence of a past history of significant withdrawal symptoms, especially seizures or hallucinations; severe comorbid psychiatric disorder, especially suicidality; medically complicating issues; a toxic home or work situation from which removal will be highly beneficial or protective of the patient or others; and persistent failure to withdraw and abstain outside.

Some patients may be helped by pharmacotherapy to prevent or manage withdrawal symptoms. Many, on the other hand, may be worsened, especially by tranquilizer therapy. Naltrexone is helpful in keeping patients in treatment and prolonging relapse. It is hepatotoxic. Disulfiram is the oldest agent – results vary enormously, and skill in its use comes from choosing that occasional patient organized and compulsive enough to use it safely. Acamprosate did not do better than placebo in the large COMBINE trial (Anton, 2006), in which naltrexone and combined behavioral treatment were roughly equivalent and not better in combination.

The general rule is not to treat with psychotropics until a patient has stopped drinking. The two exceptions to this are if the patient is showing physical signs of significant withdrawal (benzodiazepines are short-term appropriate) and if the patient is significantly depressed (beginning antidepressant treatment while still drinking is usually done and may be helpful in reducing craving).

Many patients are poorly nourished and benefit from improved nutrition and/or vitamin supplementation. A multivitamin is sensible, definitely including B vitamins and folic acid.

Where to refer and referral strategies

What to do next of course depends on the situation, the patient's strengths and risks, and severity of the crisis, if any. That said, every primary care physician should have a ready-to-hand set of alternatives for action and referral. These should include knowing a receptive, responsive, and non-exploitative treatment program, therapist, and AA group. Luckier primary care physicians know a responsive addiction specialist, who may be a psychiatrist or generalist. There are two competing specialty boards in this area, without evidence to support claims of superiority by either. Larger practices learn that having the patience, empathy, non-judgmental approach, and lack of ego needed for real effectiveness are found in a precious few practitioners. They tend not to be normatively socialized but it is well worth the effort of keeping them available to the many patients who will benefit, and to offload the difficulties of their niche on those less suited temperamentally to the work.

References

Abrams, T. W., Saitz, R. & Samet, J. H. (2003). Education of preventive medicine residents: alcohol, tobacco, and other drug abuse. *American Journal of Preventive Medicine*, **24**, 101–5.

Anton, R. F., O'Malley, S. S., Ciraulo, D. A. *et al.* (2006). Combined pharmacotherapies and behavioral interventions for alcohol dependence: the COMBINE study: a randomized, controlled trial. *Journal of the American Medical Association*, **295**, 2003–17.

Baber, T. F., Higgins-Biddle, J. C., Saunders, J. B. & Monteiro, M. G. (2001). *AUDIT: The Alcohol Use Disorders Identification Test; Guidelines for Use in Primary Care*, 2nd edn. Geneva: World Health Organization.

Barnes, H. N., Aronson, M. D. & Delbanco, T. L. (1987). *Alcoholism–A Guide for the Primary Care Physician*. New York: Springer-Verlag, pp. 1–231.

Bean, M. (1983). Clinical implications of models for recovery from alcoholism. *Advances in Alcohol & Substance Abuse*, **3**, 91–104.

Bradley, K. A., Curry, S. J., Koepsell, T. D. & Larson, E. B. (2007). Primary and secondary prevention of alcohol problems; U.S. internist attitudes and practices. *Journal of General Internal Medicine*, **10**, 67–72.

Bush, K., Kiulahun, D. R., McDonnell, M. B. *et al.* (1998). The audit alcohol consumption questions (AUDIT-C): an effective brief screening test for problem drinking. *Archives of Internal Medicine*, **158**, 1789–95.

Carroll, M. K., Ball, S. A. & Martino, S. (2004). Cognitive, behavioral, and motivational therapies. In *Textbook of Substance Abuse Treatment*, 2nd edn, eds.

M. Galanter & H. Kleber. Washington, DC: American Psychiatric Association Press, Inc.

Clark, W. (1995). Effective interviewing and intervention for alcohol problems. In *The Medical Interview: Clinical Care, Education, and Research*, eds. M. Lipkin, S. M. Putnam & A. Lazare. New York: Springer-Verlag, pp. 284–93.

Jellinek, E. M. (1952). Phases of alcohol addiction. *Quarterly Journal of Studies on Alcohol*, **13**, 673–684.

Kendler, K. S., Heath, A. C., Neale, M. C., Kessler, R. C. & Eaves, L. J. (1992). A population-based twin study of alcoholism in women. *Journal of the American Medical Association*, **268**(14), 1877–82.

Knight, J. R., Shrier, L. A., Bravender, T. D. *et al.* (1999). A new brief screen for adolescent substance abuse. *Archives of Pediatric & Adolescent Medicine*, **153**, 591–6.

Knight, J. R., Sherritt, L., Harris, S. K., Gates, E. C. & Chang, G. (2003). Validity of brief alcohol screening tests among adolescents: a comparison of the AUDIT, POSIT, CAGE, and CRAFFT. *Alcoholism: Clinical and Experimental Research*, **27**(1), 67–73.

Miller, W. R. & Rollnick, S. (1991). *Motivational Interviewing: Preparing People for Change*. New York: Guilford Press.

Miller, W. R., Zweben, A., DiClemente, C. C. & Rychtarik, R. G. (1992). *Motivational Enhancement Therapy Manual: A Clinical Research Guide for Therapists Treating Individuals with Alcohol Abuse and Dependence*. Rockville, MD: National Institute on Alcohol Abuse and Alcoholism.

National Center for Health Statistics. (2004). *Health, United States. With Chartbook on Trends in the Health of Americans*. Hyattsville, Maryland: National Center for Health Statistics.

Partanen, J., Bruun, K. & Markkanen, T. (1966). *Inheritance of Drinking Behavior*. Helsinki: Finnish Foundation for Alcohol Studies.

The Guide to Clinical Preventive Services. (2009). *Recommendations of the U.S. Preventive Services Task Force*. Washington DC: Agency for Healthcare Research and Quality. http://www.preventiveservices.ahrq.gov, accessed February 23, 2010.

Vaillant, G. (1995). *Natural History of Alcoholism, Revisited*. Cambridge: Harvard Press.

White, K. L. (2001). The ecology of medical care revisited. *New England Journal of Medicine*, **344**(26), 2021–5.

White, K. L., Williams, T. F. & Greenberg, B. G. (1961). The ecology of medical care. *New England Journal of Medicine*, **265**, 885–92.

14

Nicotine addiction and smoking cessation

Neil Hartman

The prehistory of tobacco use is undoubtedly longer than its history. Tobacco smoking was an essential ceremonial thread in the social fabric of North American indigenous populations (Hartman *et al.*, 1998). It was not until its introduction to Europe approximately 500 years ago that it became considered by some to be unhealthy or socially undesirable (Mangan & Golding, 1984), having lost its ceremonial purpose. Tobacco smoking is now widely recognized to be the leading cause of premature death in developed countries, responsible for the death of one in 10 adults worldwide, or about 5 million deaths each year. Half of the 650 million people who smoke today will eventually be killed by tobacco (Tobacco Advisory Group of the Royal College of Physicians, 2000), and this morbidity and mortality can be mostly avoided if people stop smoking (Department of Health and Human Services, 1990).

Although smoking prevalence has diminished in the US, Canada, and most western European countries, it remains high in countries such as China and India (approximately 50% and 30%, respectively, among males) and is on the rise in developing countries (Shafey *et al.*, 2003). Consequently, tobacco use is one of the few causes of death that is increasing globally.

An excellent summary of neurochemical determinants for smoking can be found in a recent review article by Le Foll and George (2007). Although tobacco smoke contains several substances, nicotine appears to be the critical reinforcing component of tobacco smoke and is responsible for most, if not all, of the addictive effects in humans. A large body of evidence implicates $\alpha_4\beta_2$-nicotinic acetylcholine receptors in the reinforcing effects of nicotine. The initial effect of nicotine is probably to activate $\alpha_4\beta_2$-nicotinic acetylcholine receptors located on dopamine neurons in the ventral tegmental area; however, it is likely that these receptors are rapidly desensitized, whereas nicotine produces a sustained effect on dopamine release in the nucleus accumbens. According to the "dopamine hypothesis" of drug dependence, the increase in dopamine levels in the nucleus accumbens produced by drugs of abuse is critical to the drugs' ability to induce motivational and reinforcing properties. Although the nucleus accumbens plays a pivotal role in drug-seeking behavior, the influence of the prefrontal cortex, the amygdala, and the hippocampus (which, through the glutamate and γ-aminobutyric acid (GABA) neurons, mediate the drive to take drugs, the influence of drug-associated cues and the memory of drug-taking) is critical.

The decline in smoking prevalence in the industrialized countries of North America and western Europe is a relatively new trend, lagging decades behind the recognition by healthcare providers of smoking-associated morbidity and mortality, mainly from pulmonary and cardiovascular disease. The delay in legislating against smoking (warning labeling, smoking bans, criminalizing sales to minors, etc.) was largely the result of the enormous economic and political influence of the tobacco industry. An hypothesis published in 1931 that the habitual nature of smoking was akin to other recognized addictions and that nicotine was a key factor (Lewin, 1931) was largely ignored in favor of behavioral explanations (McArthur *et al.*, 1958; Tomkins, 1966) which focused attention on psychogenic factors such as "oral fixation," thus enabling the industry to promulgate false claims that their products were neither harmful nor physiologically addictive. Some 40 years later, Dr. Murray E. Jarvik published his seminal paper, establishing that the addictive substance underlying tobacco smoking was nicotine. This laid the foundation for the field of nicotine research (Jarvik, 1973) and enabled recent significant progress in the clinical research, as well as legal and legislative arenas, in reducing the enormous morbidity and mortality related to smoking, as well as the economic burden to society.

The first pharmacologic breakthrough for smoking cessation research followed observations by Dr. Jarvik and his UCLA postdoctoral fellow Jed Rose, regarding "green tobacco illness," a malady afflicting tobacco harvesters. The fact that the intoxicant in tobacco was readily absorbable transdermally led Dr. Jarvik and Dr. Rose to develop the first clinically effective transdermal patch (Rose *et al.*, 1984). Anecdotally, when Dr. Jarvik and his colleagues were unable to attain approval to run experiments on human subjects, they decided to test their idea on themselves. "We put the tobacco on our skin and waited to see what would happen," Jarvik recalled. "Our heart rates increased, adrenaline began pumping, all the things that happen to smokers" (Breese, 2007). The prototypic nicotine patch, a solution containing 30% nicotine base covered by a Formula 3-cm² patch of polyethylene wrap, secured at the edges by surgical tape, was used in numerous clinical studies, such as applications for hospitalized psychiatric patients, a population known to have an unusually high smoking prevalence, at a time when hospitals were tending toward becoming smoke-free environments (Hartman *et al.*, 1991). The more sophisticated marketed patch was first available in the US by prescription for smoking cessation in 1992. Four years later, it was approved for over-the-counter sale.

The definitive mass-marketed patch, in addition to its worldwide use in smoking cessation therapy, has continued to be a valuable tool for research to reduce smoking-related morbidity and mortality in high-risk patient groups such as cardiac patients (Joseph *et al.*, 1996) and, along with subsequently developed nicotine replacements (nicotine gum, lozenge, nasal spray, and smoke-free nicotine oral inhaler), is used in more sophisticated studies to optimize the efficacy for the ever-increasing populations of smokers seeking to quit, demonstrating that the use of combinations of nicotine replacement devices is viable and needs to be made known and accessible to smokers (Schneider *et al.*, 2006; 2008). Neuroscientists have also exploited the nicotine patch in studies of the cingulate cortex, a key brain locus associated with nicotine addiction and its treatment (Hong *et al.*, 2009), as have investigators of human genetic variants as a guide for the optimal selection of smoking cessation treatment (Uhl *et al.*, 2008).

In addition to nicotine replacement, two non-nicotine-containing pharmaceuticals have been extensively studied for smoking cessation, with generally positive results. The first is the antidepressant bupropion (marketed as Zyban), studied as monotherapy (Goldstein, 1998) and in combination with the nicotine patch (Jorenby *et al.*, 1999). The other is varenicline (marketed as Chantix), a selective partial agonist at the $\alpha_4\beta_2$-nicotinic acetylcholine receptors (nAChR). One recent study concludes that "abstinence from smoking was greater, and craving, withdrawal symptoms and smoking satisfaction less, at the end of treatment with varenicline than with transdermal nicotine" (Aubin *et al.*, 2008). Four of the eight authors of this study are footnoted as being affiliated with Pfizer Global Research and Development. Because of recent revelations regarding financial ties between the pharmaceutical industry and the academic physicians who largely determine the market value of prescription drugs (Angell, 2009), in my opinion, the jury is still out on the real value of these newer smoking cessation pharmaceuticals.

With the passing of Dr. Jarvik, the pioneer in the field of nicotine addiction and smoking cessation research, the mantle has been passed to Joseph R. DiFranza (DiFranza, 2008), a family physician practising out of the University of Massachusetts Medical School in Worcester, another perennial thorn in the side of the tobacco industry, and of a bewildering national policy that offers economic incentives to an industry whose products account for 20% of US mortality while appropriating funds to reduce the carnage at only 2% of the total health research budget. Dr. DiFranza has been a vocal advocate for efforts to prevent the tobacco industry from selling its products to children, and his research and complaint to the Federal Trade Commission resulted in the demise of the notorious Joe Camel advertisements for Camel cigarettes. Dr. DiFranza's interest in the neurophysiology of nicotine addiction began with observations in treating teenage patients who were struggling to quit even though they had only recently started smoking (DiFranza, 2008). He developed the "Hooked on Nicotine Checklist" (HONC – now in use in 13 languages, and the most thoroughly validated measure of nicotine addiction) to validate his observations in clinical research (DiFranza *et al.*, 2002a, b; DiFranza & Wellman, 2005). Dr. DiFranza's findings have overturned the dogma that cigarette addiction takes years to develop. His studies of adolescent smokers show that symptoms of addiction, such as withdrawal, craving for cigarettes, and failed attempts at quitting, can appear within the first weeks of smoking. To account for these findings, Dr. DiFranza and colleagues have developed a new theory which explains why it takes such a short time for smokers to become addicted; simply put, that the brain quickly develops adaptations that counter the effects of nicotine. These adaptations lead to withdrawal symptoms when the effects of nicotine wear off. The newest and most intriguing development in the field of nicotine research is interest in smokeless nicotine as a therapeutic agent for maladies having nothing to do with nicotine addiction (Piasecki & Newhouse, 2000). These new applications for neurodegenerative diseases such as Alzheimer's and Parkinson's dementia are likely related to nicotine's well established neural cytoprotective properties in relation to prevention or postponement of symptoms in diseases involving neural tissue degeneration. Other reported beneficial effects in diseases such as schizophrenia, attention deficit hyperactivity disorder, autism, Tourette's disorder, ulcerative colitis, and even mild cognitive impairment (Newhouse, 2009) may have more to do with nicotine's complex functions in neurotransmitter receptor systems. I anticipate that the pace of definitive work in this important new field will, unfortunately, be slow because of a lack of an obvious financial incentive.

References

Angell, M. (2009). Drug companies and doctors: a story of corruption. *The New York Review of Books*, January 15, **LVI**(1), 8–12.

Aubin, H. -J., Bobak, A., Britton, J. R. *et al.* (2008). Varenicline versus transdermal nicotine patch for smoking cessation: results from a randomised, open-label trial. *Thorax*, **63**, 717–24.

Breese, K. (2007). Eureka: 25 brilliant California ideas. *UCLA Magazine*, Jan. 2007, 17.

Department of Health and Human Services. (1990). *The Health Benefits of Smoking Cessation: A Report of the Surgeon General*. Washington (DC): US Public Health Service, Office on Smoking and Health.

DiFranza, J. R. (2008). Hooked from the first cigarette. *Scientific American*, May, 82–7.

DiFranza, J. R. & Wellman, R. J. (2005). A sensitization-homeostasis model of nicotine craving, withdrawal, and tolerance: integrating the clinical and basic science literature. *Nicotine & Tobacco Research*, 7(1), 9–26.

DiFranza, J. R., Savageau, J. A., Fletcher, K. *et al.* (2002a). Measuring the loss of autonomy over nicotine use in adolescents: the DANDY (development and assessment of nicotine dependence in youths) study.

Archives of Pediatrics & Adolescent Medicine, **156**(4), 397–403.

DiFranza, J. R., Savageau, J. A., Fletcher, K. *et al.* (2002b). The development of symptoms of tobacco dependence in youths: 30-month follow-up data from the DANDY study. *Tobacco Control*, **11**(3), 228–35.

Goldstein, M. G. (1998). Bupropion sustained release and smoking cessation. *Journal of Clinical Psychiatry*, **59**(Suppl. 4), 66–72.

Hartman, N., Leong, G., Glynn, S., Wilkins, J. & Jarvik, M. (1991). Transdermal nicotine and smoking behavior in psychiatric patients. *American Journal of Psychiatry*, **148**, 374–5.

Hartman, N., Caskey, N. H., Olmstead, R. E. & Jarvik, M. E. (1998). Nicotine craving and psychiatric diagnosis: past, present, and future. *Psychiatric Annals*, **28**, 547–51.

Hong, L. E., Gu, H., Yang, Y. *et al.* (2009). Association of nicotine addiction and nicotine's actions with separate cingulate cortex functional circuits. *Archives of General Psychiatry*, **66**(4), 431–41.

Jarvik, M. E. (1973). Further observations on nicotine as the reinforcing agent in smoking. In *Smoking Behavior: Motives and Incentives*, ed. W. L. Dunn. Washington, DC: Winston and Sons.

Jorenby, D. E., Leischow, S. J., Nides, M. A. *et al.* (1999). A controlled trial of sustained-release bupropion, a nicotine patch, or both for smoking cessation. *New England Journal of Medicine*, **340**, 685–91.

Joseph, A., Norman, S., Ferry, L. *et al.* (1996). The safety of transdermal nicotine as an aid to smoking cessation in patients with cardiac disease. *New England Journal of Medicine*, **335**, 1792–8.

Le Foll, B. & George, T. P. (2007). Treatment of tobacco dependence: integrating recent progress into practice. *Canadian Medical Association Journal*, **177**(11), doi: 10.1503/cmaj.070627.

Lewin, L. (1931). *Phantastica: Narcotic and Other Stimulating Drugs: Their Use and Abuse*. London: Kegan, Paul, Trench, Trubuer.

McArthur, C., Waldron, E. & Dickinson, J. (1958). The psychology of smoking. *Journal of Abnormal Psychology*, **56**, 267–75.

Mangan, G. L. & Golding, J. F. (1984). *The Psychopharmacology of Smoking*. New York: Cambridge University Press.

Newhouse, P. (2009). Nicotine patch may be helpful in mild cognitive impairment. *American Association for Geriatric Psychiatry 2009 Annual Meeting*: Abstract NR 89. Presented March 6, 2009.

Piasecki, M. & Newhouse, P. A. (2000). *Nicotine in Psychiatry: Psychopathology and Emerging Therapeutics*. Washington DC: American Psychiatric Press.

Rose, J. E., Jarvik, M. E. & Rose, K. D. (1984). Transdermal administration of nicotine. *Drug and Alcohol Dependence*, **13**, 209–13.

Schneider, N. G., Koury, M. A., Cortner, C. *et al.* (2006). Preferences among four combination nicotine treatments. *Psychopharmacology*, **187**, 476–85.

Schneider, N. G., Cortner, C., Justice, M. *et al.* (2008). Preferences among five nicotine treatments based on information versus sampling. *Nicotine & Tobacco Research*, **10**(1), 179–86.

Shafey, O., Dolwick, S. & Guindon, G. E. (eds.) (2003). *Tobacco Control Country Profiles 2003.* Atlanta: American Cancer Society.

Tobacco Advisory Group of the Royal College of Physicians (2000). *Nicotine Addiction in Britain: A Report of the Tobacco Advisory Group of the Royal College of Physicians.* London (UK): Royal College of Physicians of London.

Tomkins, S. (1966). Psychological model for smoking behavior. *American Journal of Public Health*, **56**, 17–20.

Uhl, G. R., Liu, Q. -R. & Drgon, T. (2008). Molecular genetics & of successful smoking cessation, convergent genome-wide association study results. *Archives of General Psychiatry*, **65**(6), 683–93.

Real World

Clinical aspects of cocaine and methamphetamine dependence

Arnold Washton

Cocaine and methamphetamine are potent central nervous system (CNS) stimulants with high potential for abuse. In the early 1980s, intranasal cocaine use reached epidemic proportions in the US, especially among affluent users and others who had the financial resources to procure what was then a high-priced drug (Washton *et al.*, 1984). A variety of antecedent factors set the stage for this cocaine epidemic, including a growing social acceptance of illicit drug use that began in the 1960s, a mistaken view of intranasal cocaine use as benign and non-addictive, increased availability of cocaine supplies at reduced prices, and the glamorous image of cocaine as a "recreational" drug of the rich and famous. By the mid-1980s, cocaine use had spread to lower socioeconomic groups, especially in large urban areas as prices dropped and smokeable cocaine alkaloid ("crack") became widely available as a street drug (Washton, 1987; Washton & Gold, 1986). Cocaine-related hospital emergencies rose sharply and large numbers of cocaine users sought help at addiction treatment programs in cities and towns across the US (Rawson, 1999).

The cocaine problem in the US was further compounded by an epidemic of methamphetamine use that emerged initially in western regions of the country in the early 1990s before spreading to other geographic areas (Anglin *et al.*, 2000; Rutkowski & Maxwell, 2009). The societal costs associated with cocaine and methamphetamine use are extraordinary. They include the costs not only of treating the addiction itself, but also serious drug-related health problems, including higher rates of HIV transmission resulting from needle sharing and stimulant-induced hypersexual behaviors (Ellis *et al.*, 2003; Frosch *et al.*, 1996).

In addition to cocaine and methamphetamine use, non-medical use of prescription stimulant drugs in the US has increased substantially in recent years. The most commonly prescribed stimulant medications include methylphenidate (Ritalin and Concerta), pemoline (Cylert), modafinil (Provigil), dexedrine (amphetamine), and Adderall (a combination of amphetamine and dextroamphetamine). Over-prescribing of these medications mainly for attention deficit hyperactivity disorder (ADHD), especially in high school and college students, has created a growing illicit market for diverted supplies of these medications on school campuses (McCabe *et al.*, 2005). In general, problems associated with use of prescription stimulants are similar although substantially less prevalent in the general population and less severe than those associated with cocaine and methamphetamine abuse. The present chapter focuses exclusively on cocaine and methamphetamine dependence, and more detailed information on non-medical use of prescription stimulants can be found elsewhere (e.g. King & Ellinwood, 2005; Kroutil *et al.*, 2006).

From a treatment perspective, cocaine and methamphetamine dependence are similar in many respects to other drug dependencies, but there are certain aspects of these drugs and their unique effects that must be taken into account (Washton & Zweben, 2009), as discussed below. Clinicians treating stimulant users must be familiar, for example, with the compelling reinforcing properties of stimulant drugs, the post-stimulant dysphoria or "crash" that encourages polysubstance abuse, the progressive tolerance that sends chronic users on a futile chase to recapture the elusive high, the powerful drug cravings that accelerate the transition from use to dependence and also thwart attempts to sustain abstinence, and the powerful aphrodisiac effects of stimulant drugs that drive various types of hypersexual behaviors, including HIV-risky sex.

Preparations and route of administration

Cocaine is extracted from leaves of the coca plant (*Erythroxylon coca*), which is grown primarily in South and Central America. Cocaine hydrochloride, a white crystalline powder, is most commonly inhaled through the nostrils ("snorted"). This method of administration produces an onset of noticeable psychoactive effects approximately 10–15 minutes after inhalation which reach a peak 30–60 minutes thereafter. Since cocaine hydrochloride is soluble in water, it can be injected intravenously. Cocaine freebase or crack, a smokeable form of cocaine, produces an extremely rapid rise in plasma levels and the onset of intense but short-lived euphoric effects ("rush"). Smoking cocaine (pulmonary inhalation) produces similar effects and has essentially the same abuse liability as intravenous injection, but without the social stigma of intravenous use and the hazards associated with non-sterile use of syringes and needles.

Pharmaceutical cocaine is classified by the US Food and Drug Administration as a Schedule II controlled substance owing to its high abuse potential and limited medical usefulness. It is still sometimes used as a local anesthetic in emergency rooms and in eye surgery. Cocaine is both a CNS stimulant and a local anesthetic. Other CNS stimulants such as methamphetamine have no local anesthetic properties whereas other local anesthetics such as novocaine and lidocaine have no CNS stimulant properties.

Methamphetamine, commonly known on the street as speed, crank, crystal or meth, is made in clandestine laboratories from inexpensive and readily available precursor chemicals. Crystal methamphetamine is significantly less expensive than cocaine, but its effects are much longer lasting. It can be snorted, swallowed, or dissolved in water and injected intravenously. It can also be converted to a hard crystalline form known as "ice" for smoking.

Acute psychoactive effects

The acute psychoactive effects of cocaine and methamphetamine can be described as activated euphoria. Stimulant drugs produce increased energy, motivation, mental alertness, and a profound sense of wellbeing. Acute effects may also include sexual arousal, disinhibition, impulsivity, and various types of sexual acting out behaviors.

Although cocaine and methamphetamine are structurally dissimilar, they have very similar pharmacologic actions and subjective effects. Their psychoactive effects have been attributed to activation of neuronal activity in dopaminergic pathways, although collateral neuronal systems are also affected (Hanson & Fleckenstein, 2009). Perhaps the most significant

difference in the effects of cocaine and methamphetamine is their duration of action. Unlike cocaine, which is rapidly metabolized, methamphetamine has a long duration of action. The 10–12-hour half-life of methamphetamine is many times greater than the 30–120-minute half-life of cocaine. The cocaine-induced high typically lasts for less than 1 hour, whereas the methamphetamine-induced high can last for up to 12 hours. Dramatic differences in duration of action can produce markedly different patterns of use and also affect the likelihood of adverse consequences. For example, methamphetamine may be more likely to produce a pattern of marathon high-dose binges resulting in more profound post-drug dysphoria and other adverse effects on mood and mental state, including panic, anxiety, and paranoid psychosis. In addition to its longer duration of action, the lower street price of methamphetamine (which is domestically produced from relatively inexpensive ingredients) makes larger drug supplies and high-dose chronic use more easily accessible to a larger population of users.

The post-stimulant "crash"

When the stimulant high wears off, especially after a prolonged binge, the user's mood typically does not return to pre-drug levels, but instead plummets into a state of agitated dysphoria known as the "crash". This acute dysphoric reaction is characterized by depressed mood, anxiety, fatigue, and irritability accompanied by strong cravings, urges, and a compulsion to re-administer the drug. In general, the severity of the crash is directly related to the dose and longevity of use and also to route of administration. Smoking or injecting as compared to snorting stimulants produces a more intense high and a more severe crash. The post-stimulant crash is time-limited, often resolving without medical intervention following sleep. For some users, however, crash-induced depressive reactions can be extremely severe and may include potentially dangerous but temporary suicidal ideation requiring psychiatric intervention. This profound depressive reaction can occur even in relatively naive, non-dependent users who have no history of depressive disorders or suicidality.

Importantly, the post-stimulant crash is a major contributor to the simultaneous use and abuse of other substances. Alcohol, benzodiazepines, marijuana, and opioids are often used, sometimes in unusually large doses, to counteract the immediate post-stimulant crash and other unpleasant after-effects such as agitation and insomnia. Alcohol is often consumed before, during, and/or after stimulant use not only to cushion the crash, but also to enhance or prolong the stimulant-induced euphoria. Cocaethylene, a byproduct of combining alcohol and cocaine that produces psychoactive effects similar to cocaine but longer lasting, is thought to be an important contributor to simultaneous use of these two substances (Landry, 1992). Similarly, intravenous cocaine users sometimes mix heroin and cocaine in the same syringe (a drug combination known as a "speedball") to enhance the drug-induced euphoria and attenuate unpleasant side-effects. In recent years, snorting heroin or ingesting prescription opioids (e.g. codeine, hydrocodone, oxycodone) have become increasingly popular, especially among middle-class users, as a way to "take the edge off" or "come down" from stimulant drugs.

Substances used in combination with stimulant drugs often become relapse triggers for stimulant drug use (Carroll & Rawson, 2005; Washton & Zweben, 2009). For example, after repeatedly using cocaine and alcohol together, alcohol becomes a conditioned cue or trigger for cocaine cravings and cocaine-seeking behavior, often leading to another episode of stimulant use. Accordingly, when stimulants and alcohol have been used together extensively, abstaining from alcohol is often an important part of preventing relapse to stimulants. This is true even for stimulant users who have no prior history of serious alcohol problems, and understandably are often quite resistant to the idea of not drinking at all, citing their lack of previous problems with alcohol as justifying their intention to return to social drinking while trying to abstain from stimulants. Regrettably, this rarely works out and it often takes one or more alcohol-precipitated relapses to cocaine or methamphetamine use for these individuals to become convinced that abstaining from alcohol is going to be necessary if they want to abstain from using stimulants. A similar scenario unfolds with other substances used repeatedly to "come down" from a run on stimulants and/or alleviate the crash.

Tolerance

With chronic administration, tolerance develops to the drug-induced euphoria and other psychoactive (subjective) effects, as evidenced by the need for increasingly higher doses to achieve the same effects. Some individuals become almost totally immune to the positive psychoactive effects as their stimulant use

becomes increasingly frequent and intensive. This leads to a phenomenon known as "chasing the high," familiar to all experienced cocaine and methamphetamine users. Stimulant users caught in this vicious cycle may experience a fleeting burst of drug-induced euphoria for no more than the first few seconds or minutes after taking each dose followed by a compelling drive to readminister the drug frequently at shorter and shorter intervals. Much to the user's dismay, the desired euphoric effects remain unattainable and are rarely, if ever, recaptured except, perhaps, after a period of sustained abstinence.

Not only does chronic use of large doses cause progressive tolerance to the reinforcing effects of stimulants, but eventually with continuing use the drug may produce the opposite of its previously desired effects. Thus, euphoria can give way to depression, anhedonia, or even paranoid psychosis; sexual arousal can give way to decreased libido and sexual dysfunction; and increased energy and focus can give way to lethargy and distractibility. Continued use despite the absence of reinforcing effects concurrent with progressive accumulation of adverse effects is one of the hallmarks of stimulant dependence.

Withdrawal

Abrupt discontinuation of cocaine or methamphetamine use does not give rise to any major physiological sequelae and therefore does not require tapering or substitution with a cross-tolerant medication. Following the immediate post-drug crash, lingering symptoms of dysphoria, anhedonia, anergia, and sleep disturbance may persist for several days or weeks. These symptoms contrast sharply with the user's memory of the stimulant-induced euphoria, often eliciting intense cravings and urges and yet another cycle of drug use, especially during periods of boredom. With continued abstinence, however, these symptoms steadily improve, but in some cases may require judicious use of sedatives to alleviate persisting insomnia.

Patterns of use

Progression from initial stimulant use to full-blown dependence is not inevitable, but is difficult to predict. The beginning phase of stimulant use is typically associated with few or no identifiable problems. In fact, most who seek treatment for stimulant dependence report that at the outset their drug use facilitated rather than impaired their functioning – at least temporarily.

One factor that significantly influences the transition from initial use to dependence is route of administration. Intranasal use is often associated with a longer "honeymoon" period during which the user experiences primarily, if not exclusively, positive drug effects without any noticeable consequences. Smoking or injecting stimulants, on the other hand, often produces a much more rapid transition from initial to compulsive use. In contrast to cocaine users, methamphetamine users appear more likely to use on a daily basis and to shift from snorting or smoking methamphetamine to injecting it intravenously. This may be due in part to the fact that methamphetamine is severely irritating to both the nasal mucosa and lungs, but may also be because of financial considerations. Smoking methamphetamine requires roughly twice the volume of powder as injecting it to achieve comparable effects.

Stimulants are often used in a binge pattern characterized by periods of intensive use alternating with periods of little or no use. Binges or "runs" can last from several hours to several days until the user's drug supply or money is depleted or he or she collapses from physical exhaustion. Immediately following a binge, the user may feel guilty and remorseful, overwhelmed by negative consequences, strongly motivated to stop using altogether, and determined not to repeat this pattern again. However, with the passage of time from the last binge, the memory of drug-related consequences fades away as fantasies about returning to "occasional" or "controlled" use intensify.

Psychiatric complications

Among stimulant users who present for treatment, it is very difficult to determine whether depressive symptoms commonly associated with chronic stimulant use are caused by a drug-induced depression or an underlying (pre-existing) depressive disorder exacerbated by the stimulant use. More than 50% of stimulant users presenting for treatment meet criteria for concurrent psychiatric disorders and nearly 75% for a lifetime psychiatric diagnosis, including depressive disorders, anxiety disorders, and post-traumatic stress disorders (Ziedonis et al., 1994).

Antidepressants and/or mood stabilizers are not likely to be very effective in patients who are actively using cocaine and/or methamphetamine, but none the less may be helpful during periods of drug abstinence, especially in patients who suffer from an untreated (possibly pre-existing) mood disorder. In general, there are no contraindications in stimulant users to prescribing appropriate non-addictive psychotropic medications for co-occurring mood and other psychiatric disorders.

In addition to mood disturbances, chronic stimulant use can also lead to more severe drug-induced psychiatric problems such as paranoid psychosis, sometimes coupled with extreme agitation and aggressive or violent behavior. Drug-induced psychosis is more likely to occur with methamphetamine than cocaine use and tends to persist considerably longer after cessation of methamphetamine use. Remission of drug-induced psychotic symptoms often occurs within 1–3 days after stopping cocaine use, but may persist for several weeks or even months following cessation of methamphetamine use (Zweben et al., 2004).

Medical consequences

Stimulants produce sympathetic activation as reflected by dose-dependent increases in heart rate, blood pressure, body temperature, basal metabolic rate, muscle tone, and respiration. They also produce hyperglycemia and pupillary dilation. At high doses, especially if smoked or injected intravenously, cocaine and methamphetamine can produce pallor, cold sweat, rapid pulse, tremors, and headache (Mooney et al., 2009).

Serious medical consequences are relatively uncommon in stimulant users as compared, for example, to alcoholics. None the less, high doses can cause serious or life-threatening problems. These include cardiac arrhythmias, cerebral hemorrhage, seizures, respiratory failure, extreme hyperthermia, and sudden death. Fatal reactions to cocaine and methamphetamine, although relatively uncommon, can and do occur.

Some medical consequences are directly related to route of drug administration. Chronic intranasal use (snorting) of cocaine may be associated with chronic sinus infections, perforation of the nasal septum, and repeated nose bleeds. Smoking either cocaine or methamphetamine can cause sore throat, chronic chest congestion, lung infections, and impaired diffusion capacity as a consequence of inhaling hot vapors. Intravenous injection may be associated with abscesses at injection sites and exposure to serious infectious diseases such as HIV and hepatitis owing to sharing of unsterile needles and syringes. The risk of exposure to these and other sexually transmitted diseases is also increased by high-risk sexual behaviors (e.g.

unprotected intercourse with multiple partners) engendered by cocaine and methamphetamine use (Washton, 1989).

Cocaine use during pregnancy is associated with both prenatal and postnatal complications, especially premature delivery or miscarriage owing to drug-induced separation of the placenta – a byproduct of vasoconstriction and reduced blood flow to the uterine wall. Recent studies indicate that fetal exposure to methamphetamine is increasing and has been associated with multiple prenatal complications, such as intraventricular hemorrhage, fetal growth restriction, increased risk of preterm labor, placental abruption, decreased birth weight, cardiac defects, cleft palate, and behavioral effects in neonates (Meredith *et al.*, 2005).

Chronic methamphetamine use has been linked to significant impairments in several arenas of neuropsychological functioning (Meredith *et al.*, 2005). Methamphetamine users appear to develop different cognitive impairments than do abusers of cocaine or other types of drugs. Active users of methamphetamine and cocaine both demonstrate impaired verbal memory, but methamphetamine abusers also demonstrate deficits on tasks of perceptual speed and information processing, and on tasks that combine these skills with visual motor scanning. Additionally, as compared to users of cocaine or heroin, users of methamphetamine or amphetamine also demonstrate deficits on tests of executive function. Clinicians have noted that the cognitive deficits suffered by chronic methamphetamine users can hamper their ability initially to engage in and to benefit from psychologically oriented treatment interventions (Rawson, 1999).

Brain neuroimaging studies using PET scans in humans indicate that certain changes in brain neurotransmitter systems that underlie methamphetamine-induced cognitive deficits appear to normalize during the first year or two following cessation of drug use, but other changes persist for longer periods of time and it remains unclear whether complete reversal of these effects is attainable (Meredith *et al.*, 2005; Payer & London, 2009; Thompson *et al.*, 2004).

Stimulant drugs and hypersexual behavior

Many stimulant users experience strong aphrodisiac effects from cocaine and methamphetamine (Washton, 1989; Washton & Zweben, 2009). The combination of increased sex drive and reduced inhibitions often results in compulsive, hypersexual behaviors that may include, for example, obsessive viewing of pornography, compulsive masturbation, HIV-risky sexual encounters with multiple partners (e.g. prostitutes or other strangers), and paraphilias (e.g. cross-dressing, exhibitionism, fetishism). Other users experience no aphrodisiac effects whatsoever from stimulant drugs. Studies indicate that approximately 40–50% of male stimulant users and 20–30% of female users experience aphrodisiac effects from cocaine or methamphetamine (Washton, 1989; Rawson *et al.*, 2002). Reasons for this gender discrepancy are unknown. Once the link between stimulant use and sex is established, sexual activity of any kind can become a strong relapse trigger for stimulant use. Similarly, stimulant use can trigger a return to drug-related hypersexual behaviors. It can be very hard to break out of this "reciprocal relapse" pattern in which one addictive behavior reliably leads to engaging in the other behavior. Many stimulant users try to stop using the drug without discontinuing their previously drug-related sexual escapades – an effort likely to fail because of the extraordinarily powerful conditioned associations that develop between drug use and sex. Individuals who have acted out sexually under the influence of stimulant drugs often feel extremely embarrassed, guilty, and reluctant to discuss it without the sensitive prompting of a knowledgeable and non-judgmental clinician. Even then, it may require a few sessions to develop enough rapport and trust with the patient before he or she is willing to engage in an open dialogue about drug-related sexual behaviors. An assessment questionnaire to help clinicians identify the nature and extent of the connection between a client's drug use and sexual behavior can be found elsewhere (Washton & Zweben, 2009).

Chronic use of cocaine or methamphetamine, especially in large doses, often impairs sexual performance in both men and women, but none the less may continue to heighten sexual desire and fantasies. The resulting frustration from not being able to achieve sexual satisfaction often drives individuals to engage in increasingly intense and/or unusual sexual behaviors. Erectile dysfunction and anorgasmia are common sequelae of chronic stimulant use leading, in recent years, to increasing use of sildenafil and other PDE5 inhibitors to help alleviate stimulant-induced sexual dysfunction.

Pharmacotherapy

There is currently no effective pharmacotherapy for treating stimulant dependence. Since intense drug craving is a standard feature of stimulant dependence, a great deal of research effort has been channeled into identifying medications that may help to reduce craving and other biologically based contributors to relapse (Vocci *et al.*, 2009). Thus far, numerous medications have appeared promising in initial open trials, but have not demonstrated efficacy in controlled clinical studies. These medications include dopamine agonists (e.g. amantadine, bromocriptine, methylphenidate, pergolide), carbamazepine, and antidepressants (e.g. desipramine, fluoxetine, bupropion). A meta-analysis of 45 clinical trials concluded that these agents had no consistently positive effect on treatment outcome in stimulant users, regardless of the type or dose of medication used (Lima *et al.*, 2002).

The idea of substituting cocaine or methamphetamine with another CNS stimulant that has similar effects but less abuse potential has gained recent attention (Moeller *et al.*, 2008). Similar to buprenorphine or methadone replacement therapy for opioid dependence, the goal of stimulant replacement therapy would be to reduce cravings and other post-stimulant symptoms and thereby promote abstinence. Findings from a systematic review of controlled clinical trials evaluating the efficacy of a number of CNS stimulants (including dextroamphetamine, methylphenidate, modafinil, and bupropion) do not, however, provide strong support for using these stimulants to treat cocaine dependence (Castells *et al.*, 2007). None the less, some studies do suggest that these substitute medications, especially dextroamphetamine and modafinil, may have some potential utility in treating cocaine and methamphetamine dependence but further research is clearly needed (Dackis *et al.*, 2005; Shearer, 2008).

One pharmacological agent shown to be helpful in treating stimulant dependence is disulfiram or Antabuse (Carroll *et al.*, 1998; 2004; Vocci & Elkashef, 2005). The efficacy of disulfiram can be attributed to its ability to deter alcohol consumption – a common relapse trigger for stimulant use.

More recent pharmacological research has focused on developing anti-cocaine vaccines that may attenuate or block CNS absorption into the brain (Sofuoglu & Kosten, 2005), but to date this work remains entirely experimental. Recent studies have also been trying to identify agents that may influence mechanisms by which stimulants are absorbed, metabolized, and excreted by the body, and give rise to their characteristic reinforcing effects in the brain (Vocci *et al.*, 2009).

It appears that pharmacotherapy is unlikely to provide a "magic bullet" for stimulant dependence. Experience with medications used for treating other types of drug dependencies supports the general notion that pharmacologic agents are likely to be most effective when combined with appropriate psychosocial intervention and support.

Psychosocial treatment

Treatment for stimulant dependence, as currently practised in the US, is delivered mainly in structured outpatient treatment programs, also known as intensive outpatient programs or IOPS. Access to inpatient treatment for stimulant dependence is severely limited by third party payers owing to the absence of a stimulant withdrawal syndrome requiring medical management. In some cases, reimbursement for short-term inpatient care is approved for patients who have failed repeatedly to establish and/or sustain abstinence in structured outpatient programs. Stimulant users are more likely to qualify for reimbursement of inpatient care when there is a serious co-occurring psychiatric disorder such as psychosis and/or suicidal depression.

With the marked shift of stimulant dependence treatment into outpatient programs in recent years, considerable effort has been channeled into developing comprehensive manualized treatment approaches aimed at improving the effectiveness and consistency of treatment delivered in these programs. These approaches incorporate cognitive behavioral therapy techniques, including the relapse prevention strategies described originally by Marlatt & Gordon (1985). The matrix model, perhaps the most extensively researched approach to treating stimulant dependence to date, was developed initially for treating cocaine dependence and later adapted for treating methamphetamine dependence (Center for Substance Abuse Treatment, 2006a, b; Obert *et al.*, 1995; Rawson *et al.*, 1995). This comprehensive manualized approach incorporates not only relapse prevention strategies, but also motivational interviewing techniques, psychoeducation, family counseling, and twelve-step program involvement. Other manualized treatment approaches for stimulant dependence include contingency management (CMA; Iguchi *et al.*, 1997), community reinforcement (CRA;

Higgins *et al.*, 1993), interpersonal psychotherapy (IPT; Carroll *et al.*, 1991), and modified dynamic group psychotherapy (MDGP; Khantzian *et al.*, 1990). In addition to these approaches, developed mainly for use in agency-based addiction treatment programs, Washton & Zweben (2006; 2009) have described an integrative approach for treating stimulant dependence and other substance use disorders (SUDs) in office-based psychotherapy practice.

Therapy manuals and patient workbooks for treating stimulant dependence are available from a variety of publications (Carroll, 1998; Daley *et al.*, 2002; Mercer & Woody, 1999; Obert *et al.*, 1995; Sheets, 2003; Washton, 2008), and at no cost from government agencies (http://ncadi.samhsa.gov).

Regardless of treatment approach, patient participation in self-help programs, especially when combined with formal treatment, can enhance treatment retention and outcomes (Donovan & Wells, 2007). Twelve-step programs, including Alcoholics Anonymous (AA), Narcotics Anonymous (NA), Cocaine Anonymous (CA), and Crystal Meth Anonymous (CMA), comprise the largest and most widely available self-help system in the US and elsewhere. Several alternative support groups (e.g. SMART Recovery) have become available in recent years, albeit on a much smaller scale.

Phases of treatment

The treatment of stimulant dependence and other SUDs is often divided into four phases: engagement, abstinence initiation, relapse prevention, and ongoing or later-stage recovery.

Engagement

Perhaps the greatest challenge in treating stimulant users is to engage patients in treatment, enhance their motivation for change, and prevent them from dropping out prematurely. Often this requires the clinician to "start where the patient is" and to coax rather than pressure the patient to accept the need for change. Motivational interviewing (MI) techniques (Miller & Rollnick, 1991) provide clinicians with a useful set of interventions for accomplishing these tasks. In contrast to the traditional view that substance users become ready for change only after they have "hit bottom" owing to increasingly severe consequences, the MI approach seeks to accelerate the process of deciding to change in a gentler, more therapeutic manner. Once the clinician

has identified which stage of change the client is in, as described in the stages of change model (Prochaska *et al.*, 1992), various MI techniques can be utilized to enhance and motivate the patient's readiness for change. MI fosters a more engaging stance toward clients using a variety of client-centered (Rogerian) therapy techniques such as rolling with resistance, avoiding arguments, expressing empathy, and supporting self-efficacy.

Establishing abstinence

Stopping stimulant use completely rather than tapering gradually is the recommended strategy for initiating abstinence since there is no withdrawal syndrome to manage and continuing use at any level is likely to reignite and/or strengthen drug cravings and the impulse to use again. It is helpful to see clients frequently during the initial quitting stage to provide the needed structure, support, and guidance for breaking the recurrent pattern of stimulant use. Specific quitting strategies include, among others, breaking off contact with dealers and users, discarding drug supplies and paraphernalia, learning how to manage drug cravings and urges safely, identifying triggers and other "high risk" situations likely to re-initiate drug use, stopping the use of alcohol and other drugs, structuring and planning activities to prevent boredom and to minimize windows of opportunity for drug use, establishing a recovery support system, and implementing a schedule of urine drug testing to establish accountability and reduce the likelihood of acting on impulses to use. These strategies are described in greater detail in other publications (e.g. Carroll, 1998; Rawson, 1999; Washton & Zweben, 2009). Additional quitting strategies must be implemented when stimulant use is strongly linked with compulsive sexual behaviors (Washton & Zweben, 2009). As stated earlier, this linkage markedly amplifies the reinforcing effects of stimulant drugs, making abstinence more difficult to achieve unless pointedly addressed.

Relapse prevention

Once abstinence is firmly established, the focus of treatment shifts progressively from establishing to maintaining abstinence, i.e. toward preventing relapse (Washton, 1988; Carroll & Rawson, 2005). It has often been said that stopping cocaine or methamphetamine use is considerably easier than staying stopped over the long term. As described originally by Marlatt & Gordon (1985), relapse prevention or RP strategies are designed to help individuals who are attempting to change an addictive behavior learn how to anticipate, avoid, and cope with "high-risk situations" and other contributors to relapse. RP strategies teach clients: 1) how to anticipate and prevent the occurrence of a relapse after initial abstinence has been firmly established; 2) how to respond safely to the occurrence of a "slip" so as to short-circuit the tendency for a slip to escalate into a full-blown relapse; and 3) how to counteract an individual's desire to test control over drug use after a period of sustained abstinence. RP strategies involve a combination of psychoeducation, therapeutic confrontation, and skill development. Educating patients about the relapse process and helping them to acquire problem-solving and affect management skills are essential components of RP strategies.

Ongoing or later-stage recovery

As patients remain abstinent and the recovery process continues to unfold, psychological issues intertwined with the addiction often rise to the surface and become increasingly evident. If left unaddressed, these issues can contribute to an elevated relapse potential as "silent" generators of the desire to self-medicate intolerable moods and affects. Many individuals who become addicted to drugs are seen as "self-medicating" with these agents resulting from deficits in their ability to regulate their emotions, maintain a stable sense of self, and deal effectively with interpersonal conflict and other relationship problems (Dodes & Khantzian, 1991; Khantzian, 1997). In addition, many have unresolved psychological issues stemming from severe life traumas, including physical or sexual abuse, early parental death or abandonment, life-threatening illness, severe physical disability, etc. When appropriate and indicated, recovery-focused individual and/or group psychotherapy can be very helpful to patients in ongoing and later-stage recovery (Washton & Zweben, 2006).

Summary

Cocaine and methamphetamine use in the US continues to be a major public health problem. The pharmacology of stimulant drugs contributes to their high abuse potential and to unique behavioral effects, including stimulant-induced hypersexuality. Despite significant advances in the understanding of brain mechanisms underlying stimulant effects, no effective pharmacotherapy for stimulant dependence is currently available. Psychosocial treatment approaches rely heavily on cognitive behavioral techniques aimed at helping stimulant users establish and maintain abstinence. Psychodynamic approaches can be helpful in addressing the complex psychological and emotional issues often intertwined with stimulant dependence.

References

Anglin, M. D., Burke, C., Perrochet, B., Stamper, E. & Dawud-Noursi, S. (2000). History of the methamphetamine problem. *Journal of Psychoactive Drugs*, **32**(2), 137–41.

Carroll, K. M. (1998). *A Cognitive-Behavioral Approach: Treating Cocaine Addiction*. Rockville, MD: U.S. Department of Health and Human Services.

Carroll, K. M. & Rawson, R. A. (2005). Relapse prevention for stimulant dependence. In *Relapse Prevention: Maintenance Strategies in the Treatment of Addictive Disorders*, eds. G. A. Marlatt & D. M. Donovan. New York: Guilford Press.

Carroll, K. M., Rounsaville, B. J. & Gawin, F. H. (1991). A comparative trial of psychotherapies for ambulatory cocaine abusers: relapse prevention and interpersonal psychotherapy. *American Journal of Drug and Alcohol Abuse*, **17**(3), 229–47.

Carroll, K. M., Nich, C., Ball, S. A., McCance, E. F. & Rounsaville, B. (1998). Treatment of cocaine and alcohol dependence with psychotherapy and disulfiram. *Addiction*, **93**, 713–28.

Carroll, K. M., Fenton, L. R., Ball, S. A. *et al.* (2004). Efficacy of disulfiram and cognitive behavior therapy in cocaine-dependent outpatients: a randomized placebo-controlled trial. *Archives of General Psychiatry*, **61**(3), 264–72.

Castells, X., Casas, M., Vidal, X. *et al.* (2007). Efficacy of central nervous system stimulant treatment for cocaine dependence: a systematic review and meta-analysis of randomized controlled clinical trials. *Addiction*, **102**(12), 1871–87.

Center for Substance Abuse Treatment. (2006a). *Counselor's Treatment Manual: Matrix Intensive Outpatient Treatment for People with Stimulant Use Disorders*. Rockville, MD: Substance Abuse and Mental Health Services Administration.

Center for Substance Abuse Treatment. (2006b). *Client's Handbook: Matrix Intensive Outpatient Treatment for People with Stimulant Use Disorders*. Rockville, MD: Substance Abuse and Mental Health Services Administration.

Dackis, C. A., Kampman, K. M., Lynch, K. G., Pettinati, H. M. & O'Brien, C. P. (2005). A double-blind, placebo-controlled trial of modafinil for cocaine dependence. *Neuropsychopharmacology*, **30**(1), 205–11.

Daley, D. C., Mercer, D. & Carpenter, G. (2002). *Drug Counseling for Cocaine Addiction: The Collaborative Cocaine Treatment Study Model*. National Institute of Health Publication. No. 02–438. Available online at http://www.drugabuse.gov/pdf/Manual4.pdf.

Dodes, L. M. & Khantzian, E. J. (1991). Individual psychodynamic psychotherapy. In *Clinical Textbook of Addictive Disorders*, eds. R. J. Frances & S. I. Miller. New York: Guilford, pp. 391–405.

Donovan, D. M. & Wells, E. A. (2007). Tweaking 12-step. The potential role of 12-step self-help group involvement in methamphetamine recovery. *Addiction*, **102**(Suppl. 1), 121–9.

Ellis, R. J., Childers, M. E., Cherner, M. *et al.* (2003). Increased human immunodeficiency virus loads in active methamphetamine users are explained by reduced effectiveness of antiretroviral therapy. *Journal of Infectious Diseases*, **12**, 1820–6.

Frosch, D., Shoptaw, S., Huber, A. & Ling, W. (1996). Sexual HIV risk among gay and bisexual male methamphetamine users. *Journal of Substance Abuse Treatment*, **13**, 483–6.

Hanson, G. R. & Fleckenstein, A. E. (2009). Basic neuropharmacological mechanisms. In *Methamphetamine Addiction: from Basic Science to Treatment*, eds. J. M. Roll, R. A. Rawson, W. Ling & S. Shoptaw. New York: Guilford Press, pp. 30–60.

Higgins, S. T., Budney, A. J., Bickel, W. K. *et al.* (1993). Achieving cocaine abstinence with a behavioral approach. *American Journal of Psychiatry*, **150**, 1218–24.

Iguchi, M. Y., Belding, M. A., Morral, A. R. *et al.* (1997). Reinforcing operants other than abstinence in drug abuse treatment: an effective alternative for reducing drug use. *Journal of Consulting and Clinical Psychology*, **65**(3), 421–8.

Khantzian, E. J. (1997). The self-medication hypothesis of substance use disorders: a reconsideration and recent applications. *Harvard Review of Psychiatry*, **4**, 231–44.

Khantzian, E. J., Halliday, K. S. & McAuliffe, W. E. (1990). *Addiction and the Vulnerable Self: Modified Dynamic Group Therapy for Substance Abusers*. New York: Guilford Press.

King, G. R. & Ellinwood, E. H. (2005). Amphetamines and other stimulants. In *Substance Abuse: A Comprehensive Textbook*, eds. J. H. Lowinson, P. Ruiz, R. B. Millman & J. G. Langrod. Philadelphia: Lippincott, Williams & Wilkins, pp. 277–302.

Kroutil, L. A., Van Brunt, D. L., Herman-Stahl, M. A. *et al.* (2006). Nonmedical use of prescription stimulants in the United States. *Drug and Alcohol Dependence*, **84**(2), 135–43.

Landry, M. J. (1992). An overview of cocaethylene: an alcohol-derived, psychoactive, cocaine metabolite. *Journal of Psychoactive Drugs*, **24**(3), 273–6.

Lima, M. S., Soares, B. G., Reisser, A. & Farrell, M. (2002). Pharmacologic treatment of cocaine dependence: a systematic review. *Addiction*, **8**, 931–49.

Marlatt, G. A. & Gordon, J. R. (eds.) (1985). *Relapse Prevention*. New York: Guilford Press.

McCabe, S. E., Knight, J. R., Teter, C. J. & Wechsler, H. (2005). Non-medical use of prescription stimulants among US college students: prevalence and correlates from a national survey. *Addiction*, **100**(1), 96–106.

Mercer, D. E. & Woody, G. E. (1999). *An Individual Drug Counseling Approach to Treat Cocaine Addiction: The Collaborative Cocaine Treatment Study Model*. Rockville, MD: National Institute on Drug Abuse, NIH Publication Number 99–4380.

Meredith, C. W., Jaffe, C., Ang-Lee, K. & Saxon, A. J. (2005). Implications of chronic methamphetamine use: a literature review. *Harvard Review of Psychiatry*, **13**(3), 141–54.

Miller, W. R., Rollnick, S. (1991). *Motivational Interviewing: Preparing People to Change Addictive Behavior*. New York: Guilford Press.

Moeller, F. G., Schmitz, J. M., Herin, D. & Kjome, K. L. (2008). Use of stimulants to treat cocaine and methamphetamine abuse. *Current Psychiatry Reports*, **10**(5), 385–91.

Mooney, L., Glasner-Edwards, S., Rawson, R. A. & Ling, W. (2009). Medical effects of methamphetamine use. In *Methamphetamine Addiction: From Basic Science to Treatment*, eds J. M. Roll, R. A. Rawson, W. Ling & S. Shoptaw. New York: Guilford Press, pp. 117–42.

Obert, J. L., Rawson, R. A., McCann, M. A. & Ling, W. (1995). *Matrix Model Therapist's Manual: A 16-Week Individualized Program*. Center City, MN: Hazelden.

Payer, D. & London, E. D. (2009). Methamphetamine and the brain: findings from brain imaging studies. In *Methamphetamine Addiction: from Basic Science to Treatment*, eds. J. M. Roll, R. A. Rawson, W. Ling & S. Shoptaw. New York: Guilford Press, pp. 61–91.

Prochaska, J. O., DiClemente, C. C. & Norcross, J. C. (1992). In search of how people change: applications to addictive behaviors. *American Psychologist*, **47**, 1102–14.

Rawson, R. A. (1999). *Treatment for Stimulant Use Disorders. Treatment Improvement Protocol Series (TIP) No. 33.* DHHS Publication No. (SMA) 99–3296. Rockville, Maryland: U.S. Department of Health and Human Services.

Rawson, R. A., Shoptaw, S. J., McCann, M. J. *et al.* (1995). An intensive outpatient approach for cocaine abuse treatment: the matrix model. *Journal of Substance Abuse Treatment*, **12**(2), 117–27.

Rawson, R. A., Washton, A. M., Domier, C. P. & Reiber, C. (2002). Drugs and sexual effects: role of drug type and gender. *Journal of Substance Abuse Treatment*, **22**(2), 103–8.

Rutkowski, B. A. & Maxwell, J. C. (2009). Epidemiology of methamphetamine use: a global perspective. In *Methamphetamine Addiction: from Basic Science to Treatment*, eds. J. M. Roll, R. A. Rawson, W. Ling & S. Shoptaw. New York: Guilford Press, pp. 6–29.

Shearer, J. (2008). The principles of agonist pharmacotherapy for psychostimulant dependence. *Drug and Alcohol Review*, **27**(3), 301–8.

Sheets, M. T. (2003). *Quitting Methamphetamine: your Personal Recovery Plan*. Center City, MN: Hazelden.

Shoptaw, S., Rawson, R. A., McCann, M. J. & Obert, J. L. (1994). The matrix model of outpatient stimulant abuse treatment: evidence of efficacy. *Journal of Addictive Diseases*, **13**(4), 129–41.

Sofuoglu, M. & Kosten, T. R. (2005). Novel approaches to the treatment of cocaine addiction. *CNS Drugs*, **19**(1), 13–25.

Thompson, P. M., Hayashi, K. M., Simon, S. L. *et al.* (2004). Structural abnormalities in the brains of human subjects who use methamphetamine. *Journal of Neuroscience*, **24**(26), 6028–36.

Vocci, F. J. & Elkashef, A. (2005). Pharmacotherapy and other treatments for cocaine abuse and dependence. *Current Opinions in Psychiatry*, **18**(3), 265–70.

Vocci, F. J., Elkashef, A. & Appell, N. M. (2009). Pharmacological treatment of methamphetamine addiction. In *Methamphetamine Addiction: from Basic Science to Treatment*, eds. J. M. Roll, R. A. Rawson, W. Ling & S. Shoptaw. New York: Guilford Press, pp. 202–29.

Washton, A. M. (1987). Cocaine: drug epidemic of the 1980's. In *The Cocaine Crisis*, ed. D. Allen. New York: Plenum Press, pp. 45–64.

Washton, A. M. (1988). Preventing relapse to cocaine. *Journal of Clinical Psychiatry*, **49**, 34–8.

Washton, A. M. (1989). Cocaine and compulsive sexuality. *Medical Aspects of Human Sexuality, December*, 32–9.

Washton, A. M. (2008). *Quitting Cocaine: Your Personal Recovery Plan*. Center City, MN: Hazelden Foundation.

Washton, A. M. & Gold, M. S. (1986). Crack. *Journal of the American Medical Association*, **256**, 711.

Washton, A. M. & Zweben, J. E. (2006). *Treating Alcohol and Drug Problems in Psychotherapy Practice: Doing What Works*. New York: Guilford.

Washton, A. M. & Zweben, J. E. (2009). *Cocaine and Methamphetamine Addiction: Treatment, Recovery, and Relapse Prevention*. New York: Guilford.

Washton, A. M., Gold, M. S. & Pottash, A. C. (1984). Upper-income cocaine abusers. *Advances in Alcohol and Substance Abuse*, **4**(2), 51–7.

Ziedonis, D. M., Rayford, B.S., Bryant, K. J., Rounsaville, B. J. (1994). Psychiatric comorbidity in white and African-American cocaine addicts seeking substance abuse treatment. *Hospital and Community Psychiatry*, **45**(1), 43–9.

Zweben, J. E., Cohen, J. B., Christian, D. *et al.* (2004). Psychiatric symptomatology in methamphetamine users. *American Journal on Addiction*, **13**, 181–90.

Methadone treatment

Robert Maslansky

Review of the salient history

In 1966 two senior physicians and a first year resident in internal medicine training at Cornell Medical School's New York Hospital shifted a paradigm in the management of opioid dependence (Dole & Nyswander, 1965). Vincent Dole of the Rockefeller Institute (now Rockefeller University), a laboratory director investigating the metabolic substrates of obesity, changed the trajectory of his career. Marie Nyswander, a physician psychoanalyst, ran a walk-in storefront mental health clinic in Harlem. Her book, *The Drug Addict as a Patient*, caught Dole's eye (Nyswander, 1957). The third of the triumvirate was Mary Jeanne Kreek, the first year resident. At that time, New York City was being assailed by yet another heroin epidemic. There were many heroin overdose deaths. Insidiously, it crept into every socio-economic, ethnic, and geographic niche of New York. Arrests for violating any aspect of the complicated drug offense laws were at an all-time high. And most distressing, the age of the offenders and those who died was declining.

John Vliet Lindsey took office as mayor on New Year's Day, 1966. Among his first promises to the city was to address the heroin epidemic now raging. His options were to increase enforcement personnel assigned to containing supply. This meant more police on the street, more judges, and for those indicted and going to trial more years behind bars and more, much more, alienation for an ever larger segment of the population.

The other approach was to reduce demand. This meant rethinking treatment options for heroin dependency and addiction. Since the 1920s and early 1930s the concept of maintenance therapy for the disease of opiate addiction had not been a consideration (Musto, 1987). The body of law developed around the Harrison Narcotics Tax Act of December 1914 ruled out open-ended use of an opiate or opioid solely for the purposes of sustaining dependency. Under the fierce and combative leadership of Harry Anslinger, the Federal Bureau of Narcotics closed clinics in the US whose

purpose was to use narcotics only for maintaining the dependency. Many of these physicians were taken into custody, indicted, tried, and sentenced to long prison terms. This was the law when Mayor Lindsey took office. The rethinking challenge was given to Vincent Dole. He and his colleagues Nyswander and Kreek created rigorously designed experiments to establish the effectiveness and the efficacy of opiate maintenance for *the disease* of opiate/opioid dependency and addiction. Given the chronic and relapsing nature of the disease, all measures taken to detoxify, rehabilitate, and then maintain recovery without medication assistance had a disappointingly low success profile.

Review of the practical pharmacology of methadone

The success pharmacologically (and legally) turned on the selection of a pure μ-agonist meeting specific goals.

1. It needed to be long-action. The pharmacokinetics (what the body does to the drug) must be such that a dosing schedule of once a day orally would be feasible.
2. It must have a safety profile established by its use as a pain-relieving agonist. It should have years of clinical use without a negative impact on the kidneys, the heart, the liver, the lungs, skeletal system, the central and the peripheral nervous systems, the blood, and the immune capacity.
3. It should not be prohibitively expensive to scale up production.
4. Its oral route of administration should have approximately one half the bioavailability of the parenteral route. This should be recalled when there is a switch to the oral route of administration. Because of its high lipid solubility, its functional half-life should be longer than morphine-based drugs.

In Vancouver, Canada, as early as 1959, the physicians at the Narcotic Addiction Foundation were interested in methadone for short-term treatment. The position of precedence belongs to this group for having introduced long-term maintenance in 1963. It was at the prestigious Rockefeller Institute, however, where the definitive clinical investigations established open-ended treatment with methadone. Please note that the Dole protocol was tightly coupled to psychosocial interventions (Dole *et al.*, 1966).

The pharmacodynamics (what the drug does to the body) must be as specific as possible to substitute for diacetylmorphine (heroin) and, perhaps, be preferred to heroin. Methadone is almost a perfect fit. The mu (mu for morphine) receptor avidly binds methadone. When this occurs it is designated as having intrinsic activity at that receptor and a cascade of neurochemical events follow: 1) relief of withdrawal sickness; 2) there is a realistic feeling of wellbeing consistent with pursuing a crime-free style of living; 3) a blockade is established, to a degree, to the use of heroin. The latter is dose-dependent (Code of Federal Regulations, 2010).

Methadone is a DEA Schedule II medication. Its use for pain relief is well established. Among the facts mixed with apocrypha is that it was the product of the German pharmaceutical industry, I Farben, Hoechst-Am-Main shortly before World War 2 (1937). On September 11, 1941, Bockmuhl and Erhardt patented the formula for Polamidon, now known as methadone, the name given to this new chemical entity. Its structure was unrelated to morphine or its derivatives but it had almost all of the pharmacodynamic properties of morphine.

In part its invention was mothered by necessity. Opium-derived analgesics were not available to the Third Reich. No country where the opium poppy was grown was under Germany's hegemony. Those are facts. That its proprietary name, *Doloph*ine, *was* in honor of Adolph (The Führer) Hitler is apocryphal. "*Dolo*" is derived from the Latin, *dolor*, that translates as "pain" in English. Eli Lilly introduced the medication to the US in 1947.

Its use for maintenance at the outset was not encumbered by threats of prosecution. It became a tightly regulated drug, however, when it was used for open-ended treatment of dependency and addiction.

Running a methadone treatment program

Regulations and rules

Local, state, and federal agencies have, over the years, created a web of regulations for the methadone

treatment community that is daunting. Not adhering to them will cause practitioners to answer for their lapses. Under the threat of sanctions, clinics expend energy and money to gain and, if required, regain their good name and the community's trust.

Fortunately, the governance over methadone clinics recognizes the dynamics of treatment. The rules are changed, most often for the better, when change is needed. As an example: permission to take doses of methadone away from the clinic to be used later that day (this is called "split dosing") is now permitted. More leniency for "take-home" bottles has evolved over the years. Patients who have stabilized their lives, who have legitimate employment, or who have childcare obligations and who have demonstrated by toxicological examinations, often supervised (observed while urinating), a profile of non-use of *any* other inappropriate and/or illegal drugs may take home as much as 4 weeks' medication. In many places throughout the treatment program community, substituting saliva toxicological examination is now permitted, easing the burden on staff as well as eliminating a potentially humiliating experience, the taking of observed urine specimens.

Though agencies try to create an environment sympathetic to a clinic's location in populated parts of the community, NIMBY (Not In My Back Yard) often carries the day when plans for a new treatment center are announced.

In 1996 the Federal Department of Health and Human Services (DHHS) codified patient confidentiality, announcing the Health Insurance Portability & Accountability Act (HIPAA). One of its important corollaries is the strict enforcement of patient confidentiality (Code of Federal Regulations). It is settled law noted in the Code of Federal Regulations (CFR 42, Part 2). This is of significance to methadone-treated patients. Many have had involvements with the law. Some are on parole from unfinished prison terms. Some are on probation. Some have outstanding warrants for arrest. A patient coming to an institutional setting such as a treatment facility worries about privacy and the possibility that the clinic will report his or her presence to the police. The HIPAA regulations abide in a methadone treatment clinic. With this assurance of confidentiality, the work of rehabilitation can commence.

Staffing

There are more than 1200 methadone treatment facilities in the US. The pattern of staffing varies widely throughout the treatment community. A maximum caseload of 50 clients per counselor meets all regulatory constraints (Fuller *et al.*, 2006). If manageable, each counselor should be limited to 40 clients. The funding stream dictates staffing. If a clinic depends solely on reimbursement from Medicaid or any other entitlement program, then a problem emerges. Motivation to enjoin patients to find work "on the books" would run counter to the clinic's "*Business Plan.*" When a patient becomes employed the Medicaid payments stop. The clinic is starved for operating capital. What a paradox! Treat someone successfully and there will be less money to treat others. Services will be compromised. Creative Arts therapy, a dynamic part of the treatment landscape, may be the first to go. Next on the block would be vocational services, an essential for uncompromised recovery. Sadly, such clinics must abandon the Dole–Nyswander vision of 40 years ago (Dole & Nyswander, 1965).

> This treatment (op. cit.) requires careful medical supervision and many social services. In our opinion, both the medication and the supporting program are essential.

Administrators, those not directly concerned with patient care, must be chosen carefully. Often, if the clinic is part of a larger healthcare provider, i.e. a community hospital, selecting new hires is not within the province of the clinic leadership. It must take what it gets. The cautionary note to be struck has to do with staff attitudes toward patients. The administrative staff is the first to greet the new patient. They must create a climate of hope, not judgment. They must be professional in their demeanor but demonstrate genuine concern. This means listening creatively. The mean streets from which most patients have come take their toll. New patients are giving away a lot of pseudo-freedom when they come to a place that is known by some as "the clinic with liquid handcuffs." There is a crude semi-truth to the utterance by a rock star from long ago, "(F)reedom's when you ain't got nothing more to lose" (Hartnoll, 1994). Persons who come to the door of a methadone treatment facility often, but not always, are down to their last dimes. There is nothing else for them to lose other than their lives. Many are angry, furious in fact, at the prospect of losing their only friend … a bag of heroin. Those that man the front gate need to understand that the fury they see from time to time is the profound ambivalence a new patient brings to that gate.

Governance

Clinics establish a clear division of labor. The nurses are responsible for medicating patients. This includes preparing take-home medication for Sundays if the clinic is not open on Sundays and for patients granted additional "*off*" days.

The final authority is the individual who writes the orders for medication, the physician, or in some locations a physician's assistant or a nurse practitioner under the supervision of the licensed physician. Well run clinics have, it has been noted, one striking commonality – responsibility for certain aspects of treatment, as much as possible, should not be split away from the authority to carry out those therapeutic decisions. Though there are rare instances where the physician or his surrogate must make the final judgment, the staff must be given agency to carry out their jobs.

Clinics can run aground. There are layers of officialdom with the charge to examine all aspects of the operation and impose sanctions if there are deficiencies. The examinations by the Joint Commission for Health Care Accreditation (JCAHO), the Food & Drug Administration (FDA), the Drug Enforcement Administration (DEA), and the local and state authorities can be daunting. They are an imperative, however. They must go forward. The well-advised clinic takes them in its stride and goes on with its work.

Now that opiate substitution therapy is accepted as the gold standard for the management of most people suffering, and indeed it is suffering, from relapsing, chronic opiate addiction, clinics can be found throughout western and central Europe, Israel, Australia, South Africa, and China. How clinics are governed, how they are organized, varies widely. The American standards of care are not necessarily the model for other countries. It should be noted that some countries with well known heroin addiction problems are shockingly absent from this list.

Who pays the bills?

It is assumed that a life (anyone's life, to be valued, especially by the one who is living it) must have as one of its components a way of spending days meaningfully. Most, if they are not impaired so as to pre-empt it, feel that work in one form or other brings this value. The heroin user on the street needs to be fully occupied with his job. His full-time employment, with much overtime, is to bring in sufficient income so that for most of the hours of the day he feels well enough to carry on until the next time he purchases and uses heroin. Giving up this pursuit must have a compelling reason or, indeed, reasons. Many heroin users are in the heroin business. There are specialties in the "trade."

All specialties provide a reasonable income, some with only modest risk. Street sales have the most liabilities and, in the short term, the biggest margin. The ubiquitous cell phone now leads to anonymous home deliveries, thus making street sales less complicated. Free product is often one of the perks.

Preparation of the product for market employs many who are risk-aversive. This requires several specialties. Cutting the heroin with an additive, thus increasing the margin of profit, is one such specialty. Packaging is another. Delivery to the large markets, western Europe and the US, is yet another. Getting raw material out of the poppy fields of Afghanistan, Mexico, Kazakhstan, Colombia, and many other producing countries, and processing it to diacetylmorphine (heroin) are specialties as well. Delivering product from laboratories in Afghanistan, Turkey, Syria, Myanmar, and other producers is done in a variety of ways, some ingenious, some lethal if something goes wrong. Heroin is packaged in a contraceptive rubber and then swallowed, perhaps five or six to a person (called "mules" in the trade); when delivered to its destination this may realize US$10 000 or more for the pure wholesale merchandize. This, in turn, may turn around and be sold on the street for US$100 000 properly cut and bagged. For many merchants this is a pot of gold!

The answer, indeed "answers" to the question, "(W)hy are you coming into treatment *now* rather than yesterday or tomorrow or a year from now?" Most say in various ways, "I'm tired of the streets. I'm tired of spending every last dollar on dope." "I'm sick and tired of being sick and tired."

In the US the complicated healthcare payment structure for medical services and for medication does not reduce to a manageable formula. Most patients in most methadone treatment clinics arrive impoverished. If a new patient brings with him entitlements such as Medicaid, the state and federally funded programs for the payment of medical services and for medications, then Medicaid may apply, but not always, and not everywhere. According to data updated to 1994, approximately 45% of the patients have Medicaid (Hartnoll, 1994). Some insurance carriers will cover the cost of opiate substitution therapy with a deductible and a co-pay. Self-pay patients represent 10–15% of the treated population. Self-pay patients are charged according to their means. Whatever they are charged, it rarely covers the cost of their treatment. Most clinics survive fiscally only if the patients with entitlements (insurance, Medicaid, and Medicare) far outnumber the self-pay population. Some clinics are fortunate enough to have grants that cover part of the operating cost. When the US joins most of the nations of western Europe and Canada with a single party payer healthcare system with universal coverage then, and only then, will there be certainty that people in need of opiate substitution therapy will get it, hassle-free.

Who are the patients and what do they want?

The demographics of age and ethnicity for opiate addiction are a reflection of the community the particular clinic serves (Gossop *et al.*, 2003). This may come as a surprise to some preferring to think that the middle and wealthy classes are rarely heroin and/or opiate/opioid medication misusers. It has not been true in the past nor is it now. Dependency leading to addiction cuts a broad swathe through communities. It has little regard for economic means or/and social status. It is true that people with resources may be able to sidestep methadone treatment and sustain their dependency in other ways. Now that buprenorphine treatment is an option this becomes as easy as finding a physician who is certified to prescribe the two formulations of buprenorphine (more about this below).

It is essential that clinic personnel not overestimate a new patient's desire to change. Nor should they underestimate a patient's capacity to change once this chronic relapsing disease is brought under control. The medical and social services literature regularly reviews recovery goals and the percentages of patients achieving these goals. Some of the markers are: 1) staying out of trouble with the law; 2) entering the tax-paying workforce; 3) maintaining employment; 4) structuring or restructuring connections with family and friends; and 5) addressing serious health issues with consistency, i.e. HIV/AIDS, hepatitis C & B, diabetes, and hypertension.

If a patient is determined to end methadone dependency irrespective of not having achieved success, especially success in eliminating heroin use, the regulations require that the staff proceed with a tapering schedule. This should *not* be referred to as a methadone detox. Methadone used as part of a complete therapeutic strategy is not toxic. The term taper is to be used just as it is when any medication is discontinued slowly.

Other drugs used by patients in methadone treatment programs

Methadone's pharmacodynamics substitute for those dependent and addicted to pure μ-agonists. In a year, 80% of methadone patients stop using opiates (heroin and pharmaceutical opioids) (Shi *et al.*, 2008). The ambience of a clinic with its emphasis on recovery takes patients' use of other abusable drugs, licit or illicit, as a treatment issue. Manifest evidence for use, i.e. obvious impairment or, indeed, a patient's acknowledgment of the use of cocaine or benzodiazepines or alcohol, is one way. The use of toxicological examinations, though costly and fraught with technical difficulties, is another. Regulatory bodies require this. How often and what technology is used is dependent on the clinic's financial resources. Saliva testing using a mouth swab is reliable but costly. The issue of observed urine specimen accession with its attendant privacy issues is obviated. Most clinics in most countries use urine toxicologies for case finding. Some clinicians in this field have troubled feelings about doing any kind of assessment for the use of other abusable drugs, licit or illicit. A libertarian mindset requires complete personal agency over our lives. Patients in a treatment setting using substitution therapy for opiate addiction are included. They should not be harassed over their *choices* to use other substances. This is *not* the prevailing view. Regularly, it is observed that a putative *choice* is not a choice at all. And that is the essence of the disease of addiction: loss of agency over the unmanageable craving to use. Sophisticated imaging with functional MRI and third generation PET scanning has confirmed the microneuroanatomic and functional changes wrought by drugs of potential abuse used to the point of dependency and addiction.

Testing for other substances using either saliva or urine should be part of the treatment protocol. It should be done in a laboratory that is certified, frequently inspected, accessible to the clinical staff, and with a swift turn-around time. Treatment responses to so-called "*dirty*" urines, a word that is an anathema to many addiction specialists, is broad and variable from patient to another patient, from time to another time, from clinic to another clinic. The use of a contingency model(s) is receiving much attention these days. Rewards and punishments are issued in the context of Skinnerian behaviorism: do the right things and get additional days off or a card to a local store loaded with a known amount of credit. Do the wrong things,

i.e. present urine or saliva that on toxicological examination show "positive for banned substances" (the preferred terminology) and privileges such as methadone for days off from the clinic are lost.

The future

Maintenance therapy with other opiates or opioids

Buprenorphine, an analgesic, has been approved for maintenance therapy. It is an agonist/antagonist opioid with distinct pharmacodynamic effects, making it less abusable and only rarely producing a dysfunctional hyperphoria (high). In fact, because of its antagonist component, if taken in excess it precipitates withdrawal.

Suboxone comes in two formulations: 2 mg buprenorphine 5 mg naloxone, and 8 mg buprenorphine 2 mg naloxone. The naloxone is compounded with buprenorphine in Suboxone to precipitate withdrawal if used intravenously. Of the patients using this compounded formulation, 10% absorb a sufficient amount of naloxone when Suboxone is used sublingually to have significant withdrawal manifestations. The Drug Enforcement Agency of the US suggested the combined preparation. Reckitt Benckiser, vendors of buprenorphine, have acceded to this request. Knowing their patients beyond the context of their substance abuse, unarguably, is the best way to prevent untoward intravenous use of these preparations. The DEA has made a worthy effort to forestall intravenous use by lacing buprenorphine with naloxone in the Suboxone formulation. The one in ten patients who absorb naloxone sublingually may be turned away from a valuable pharmacotherapeutic intervention if this precipitates uncomfortable withdrawal symptoms. This may be another instance of assuming all "junkies" are the same and none can be trusted to do the right thing.

Oral preparations of pure antagonist have been available for maintenance after achieving abstinence. Repository naloxone subcutaneously injected lasting perhaps 4 weeks is yet another way to sustain narcotic freedom. This approach has not found great favor amongst opiate-dependent patients. In a carefully selected few this intervention may be effective. In some patients a pure opiate antagonist will produce dysphoria. These patients will quit the naloxone as quickly as possible.

In Australia, Switzerland, and, for a short time, Canada and perhaps Thailand and Sweden there has been interest in establishing injecting rooms for that group of heroin users who will not enter any other therapy. Reports from Switzerland and Australia are encouraging (Shi *et al.*, 2008). The general public will need to acclimatize to this profound departure from the conventional thinking on the matter of legally sanctioning injection delivery of heroin.

Will there be methadone clinics in 50 years?

For speculations on the future of any particular therapy, looking at the past may be helpful. The medicine cabinets of patients, metaphorically speaking, are littered with medications that have seen their "moments" in the sun only to be retired, occasionally ignominiously, because of unexpected toxicity, or inefficacy, or a new product doing the therapeutic job as well, if not less expensively, and thus improving the share price of the parent pharmaceutical company.

Except for a brief flirtation with LAAM (*levo*-alpha-acetylmethadol, the longest-acting enantiomer of methadyl acetate), nothing yet has filled methadone's shoes. LAAM's "moments" lasted approximately 20 years. Its virtue was its duration of action; 72 hours of effective pharmacodynamics, largely the result of the bioactivity of its metabolites. Its value according to the final regulatory authority, the DEA, was that the patient could be medicated three times weekly in the clinic, obviating the need to give anyone medication to take home – and possibly sell. The end of LAAM's utility came when several instances of the rare but often fatal tachyarrhythmia, torsades de pointes, occurred. LAAM prolongs the depolarization–repolarization time, the QT interval. It was this effect on the electro-mechanical aspect of cardiac function which made the heart susceptible to torsades. LAAM's end came swiftly after the publication of these cases. Several European drug control agencies struck it from the approved list of pharmaceuticals. At the time of writing it is still available in the US but is infrequently used.

Because *levo*-alpha-acetylmethadol is a congener of methadone HCl, methadone became suspect (Ehret *et al.*, 2007). Nothing of consequence came from this new scrutiny. Though several instances of prolonged QT interval were reported in patients on doses over 300 mg per diem, no convincing argument was made to discontinue the practice of methadone maintenance.

Interestingly, the work of Garrett Gross and others may provide animal model support for what appears to be a striking cardioprotective effect for long-term methadone use. The opiates in general and methadone specifically simulate the phenomenon of ischemic preconditioning, thus improving the energetics of the mass of cardiomyocytes downstream from the interruption of blood supply. Despite risk factors such as cigarette smoking, cocaine use, untreated hypertension, and poorly controlled diabetes mellitus that are common in this population, manifestations of cardiac ischemia represented as angina pectoris or myocardial infarction may rarely be seen (Peart *et al.*, 2005).

To end on this upbeat note: treating opiate/opioid addiction with substitution therapy is the gold standard for the disease of chemical dependency of the opioid type. The pure μ-agonist methadone, that has an accommodating pharmacokinetic profile, that has an outstanding safety profile borne out of 40 years of steady use, that has a record of efficacy and effectiveness derived from observations on the million or more patients who have been or are on a regulated program, that has a patient acceptance level higher than any other opiate or opioid used for maintenance, will be with us into the foreseeable future. The only variable impacting on methadone maintenance as a gold standard of treatment is the remote possibility of some kind of psychosocial or political intervention which renders young people immune to the compelling experience of opiate ingestion.

What we know of the chemical signaling at the μ receptor when the intrinsic activity of the cell begins makes it difficult to imagine a drug substituting for methadone. The neurochemical initiation of a cascade of central nervous system events is a profoundly rewarding experience for the mammalian brain.

Methadone treatment will be here for a long time. When healthcare delivery is re-tooled and made rational for all the people living in the US, most of the problems experienced in treatment programs will fade away.

References

Code of Federal Regulations (2010). (CFR 42, Part 160 & 164) Title 21. *Food and Drugs*. Revised April 2010. Washington DC: Food and Drug Administration, DHHS.

Dole, V. P. & Nyswander, M. (1965). A medical treatment for diacetylmorphine (heroin) addiction, a clinical trial with methadone HCl. *Journal of the American Medical Association*, **1931**, 646–50.

Dole, V. P., Nyswander, M. & Kreek, M. J. (1966). Narcotic blockade. *Archives of Internal Medicine*, **118**, 304–9.

Ehret, G. B., Desmueles, J. A. *et al.* (2007). Methadone-associated long QT syndrome: improving pharmacotherapy for dependence on illegal opioids and lessons learned for pharmacology. *Expert Opinions on Drug Safety,* **6**(3), 289–303.

Fuller, B. E., Rieckman, T. R., McCarty, D. J. *et al.* (2006). Elimination of benefits in the Oregon health plan and its effects on patients. *Psychiatric Services,* **57**(5), 686–91.

Gossop, M., Stewart, D. & Marsden, J. (2003). Treatment process components and heroin use outcome among methadone patients. *Drug and Alcohol Dependence,* **71**, 93–104.

Hartnoll, R. I. (1994). Opiates: prevalence and demographic factors. *Addiction,* **89**, 1377–83.

Musto, D. F. (1987). *The American Disease; Origin of Narcotic Control.* New York: Oxford University Press.

Nyswander, M. (1957). *The Drug Addict as a Patient.* New York: Grune and Stratton.

Peart, J. N., Gross, E. R. *et al.* (2005). Opioid-induced preconditioning: recent advances and future perspectives. *Vascular Pharmacology,* **42**(5–6), 211–18.

Puigdollers, E., Cots, F., Brugal, M. T. *et al.* (2003). Methadone maintenance programs with supplementary services: a cost-effectiveness study. *Gaceta Sanitaria,* **17**, 123–30.

Shi, J., Copersino, M. L., Fang, Y. X. *et al.* (2008). PET imaging and dopamine transporter and drug craving during methadone maintenance treatment and after prolonged abstinence in heroin users. *European Journal of Pharmacology,* **579**(1–3), 160–6.

Psychoactive prescription drug abuse

Bernard Salzman & Peter Micheels

Introduction

Prescription psychoactive drug abuse is a twenty-first century epidemic. Prescription psychoactive drug abuse is defined by the National Institute on Drug Abuse (NIDA) as the use of approved prescription medication without a prescription, use for purposes other than prescribed, or use simply for the experience or feeling that the drug can cause (Volkow, 2006). Commonly abused classes of these drugs include opioids (often prescribed to treat pain), central nervous system (CNS) depressants (often prescribed to treat anxiety and sleep disorders), and stimulants (prescribed to treat narcolepsy, attention deficit hyperactivity disorder, and obesity).

The Substance Abuse and Mental Health Service Administration's 2005 *National Survey on Drug Use* found that 6.4 million people, aged 12 or older, reported having misused prescription drugs in the month prior to participating in the survey. The largest portion of this population, 4.7 million people, claimed to have abused pain relievers, whereas 1.8 million abused tranquilizers, 1.1 million abused stimulants, and 272 000 abused sedatives.

In 2006, the incidence of prescription drug abuse was second only to marijuana abuse. The most recent household survey, at that time, indicated that most initiates to drug abuse started with prescription drugs (particularly pain medications) more often than with marijuana. Prescription drug abuse is facilitated by easy access (via physicians, the internet, and the medicine cabinet) and a perception of safety (since the drugs are FDA-approved) (Manchikanti, 2006).

In her testimony before the United States Senate in 2008, Doctor Nora Volkow, the Director of NIDA, stated that several factors have recently contributed to the severity of prescription drug abuse, including drastic increases in the number of prescriptions written, greater social acceptance of using medications, and aggressive marketing by pharmaceutical companies.

To illustrate, the total number of stimulant prescriptions in the US soared from around 5 million in 1991 to nearly 35 million in 2007. Prescriptions for opiates (hydrocodone and oxycodone) have escalated from around 40 million in 1991 to nearly 180 million in 2007, with the US their biggest consumer. The US is supplied with 99% of the world total for hydrocodone (e.g. Vicodin) and 71% of oxycodone (e.g. OxyContin).

By 2002, 31 million prescriptions for sedative hypnotics were filled in the US, jumping to 54 million in 2007 according to the US Department of Health and Human Services (Manchikanti, 2006).

People who abuse medications are not a single monolithic group. Some people borrow or exchange medications with friends or relatives, assuming that their medical conditions are similar, an often dangerous assumption. Others unilaterally escalate or mix medications, increasing the likelihood of side-effects, overdoses, or drug dependence.

A common misuse is seen in patients who are not primary drug abusers, but suffer from severe symptoms of depression and pain or anxiety. These prescription drug users change the dose or frequency of medication silently, which can inadvertently lead to dependence. At this point the use becomes self-perpetuating to stave off the discomfort of withdrawal.

There is also a concomitant subgroup of drug abusers, who dangerously use prescription drugs to expand, extend, and heighten the effect of illegal drugs and alcohol. Alcohol is the universal mixer that enhances and prolongs the effects of prescription and non-prescription drugs. Unfortunately, mixing drugs compounds their effects and their side-effects, leading to potentially fatal combinations, as does changing their route of administration by crushing the pills and then snorting or injecting them.

In a study examining the relationship between past-year drinking behavior and the abuse of prescription drugs, McCabe *et al.* (2006) found that prescription abuse of opioids, stimulants, tranquilizers, and sedatives was 18 times higher among dependent alcoholics than past-year abstainers. Furthermore, one in every four young adults aged 18–24 diagnosed with DSM-IV alcohol dependence also reported abusing prescription drugs. This suggests that young adult alcoholics should also be screened for prescription drug abuse, and prescription drug abusers should be screened for alcohol abuse.

Opioids

Pain is one of the most ubiquitous and complex of human experiences. In its acute form it is the body's response to a peripheral injury. It can be sharp, circumscribed, and persistent. Treatment often includes simple analgesics, applied heat or warmth, and somatic treatment, if necessary.

For more severe pain, beyond the common analgesics, opioids or morphine are prescribed. Codeine derivatives are often compounded with aspirin or acetaminophen. These drugs, oxycodone and hydrocodone, are commonly given for acute pain. Because of the rapid relief of pain, and their short action, they are extremely seductive. These drugs, like other members of the family, not only reduce pain but produce mood changes. These include euphoria and tranquility which become more prominent as the dose is increased. If you change the route of administration from oral to parenteral, the drug concentration to the brain increases. The psychotropic effects are heightened but the discomfort of drug withdrawal increases, reinforcing re-use. This can create a cycle leading to drug dependence.

Chronic pain represents a serious problem. According to NIDA (2007) it is estimated that more than 50 million Americans suffer from chronic pain. Pain is now the "fifth vital sign" and physicians face disciplinary action for failure to relieve pain adequately (Mendelson et al., 2008). When treating pain, however, healthcare providers wrestle with a dilemma: how to relieve a patient's suffering adequately while avoiding the potential for the patient to become addicted to the pain medication.

Consequently, many healthcare providers under-prescribe opioid pain relievers, such as morphine and codeine, because they overestimate the potential for patients becoming addicted. This fear of prescribing opioid pain medication is known as "opiophobia." Although these drugs carry a risk for addiction and physicians should watch for signs of abuse and addiction in their patients, the likelihood of patients with chronic pain becoming addicted to the opioids is low

(with the exception of those with a personal or family history of drug abuse or mental illness). The risk of becoming addicted to prescription pain medication is also minimal in those who are treated on a short-term basis.

Those suffering with chronic intermittent pain, however, will sometimes increase the amount and frequency of the medication prescribed for them without consulting their healthcare provider. This may lead to physical dependence, drug-seeking preoccupation, and other dissocial behaviors. This includes the use of multiple medications, including over-the-counter medications and abuse of alcohol.

Signs of opioid abuse include constipation, low blood pressure, respiratory depression, depressed mood, and confusion.

Legitimate pain management for patients who are substance abusers is particularly challenging, but these patients can be treated successfully with opioid pain medications, although it might be best if they are treated by a pain management professional.

The immediate release forms of oxycodone and hydrocodone are commonly abused. However, beginning in 2000 there were widespread reports of the diversion and abuse of a sustained release form of oxycodone prescribed as OxyContin. There has been a general increase in the abuse of analgesics in general, but this new product is now the most frequently abused (Cicero et al., 2005).

The abuse of OxyContin has gone beyond its medical use, into street and recreational abuse. Most of the drugs were obtained from friends (70%) and 14% directly from physicians (Mendelson et al., 2008).The vast majority of the oxycodone abusers had a prior history of drug abuse and some migrated to using heroin. There is an increasing rate of use, beginning with eighth grade and progressing to college students and young adults.

Anxiolytics

Anxiety, one of the most common symptoms, is often manifested as feelings of eminent dread or panic. It can be experienced in somatic terms as transient chest pains, shortness of breath, or inability to swallow. In its acute form it can lead to suicidal thoughts and behaviors.

The first of the modern anxiolytics, developed after World War 2, were the meprobamates which quickly calmed and mildly sedated the anxious patient. The use of meprobamates rapidly increased.

Physicians distributed the medication as if it were candy, and drug dependence became an increasing public problem. Short- and rapid-acting, tolerance developed quickly and increased amounts were needed to achieve the same degree of tranquility.

The second family of anxiolytics was the benzodiazepines. Popularized in the 1960s, the first two drugs of this class were diazepam and chlordiazepoxide. Diazepam was rapid- and long-acting and thought to be relatively safe. The drug provided quick relief of anxiety and was, and is, an effective muscle relaxant. The drug quickly became popular as the medical indications became broader, and the number of prescriptions increased geometrically. Even the slightest stress led to escalating use and increased tolerance. The quantity of medication taken was immense because the drug was difficult to overdose on – even doses as high as 3000 mg were tolerated, although the conventional dose was only 5 mg.

Like its predecessor meprobamate, drug dependence became more common. Abrupt withdrawal led to painful muscle pain and often culminated in grand mal seizures. Most insidious was the combination of alcohol and diazepam, which, unknowingly, becomes a fatal cocktail. The two drugs have similar and addictive effects, leading to increasing CNS depression, coma, and death.

The next generation of benzodiazepines arose in an attempt to diminish the addiction liability of the longer acting benzodiazepines. The short transit time and rapid effect was thought to decrease the drugs' potential for abuse.

The two most popular short-acting benzodiazepines are alprazolam and lorazepam. They both provide short-term relief of anxiety symptoms. They do, however, add to the CNS effect of depressants such as alcohol, narcotic analgesics, and sedative hypnotics.

They are efficacious, short-acting, and extremely sedative. Their abuse liability is greater than Valium, although these two drugs were seen as benign and given out in large open prescriptions, which promoted their abuse and liability. They are known to cause "a buzz," increasing their use beyond relief of stress, particularly with adolescents. More dangerously, they act adjunctively with alcohol or other CNS depressants for an addictive effect or with stimulants to take the edge off their jagged side-effects. The use of benzodiazepines has been made famous by contributing to the deaths of a number of prominent entertainers.

Often the short-acting benzodiazepines are diverted from legitimate use (symptom relief) and traded or borrowed by contemporaries for other uses, such as "coming down" from hard drugs.

Sedative hypnotics

A second common disorder that plagues humankind is insomnia – difficulty falling or staying asleep. Pharmaceuticals have produced cures, from opiates to barbiturates to synthetic hypnotics to benzodiazepines and beyond. All classes of drugs have been effective, but also potentially addicting, and in some cases fatal. Overdoses were common with opiates and barbiturates, and these drugs were commonly used with alcohol in suicide attempts.

In the 1960s and 1970s synthetic hypnotics, such as glutethimide and ethchlorvynol, were developed. If the sedative effect were fought off, the drugs would produce a state of intoxication and were more likely to be abused. These drugs had a narrow margin of safety between the effective and lethal dose, and overdose and death were common.

When the benzodiazepines were developed, some members of the family were marketed as hypnotics rather than anxiolytics. These included flurazepam, diazepam, and triazolam. Like other hypnotics, individuals would be refractory to the hypnotic sedative effect and would escalate the dose, creating a possible addiction paradigm.

The newest and related form of the hypnotic sedatives are thought to be less addicting and more effective. They include zolpidem and zaleplon. Zaleplon's infamous side-effects include sleep walking, hallucinations, and hangover. They too are subject to refractoriness and dependence as the drug effect tapers off.

Factors that contribute to substance dependence, in general, such as personal and family history of addiction, are likely to play a role in the development of sedative hypnotic dependence (Caplan et al., 2007).

The abrupt discontinuation of barbiturates or benzodiazepines can produce a withdrawal syndrome, like that seen in chronic alcoholics, which can include delirium, seizures, and possibly death if left untreated (Morgan, 1990).

The neuropsychiatric effects of sedative hypnotic addiction include deficits in memory, motor coordination, visuospatial learning, processing speed, and verbal learning, even after drug discontinuation (Caplan et al., 2007).

Signs of anxiolytic and sedative hypnotic abuse include impaired judgment, unsteady gait, rapid involuntary eye movement, confusion, and drowsiness.

Stimulants

Stimulant abuse is not new. They have been used classically by college students to avoid sleep and to complete assignments. Similarly, stimulants have been used by shift workers and long distance truckers to stave off sleep and to be able to concentrate.

All stimulants work by increasing the neurotransmitter dopamine, which is associated with pleasure, movement, and attention. However, when taken in doses and routes other than prescribed, stimulants can increase dopamine in a rapid and amplified manner, producing euphoria and increasing the risk of addiction.

The major family of stimulants is amphetamines and amphetamine-like compounds. The misuse of amphetamines in various forms reached epidemic proportion in the 1960s, when they were used as anorectics. Used alone, or in combination with diuretics and thyroid stimulants, they become part of a formula for quick weight reduction. Some physicians prescribed stimulants promiscuously. The drugs were easily diverted and entered the world of drug abusers.

The problem became so bad that in the 1970s New York State introduced triplicate prescriptions to keep count of the drugs and also the prescribers. This tactic worked as physicians were deterred from reckless prescribing, and the number of prescriptions for amphetamines and its derivatives dropped precipitously. However, currently, the rate of abuse in the nation is significant.

In the 1930s the condition ADHD (attention deficit hyperactivity disorder) was first described, predominantly in boys, manifested by a persistent pattern of inattention and/or hyperactivity–impulsivity that is more frequently displayed and more severe than is typically observed in individuals at a comparable level of development. In the 1990s, with better screening and diagnosis, more children and adolescents were placed on the treatment of choice, stimulants. Rather than causing "a high," the medication allowed students to concentrate, read, and adjust their behavior in the classroom. The number of prescriptions has increased dramatically over the past 10 years, as has the amount of diversion for abuse. Adolescents traded their stimulants, amphetamines

or methylphenidate, to their friends. The stimulants were not only diverted but were often altered, so the drug can be inhaled or injected. Many abusers went on to use the so-called hard drugs: cocaine and meth-amphetamines.

Results from the 2007 National Survey on Drug Use and Health (The NDUH Report, 2009) demonstrated a higher rate of non-medical use of the amphetamine Adderall® (a mixture of amphetamine salts) among full-time college students than among others in the same age range (18–22 years). This is a public health concern because of this drug's very high potential for dependence and abuse. Healthcare providers, educators, and counselors who work with students need to be aware that polydrug use was prevalent among full-time college students who used Adderall® non-medically in the past year. Furthermore, both cocaine and stimulants such as Adderall® increase a person's risk for a heart attack or stroke. Students who use Adderall® non-medically may also need to take CNS depressants such as pain relievers or tranquilizers (which carry their own risk of dependence or abuse) to counteract the stimulant effects of Adderall®. Moreover, high rates of binge and heavy alcohol use among full-time college students who used Adderall® non-medically in the past year are a cause for concern because of the well documented associations between excessive drinking among college students and the adverse consequences for students' physical and mental health, and safety (NDUH Report, 2009).

Non-ADHD users often develop acute tolerance to the subjective effects of stimulants (euphoria, alertness, and increased arousal); this can play a major role in dose escalation and subsequent toxicity. In acute intoxication and with long-term use, stimulants may cause insomnia, irritability, aggressive behavior, and psychosis, especially paranoia. Medical complications of acute intoxication with stimulants include an altered mental status, autonomic instability (including elevated blood pressure, heart rate, and hyperthermia), decreased sleep and appetite, along with seizures, or the development of a serotonin syndrome. These drugs now carry a "black box warning" that "misuse of amphetamine may cause sudden death and serious cardiovascular adverse events." In general, the use of additional substances, including alcohol, with prescription stimulants is associated with increased morbidity and mortality (Caplan *et al.*, 2007).

Vulnerable populations

Adolescents

Adolescents are the most vulnerable for both street drug and prescription drug abuse. Like their prefrontal cortex, their executive judgment is not fully developed yet, leading to reckless and impulsive behavior.

Adolescents' interest turns outward toward their peers, subject to their pressure and substituted judgment. The need for novelty, danger, autonomy, and social acceptance becomes more prominent. This is a set-up for prescription and street drugs, and alcohol abuse.

The major source of adolescent prescription drugs is the adolescent's family and friends. The medications are stolen from family members or discarded by them. Older friends and peers share or sell these unused drugs, and misusing them becomes part of a bonding ritual.

In one study of 2.3 million adolescents, 9.3% reported non-medical prescription drug use. The reason for use included sleep aid, pain relief, and increased alertness. All the drug groups, including pain analgesics, stimulants, and CNS depressants, were abused. Opioid analgesics were the most commonly abused, particularly amongst female adolescents. There are racial and economic differences in prescription drug abusers which reflect availability rather than preference. Also alarming is that 60% of these prescription drug abusers went on to use illicit drugs (Substance Abuse and Mental Health Administration, 2006).

Research also shows that adolescents who abuse prescription drugs are twice as likely to engage in delinquent behavior and nearly three times as likely to experience an episode of major depression compared to teens who did not abuse prescription medication over the previous year (Volkow, 2005).

As noted, the consequences of non-medical prescription use are potentially lethal, with risks of violence, trauma, overdose, and life-threatening withdrawal.

The increased availability of prescription drugs and the trivialization of their use is a threat for not only this generation, but also generations to come.

Elderly

The older population, 65-plus, is particularly vulnerable to drug misuse and abuse. They have a number of predisposing factors – in general their metabolism is slow, so that the medication breaks down more slowly and has a longer transit time. Consequently, medication may accumulate and dosages overlap. Short-acting benzodiazepines are one example of this phenomenon. After a single dose, a second dose in the same day would have the same effect as one and a half doses. In this particular example, the effect would be increased sedation and greater risk for falls, or other accidents.

Often the elderly are suffering from multiple chronic medical conditions such as hypertension, diabetes, and arthritis. They commonly take as many as five or six different medications. This could further increase the slowing of their metabolism, leading to confusion and an inadvertent overdose.

Perhaps the most common disorder in the elderly is insomnia. There are physiological changes in the sleep patterns of the elderly, including increase in sleep latency, more frequent awakenings, and decrease in total sleep. The sleep is also disrupted by frequent awakenings for evacuation. The elderly often resort to over-the-counter supplements or hypnotic sedatives with unpredictable effects. They forget how much they have taken, how long ago they took it, and compound the effect by adding late-night alcohol. The net effect is confusion, disorientation, and clumsiness, again leading to serious accidents.

According to Kirsh and Smith (2008), older patients who have pain present unique challenges for clinicians. On the one hand, care must be taken to treat pain aggressively, while preventing excessive side-effects such as drowsiness, nausea, vomiting, and constipation. On the other hand, the clinician must not only assess the patient, but also the patient's family, who may not have the patient's interest at heart when it comes to pain medications. Furthermore, the clinician may have the burden of convincing some patients that they would benefit from pain medication.

Culberson and Ziska (2008) report that one-quarter of the prescription drugs sold in the US are used by the elderly, often for problems such as chronic pain, insomnia, and anxiety. The prevalence of abuse may be as high as 11%, with female gender, social isolation, depression, and a history of substance abuse increasing the risk. Although tolerance, withdrawal syndrome, and dose escalation may be less common in older patients, some clinicians' fear of abuse often results in a failure to treat symptoms such as anxiety, pain, and insomnia adequately.

Preventing prescription drug abuse

NIDA (2009) maintains that about 70% of Americans – approximately 191 million people – visit a healthcare provider, such as a primary care physician, physician's assistant, or nurse practitioner, at least once every 2 years. Thus healthcare providers are in a unique position not only to prescribe needed medications appropriately, but also to identify prescription drug abuse when it exists and help the patient recognize the problem, set goals for recovery, and seek appropriate treatment when necessary. Screening for any type of substance abuse can be incorporated into routine history-taking with questions about what prescriptions and over-the-counter medicines the patient is taking and why. Screening can also be performed if a patient presents with specific symptoms associated with problem use of a substance. NIDA has developed a clinician's screening tool (NIDA, 2009). This web-based interactive tool guides clinicians through a short series of screening questions and, based on the patient's responses, generates a substance involvement score that suggests the level of intervention needed.

Over time, providers should note any rapid increases in the amount of medication needed – which may indicate the development of tolerance – or frequent requests for refills before the quantity prescribed should have been used. They should also be alert to the fact that those addicted to prescription medication may engage in "doctor shopping," moving from provider to provider in an effort to get multiple prescriptions for the drug(s) they abuse, or that the patient is exhibiting excessive mood swings.

To reduce rates of non-medical use of pain relievers and other prescription drugs, medical practitioners must not only continue to exercise care in prescribing and monitoring their patients for signs of misuse, but should also counsel them about not sharing their prescription medications, preventing others from having access to their medications, and properly disposing of remaining dosage units once the need for the medication has passed (The NDUH Report, 2009).

Treatment of prescription drug addiction

Addiction to any drug, whether illicit or prescribed, is a brain disease caused by the effects of prolonged drug exposure on brain functioning. However, like other chronic diseases, addiction can be effectively treated. However, successful treatment may need to incorporate several evidence-based components, including detoxification, behavioral interventions, and the use of pharmacological therapies. Moreover, multiple courses of treatment may be needed for the patient to make a full recovery.

Opioid addiction

Several options are available for treating prescription opioid addiction. These options include medications such as methadone, buprenorphine, and naltrexone, along with behavioral counseling approaches.

Methadone (a long-acting synthetic opioid) maintenance programs have been used for over 30 years to treat heroin addicts. According to NIDA (2009), the most effective methadone maintenance programs included individual and/or group counseling in their treatment regime.

The Food and Drug Administration approved buprenorphine in October 2002, after more than a decade of research supported by NIDA. Buprenorphine is a partial agonist (having both agonist and antagonist properties) at the opioid receptors, and carries a low risk of overdose. It reduces or eliminates withdrawal symptoms associated with opioid dependence, but does not produce euphoria and sedation. The drug is available in two formulations: Subutex® (a pure form of buprenorphine) and the more commonly prescribed Suboxone® (a combination of buprenorphine and the opioid antagonist naloxone). This latter formulation produces severe withdrawal symptoms when addicted individuals inject it to get high, lessening the likelihood of diversion. Buprenorphine, which can be prescribed by certified physicians in an office setting, is long-lasting, less likely to cause respiratory depression than other drugs, and is well tolerated. Furthermore, patients stabilized on these medications can engage more readily in counseling and other behavioral interventions essential to recovery and rehabilitation.

A useful precursor to long-term treatment of opioid addiction is detoxification. Detoxification in itself is not treatment. Rather its primary objective is to relieve withdrawal symptoms while the patient adjusts to being drug-free. To be effective, detoxification must precede long-term treatment that requires either complete abstinence or incorporates a medication, such as methadone or buprenorphine, into the treatment program.

Sedative hypnotics

Patients addicted to barbiturates and benzodiazepines should undergo medically supervised detoxification, because the treatment dose must be gradually tapered due to the potentially life-threatening side-effects of a too-rapid discontinuation of the drugs. Inpatient or outpatient counseling can help patients during this process. Cognitive behavioral therapy, which focuses on modifying the patient's thinking, expectations, and behaviors while at the same time increasing skills for coping with various life stressors, has also been used successfully to help individuals adapt to the discontinuation of benzodiazepines.

Often barbiturate and benzodiazepine abuse occurs in conjunction with abuse of another substance or drug, such as alcohol or cocaine. In these cases of polydrug abuse, the treatment approach must address the multiple addictions.

Prescription stimulants

Depending on the patient's situation, the first step in treating prescription stimulant addiction may be tapering the drug dosage and attempting to ease withdrawal symptoms. The detoxification process could then be followed by one of many behavioral therapies, e.g. contingency management, which uses a system that enables patients to earn vouchers for drug-free urine tests. These vouchers can then be exchanged for items that promote healthy living. Cognitive behavioral therapy may also be effective in conjunction with recovery support groups.

References

Caplan, J., Epstein, L. A., Quinn, D. K. *et al.* (2007). Neuropsychiatric effects of prescription drug abuse. *Neuropsychological Review*, **17**, 363–80.

Cicero, T., Inciardi, J. A. & Munoz, S. (2005). Trends in abuse of OxyContin and other opioid analgesics in the United States, 2002–2004. *Journal of Pain*, **6**, 662.

Culberson, J. W. and Ziska, M. (2008). Prescription drug misuse/abuse in the elderly. *Geriatrics*, **63**(9), 22–31.

Kirsh, K. L. & Smith, H. S. (2008). Special issues and concerns in the evaluation of older adults who have pain. *Clinics in Geriatric Medicine*, **24**, 2.

Macabe, S. E., Cranford, J. A. & Byd, C. J. (2006). The relationship between past year drinking behaviors and nonmedical use of prescription drugs: prevalence of co-occurrence in a national sample. *Drug and Alcohol Dependence*, **84**(3), 281–8.

Manchikanti, L. (2006). Prescription drug abuse: what is being done to address this new drug epidemic? Testimony before the Subcommittee on Criminal Justice, Drug Policy and Human Resources. *Pain Physician*, **9**(4), 287–321.

Mendelson, J., Flower, K., Pletcher, M. J., & Galloway, G. P. (2008). Addiction to prescription opioids: characteristics of the emerging epidemic and treatment with buprenorphine. *Experimental Clinical Psychopharmacology*, **16**(5), 435–41.

Morgan, W. (1990). Abuse liability of barbiturates and other sedative-hypnotics. *Advances in Alcohol and Substance Abuse*, **9**, 67–82.

National Institute on Drug Abuse. (2007). Bulletin board. Meeting reviews progress on prescription opioid misuse, **21**(3).

National Institute on Drug Abuse. (2009). *Screening for drug abuse in general medical settings: quick reference guide.* NIH Publication No. 09–7384.

The NDUH Report (2009). Nonmedical use of Adderall® among full-time college students. *The NSDUH Report.* February 5, 2009.

Substance Abuse and Mental Health Administration (2006). *2005 National Survey on Drug Use.* http://www.oos.samhsa.gov/nsduh, accessed 10 June 2010

Volkow, N. D. (2005). What do we know about drug addiction? (Editorial). *American Journal of Psychiatry*, **162**, 1401–2.

Part 3 | Praxis

Praxis

Pain management and addiction treatment

Robert Maslansky

Pain management's professional societies

A group of dedicated physicians oversaw the creation of The American Pain Society (APS) in Chicago on March 6, 1977. The first Annual Scientific meeting was held in San Diego in September of 1979 and by all accounts it was a bit rancorous but immensely successful. As is the case with new professional societies, the gestation and the birthing were not easy. The notion that *pain* requires a special organization was novel and in some ways troublesome. Pain management often involves prescribing scheduled drugs and this means close attention to regulations established by the Drug Enforcement Administration (DEA). Failure to do so may have unpleasant consequences: censure, DEA certification suspension, state license jeopardy, and criminal indictment.

The mission statement of the APS is concise and to the point:

> The American Pain Society is a multidisciplinary community that brings together a diverse group of scientists, clinicians and other professionals to increase the knowledge of pain and transform public policy and clinical practice to reduce pain related suffering.

> (http://www.ampainsoc.org/ce/cme_mission.htm, accessed March 4, 2010)

In 1983, the American Academy of Pain Medicine (AAPM) had its first annual meeting. Its purpose was to meet the challenge of increasing numbers of clinicians devoted to the diagnosis and treatment of acute and chronic pain. Their statement of mission broadens the scope of pain treatment.

> The practice of Pain Medicine is multi-dimensional in approach incorporating modalities from various specialties to ensure the comprehensive evaluation and treatment of the pain patient. AAPM represents the diverse scope of the field through membership from a variety of origins, including such specialties as anesthesiology,

internal medicine, neurology, neurosurgery, orthopedics, physiatry, and psychiatry.

> (http://www.painmed.org/, accessed March 4, 2010).

Physicians who thought about pain, who wanted to construct a foundation (a philosophy, if you will) supporting the management of pain, had a daunting task. From Hippocrates to Maimonides to the founding fathers of scientific medicine pain was a paramount clinical consideration. With the development of scientific medicine it became subordinate to precise diagnosis and the biological specificities of treatment. That the patient suffered pain was but one among other concerns. Devotion to curing or ameliorating the disease was primary. If this happens, the pain associated with it would disappear. Thus, pain was a secondary issue.

This has changed. Once again, pain is at the forefront of clinical thinking. Pain is assessed and graded on a semi-objective scale of ten along with the blood pressure, pulse rate, and temperature (Ritter *et al.*, 2006). For a patient suffering chronic and relentless physical pain, often along with anguish (anxiety) and depression, there are experts who have shaped their professional lives around the treatment of pain.

The American Society of Addiction Medicine: its mission statement

The timeline for the organization now known as the American Society of Addiction Medicine (ASAM) begins in 1951 with the creation of The New York City Medical Committee on Alcoholism (NYCMCA). In 1988 ASAM was accepted as a participating member by the House of Delegates of the American Medical Association (AMA). A certifying examination instituted in the mid 1980s created a body of information that should be acquired by an addiction specialist. The mission statement for the ASAM reads as follows:

(I)ncrease access to and improve the quality of addiction treatment; to educate physicians and other health care providers and promote the appropriate role of the physician in the care of patients with addictions; and to establish addiction medicine as a specialty recognized by professional organizations, governments, physicians, purchasers and consumers of health care services and the general public.

(http://www.asam.org/, accessed March 4, 2010)

When does pain management become addiction treatment? When does addiction treatment become pain management?

These two admirable expressions of humanistic medicine, the AAPM and the ASAM, were set on a collision course at the mu and delta receptors of a neural pathway euphemistically called "the river of reward." To avoid mixing a metaphor, it can be called, with greater accuracy "the highway to reward." This neural pathway (highway) is the locus of pharmacologically induced reward systems activated by its dopaminergic response to circulating endogenous or exogenous ligands. Substances of potential misuse as well as certain aberrant behaviors such as eating to the point of morbid obesity, gambling to penury, and predatory sex are activities that initiate this neurochemical cascade (Saal *et al.*, 2003).

The early recognition that opiates used for non-terminal but chronic pain were an appropriate therapeutic choice in selected patients was accompanied by a set of rules for their use in such a setting. These rules undergo periodic modifications to reflect new developments in pain management.

That branch of philosophy called epistemology asks, "(H)ow and what do we know?" Among other ways, how we know is the use of words with intelligible and stable meaning. The distinction between addiction and dependency must be clear. What we know in this instance is that dependency is a neurophysiological phenomenon having these characteristics:

1. Development of variable degrees of tolerance. Often, but not always, there is the need to escalate the rewarding stimulus.
2. If the dependency-producing substance or activity is abruptly taken away then a state of dysphoria occurs. This may start within hours of the deprivation. With certain dependency states,

it may occur days or even weeks following the abrupt discontinuance (Christie, 2008). It can be seen following the use of drug-specific antagonists.

3. With current imaging technology, dependency can be identified within certain receptor sites and neural pathways (Goldstein & Volkow, 2002).

Behavior defines addiction. If dependency leads to activities either inimical to the individual's health and/or life or, as currently codified, criminal behavior, or behavior inconsistent with normative conduct in contemporary society, this is called addiction. Brain imaging has provided evidence for specific neural events occurring with addiction.

The subjective state of irrepressible craving is a neurobiological event in the time–space continuum of the central nervous system. In the radiations from the median forebrain bundle to the nucleus accumbens (Jones *et al.*, 2008), dopaminergic synaptic transfer systems modulate the intensity of the neural messages. They are responsible for the explicit subjective report of craving.

Addiction treatment and pain management: two cases with interesting outcomes

Case 1

L. B. is a 26-year-old web designer currently employed in a management level at a local web design firm. He sustained a sports career-ending injury in a downfield tackle 6 years ago as a running back for an Ivy League football team. An MRI at that time showed compression fractures of L_3, L_4, L_5, and a fracture of the transverse process of L_4 on the left side. He had lancinating pain in the distribution of sciatic nerve, spinal roots 3, 4, and 5. The pain was constant but bearable. Surgery was advised more than once. He refused each time. He states that he watched his father die postoperatively from a pulmonary embolism after a back operation.

He pursued prescribed physical therapy diligently. For pain he took only ibuprofen 800 mg three times a day. He stated he never took more than the appropriate dose. Gradually, he improved. He finished college a year later. He settled into an excellent job with a software company. Then at his early morning jog he fell to the ground with severe pain in his low back that radiated down the right side in the distribution of the L_4, L_5 nerve root. As noted, his prior radiculopathy was on the left side. The right-sided pain did not improve after 3 weeks of conservative treatment. Imaging revealed the same structural pathology noted 2 years ago. Now in addition, the nerve root foramen on the right side was compromised, fitting the neurological findings of pain in the distribution of right-sided L_4, L_5.

Because of job time constraints he was unable to fit in the rigorous physical therapy program he had before. His orthopedist referred him to a neurologist, who in turn suggested that he see a neurological surgeon. His lumbar spine pathology was thought to be surgically remediable. He refused surgery. That his first episode diminished with time and physical therapy was enough for him to refuse surgery again. But this time he did not improve and, in fact, he got worse. Now there was motor involvement. He developed a slight foot drop. The pain became formidable, disturbing his sleep, his social life, his bladder function, his work, and his erectile capacity.

The neurosurgeon felt that although surgery may help it could make things worse. He suggested that he see a pain specialist on faculty at his University Hospital. The one chosen was part of the University Hospital pain clinic. Her credentials were impeccable. In her care he had three carefully performed epidural injections guided by fluoroscopy. There was little relief. His pain management physician tried several NSAIDS to no avail. Lidocaine patches, acupuncture, and exterior bracing were introduced, and transcutaneous electrical nerve stimulation (TENS) all effected minimal but transient improvement. Finally, after more than 2 years the patient (with some resistance on his part) was started on tramadol HCl 100 mg three times daily along with gabapentin 600 mg also three times daily. For the first time he had relief, certainly far from complete remission.

Now, tragically, the fabric of his life unraveled. The woman he wanted to marry threatened to break off their relationship because of his perpetual gloominess. For the first time in his life he became melancholic. He had a poor sleep pattern with early morning awakening, compromised work performance, anhedonia, and intrusive suicidal ruminations.

He related all this to his relentless pain. With misgivings, his pain physician stopped the tramadol and started Vicodin ES[R] (10 mg hydrocodone/660 mg acetaminophen) every 6 hours. Accompanying the prescription was a carefully worded contract signed by the doctor and the patient. It stipulated the nature of the medication, its locus of action, and its side-effects. It spelled out dependency and addictive liability. Carefully, it described "addiction." The contract made clear the expectations on the contractual participants.

When the patient reported to his doctor 3 days later, he declared "I haven't felt this well since my injury 6 years ago!" After some weeks he stated that his mood had improved. His performance at work turned around dramatically, and he believed his relationship with the woman in his life was heading toward marriage. However, there was a problem. He was keenly aware of it. Though he did not articulate it exactly this way he felt he had become physiologically dependent on the Vicodin. He reported that on two occasions he missed 2 days of medication. Not only did the pain become intense but his melancholy returned and he felt as if he had the flu. His ending-of-life ruminations returned. Soon he convinced his physician that he needed additional medication and was given a prescription that he filled immediately (*in a different drugstore*). He swallowed three pills. The pain diminished, good feelings returned. Over the next few months, without telling the pain management team, he went to a second physician, not a pain specialist, and was able to get a prescription from him by lying and claiming a severe toothache that he thought may be an abscess. He went one evening to a part of town known as a "drug market." He found a "vendor of pharmaceuticals." He bought some OxyContin (oxycodone HCl). In fact, he bought a lot of OxyContin. The pharmacology had taken over.

Finally, guiltily, and with much shame he went to his pain physician. After a long discussion and tears and with the utmost sensitivity on his doctor's part he accepted a referral to an addiction specialist.

The addiction expert agreed that he had become dependent on the hydromorphine. Further, he understood that his dependency resulted in characteristically addictive behavior (Jones *et al.*, 2008). The plan of treatment was as follows: he must reduce his Vicodin dose to a level that resulted in withdrawal symptoms then he was to start a buprenorphine preparation marketed as Suboxone (a combination of buprenorphine and naloxone 8 mg/2 mg that, administered by the sublingual route, would assuage withdrawal and provide significant relief of his pain). He did this. It worked. He needed 16 mg per diem. It should be added that there was a thorough exchange of ideas between the treating physicians.

The most irksome side-effect was constipation. Stool softeners, fiber supplements, increased water intake, and the occasional enema made this manageable.

He has continued this dosage schedule until today. His life seems to be on track.

Case 2

K. L. is 36-year-old woman. Her childhood was chaotic in the extreme. She was an only child. She describes her father as a brutal alcoholic who beat her mother often. As she grew older and her father became weaker, she defended her mother against his unprovoked attacks. Finally, her father died of end-stage liver disease. When she was 13 her mother died. Child Protective Services placed her in a licensed foster home. Surprisingly, she thrived. She describes her foster parents as strict but kind. Where in her parents' home, school was an afterthought, in the foster setting it was a condition clearly set forth by her caretakers. The streets were alluring, however. After 4 years and having finished high school with excellent grades, she began "hanging out." College was an option and, though eligible for financial aide, she went to work in a factory making toy soldiers. She started a relationship with a co-worker who, it turns out, sold heroin as a sideline. He introduced her to it and she, as she states, *truly* "fell in love." She became dependent rapidly. She used intravenously from the very beginning. Her habit, supported by her boyfriend, was large.

Shortly thereafter, she had an unusual accident with grave consequences. She fell into an uncovered manhole, fracturing both femurs, the right one compound, the left one comminuted with several fragments. She fractured the third, fourth, and fifth ribs on the right side anteriorly, causing a pneumothorax. Fortunately, though late at night, the accident was observed. She was taken to a nearby hospital in a critical condition with significant blood loss. The pneumothorax compromised her oxygenation. Rapidly, she went into hypovolemic shock. She was treated aggressively. She survived the acute life-threatening problems thanks to superb care.

Then came an extended stay in the hospital with several operations to repair her shattered legs. When discharged after 3 months, her whole life needed re-tooling. She was drug-free for 3 whole months in the hospital. When discharged she was determined to "stay clean" and, indeed she did, but

the pain in her legs, particularly the left one which required a lot of hardware to proximate the fragments, left her in constant distress, some of it clearly neuropathic. Her physiatrist started her on an opiate pain management regimen. It was helpful but she always felt seriously underdosed.

She did what she knew would help. She went to her old neighborhood, found a dealer easily, and bought heroin. What happened next is not entirely clear. Several days after she started what she thought was a measured amount of heroin she overdosed. Unlike before, now she used alone. Fortunately, her landlady on her rounds to collect rent, knowing that she was home, entered her apartment with a pass key and found her unconscious with a needle still in her arm. Her physiatrist was called because she had his card in her wallet. She recovered immediately after the ambulance team administered Narcan (naloxone). With her permission, the physiatrist referred her to an addiction specialist. After a careful assessment, including the story of her addiction, he concluded that her condition was a pain management problem. She characterized her pain as a constant eight on the pain scale of ten.

When seen in the pain clinic she was kept on a regimen of OxyContin escalating to 60 mg twice a day. To this gabapentin 800 mg three times a day was added. There were lidocaine infiltrations and continued physiotherapy. In the middle of her treatment her lawyer informed her that her lawsuit with the city as defendant offered to settle for a sum that, if properly managed, should last her a lifetime. Her opiate regimen continued without interruption, with no escalation of dose.

Her plan was to start college in the fall term. This she did. She finished college in less than 4 years. She went to graduate school, gained a masters in oceanography. She went on to complete her PhD. She married a co-worker at the laboratory. They had two boys.

Treatment and management issues: when does pain management become addiction treatment? When does addiction treatment become pain management?

These two clinical scenarios (both actual) are representative of careful assessment and appropriate referral to an alternative system of care that seemed essential for the best outcomes. In short, this was practising medicine competently and humanely. Clearly, in both instances this is arguable. Others, with at least their own justifications, would pursue a different set of interventions. That elusive concept "quality of life" figures here. Whose quality of life, the patient's or the physician's? In the case of the young athlete, pain management with an opiate was heading down into dangerous territory. Desperately, this highly motivated young man saw no other way out but to take matters into his own hands and supplement his opiate use any way he could. That he found a path to buprenorphine was a matter of timing and the wise recommendation of his pain doctor referring him to an addiction specialist. Before the year 2000 that option was not available. Attitudes 25 years ago concerning long-term pain management with an opiate or an opioid in a non-terminally ill person with his intensity of relentless pain might have made L. B. seek a dangerous and unlawful way to relief. This would end his dreams of rising to the highest levels in his chosen field, marrying the woman he loved, and living a pain-modified life. Fortunately, the pendulum swings these days toward a clearer understanding of both pain and addiction.

Ominously, it is possible that the pendulum has swung too far. The ease with which narcotic pain relief has become a "standard of care" has produced a small cadre of physicians with a license to prescribe these powerful medications but whose knowledge of pain management and the treatment of patients with an addictive pattern of behavior is at best incomplete, at worst, non-existent, and occasionally with motivations that are exclusively pecuniary.

Buprenorphine is a DEA Schedule III medication. To prescribe it for the treatment of opiate dependency and/or addiction, a special certifying process is required. No such special certifying process is needed to issue prescriptions for Schedule II drugs with a much higher liability for abuse and, one must add, diversion to illicit places. All one must have is a license to practise medicine in a state, a territory, or a protectorate of the USA and submit an acceptable application to the DEA.

It is true that physicians who have misapplied this privilege are in jeopardy for legal sanctions: loss of DEA certification, loss of license to practise, and, in rare cases, incarceration. A practitioner may have a patient with chronic pain who has had a thorough assessment and various modalities of treatment but still has not responded with a manageable degree of

pain modification. He starts an opiate, OxyContin, for example. The physician may become known in the neighborhood as someone from whom one can obtain an endless supply of these potentially misused medications. This does a disservice to the pain treatment community. It could lead to overdose deaths from these potentially lethal medications in opiate-naïve individuals. In fact, there have been prominently reported news items that turned out to be damaging to the methadone treatment community. There has been a serious up-tick in the number of methadone overdose deaths reported by medical examiners' offices throughout the country. Legally operating methadone treatment clinics were accused of laxity in the safeguards used to thwart diversion. Subsequently, it was established that almost all the methadone used in the overdose deaths came from the offices of individual practitioners who called themselves "pain specialists." The victims were for the most part non-users of opiates, thus unprepared for the large doses of methadone they purchased from people who were prescribed methadone for their putative pain. Evidence is accumulating that a genomic configuration predicates the biochemical architecture of the corticolimbic radiations. These transmit reward messages. This codes for phenotypes susceptible to drug abuse (Xuei *et al.*, 2008). Whether these phenotypes are especially interested in experimenting with drugs of potential misuse is not yet clear. If they do and the population of "tryers" are enticed by peers and dealers, the drug-naïve amongst them will try the new drug for sale and some may die of an overdose. Alternatively, they may find the new drug so rewarding they will continue to buy it and use it until they become dependent on it (Takahashi *et al.*, 2009). And this does not take long. Addictive behavior, starting with the first purchase, now enters a malignant phase. It may end with an arrest. Along the way comes alienation from family and non-using friends, loss of job, of self-respect. This is a path all too familiar to the addiction specialist.

Thus there is a dilemma. One horn is the clear need for a cadre of well trained pain specialists who have certification by a governing body. On the other horn are those physicians who see an occasional patient with chronic pain in non-fatal disorders but who are not trained to use opiates for its relief in a way consistent with "best practices." These include: 1) careful monitoring of supply: this means that lost, stolen, or "the dog ate my prescription" excuses cannot be tolerated; 2) if there is a suspicion that more than one physician is prescribing then this too is a warning that all is not well with this patient; 3) reassessment of the pain at regular intervals to determine continued need for opiates.

Finally, there is the patient who stands between these two valuable assets which are now an important part of the practice of medicine: pain management and addiction treatment. This is the person in pain.

It has been said, wisely, "Anger, one can overcome. Fear will dissipate. But pain. . . . One obeys."

References

Christie, M. J. (2008). Cellular neuroadaptations to chronic opioids: tolerance, withdrawal & addiction. *British Journal of Pharmacology*, **154**(2), 384–96.

Goldstein, R. G. & Volkow, N. D. (2002). Drug addiction and its underlying neurobiological basis: neuroimaging and evidence for involvement of the frontal cortex. *American Journal of Psychiatry*, **159**(10), 1642–52.

Gross, E. R., Hsu, A. K., Gross, G. J. (2009). Acute methadone treatment reduces myocardial infarct size via the δ-opioid receptor in rats during reperfusion. *Anesthesia and Analgesia*, **109**(5), 1395–402.

Jones, J. L., Wheeler, R. A. & Carelli, R. M. (2008). Behavioral responding and nucleus accumbens cell firing are unaltered following periods of absence from sucrose. *Synapse*, **62**(3), 219–28.

Ritter, P. L., Gonzalez, P. M., Laurent, D. D. & Lorig, K. R. (2006). Measurement of pain using the visual numeric scale. *Journal of Rheumatology*, **33**(3), 574–80.

Saal, D., Dong, Y., Bonci, A. & Malenka, R. C. (2003). Drugs of abuse and stress trigger a common synaptic adaptation in dopamine neurons. *Neuron* **37**(4), 577–82.

Takahashi, H., Mitochiro, D., Matsuura, M. *et al.* (2009). When your gain is my pain and your pain is my gain: neural correlates of envy and shadenfreude. *Science*, **13**(323), 937–9.

Xuei, X., Flury-Wetherill, L., Almasy, L. *et al.* (2008). Associated analysis of genes encoding the nocioreceptin receptor (OPRL-1). *Addiction Biology*, **13**(1), 80–7.

EEG neurofeedback therapy

Siegfried Othmer & Mark Steinberg

Introduction and foundation

This chapter describes a novel approach to understanding and treating addictions. This approach involves the use of EEG biofeedback (neurofeedback) as a modality for treating addictions. In the case of EEG biofeedback, the data generated the model. It is preferable, however, for an explanation of the model to precede the data. Addictions can result from both psychological and physiological factors. Neurofeedback lies at the nexus between them.

Though it is tempting (and perhaps traditional) to leave the realm of brain behavior entirely to neurophysiology, doing so could omit or minimize some critical elements. Medical science has supplied a great deal of knowledge about structural deficits in brain function; additionally, however, the *functional* domain of brain behavior is crucially relevant. Cognitive neuroscience – which concerns itself with brain function – has only begun to engage the challenge of psychopathology.

Neuronal networks organize behavioral repertoires. These networks exhibit a high level of integration and hierarchical organization. On the operational level, as in all communication networks, timing is crucial. Whenever a system is compelled to operate under tight constraints, there is opportunity for departure from functional integrity.

A key assumption is that psychopathology in general, and addiction in particular, arises from deficits in *network relations*. Recent thinking posits "connectivity deficits" as central to disorders such as schizophrenia, autism, and Alzheimer's disease. These clinical syndromes aside, this model may also help explain less acute or more "characterological" problems.

Pharmacologic interventions may not exhaust all therapeutic options. Neurophysiologic interventions, based on EEG data, afford additional and complementary treatment. Operant conditioning of EEG parameters is known as EEG biofeedback – more recently termed neurofeedback to distinguish it from its predecessor, biofeedback applied to peripheral physiology. Though clinical applications of EEG feedback have been extensive with childhood behavioral disorders, numerous other applications have been reported in clinical research.

Origins of EEG biofeedback for addiction treatment

In 1989, Eugene Peniston published a controlled study using EEG feedback with treatment-resistant Vietnam veterans suffering from alcohol dependence and post-traumatic stress disorder (PTSD) (Peniston and Kulkosky, 1989). The EEG feedback was an adjunct to standard treatment at the time – individual and group psychotherapy. Ten subjects in the treatment group had good outcomes, while control subjects remained alcohol-dependent. Small replication studies appeared in subsequent years; most of these supported the original finding. Peniston also followed up with additional confirming studies (vide infra). One subsequent large-scale controlled study, undertaken at a residential treatment center in Los Angeles, replicated the previous Peniston findings; the neurofeedback intervention was also applied to patients with substance dependencies other than alcohol. Participant outcomes did not depend on the drug of choice; at 1-year follow-up, three out of four subjects maintained sobriety. At 3-year follow-up, most experimental subjects continued to maintain sobriety, while controls continued to revert to pretreatment status.

Since that time, a small number of addiction treatment programs have incorporated neurofeedback. The lack of more robust growth of the technology in addictions treatment is puzzling. Perhaps this is a result of lack of familiarity with neurofeedback within the addictions treatment community.

The larger context of addiction

The following comorbid conditions may accompany addictive diseases:

- Anxiety or depressive disorder
- Undetected learning disabilities that diminish self-esteem and coping capacities
- Personality disorder, including compulsive or antisocial behavior
- "Organic" personality disorder concurrent with addictive disease
- Unrecognized traumatic brain injury or psychological trauma that limits functionality.

EEG biofeedback training can influence and modify each of the potential accompanying dysfunctions (each is regulated by particular and accessible brain networks).

In neurofeedback, the key intervention is *self-regulation* of impaired, or disregulated, neuronal systems. Because the technique is non-verbal and targets brain behavior directly, it bypasses the usual (verbal) resistances often encountered in therapeutic practice. Since biofeedback aims for improvements in self-regulatory function, this technique could well be considered the *self-regulation remedy*.

The self-regulation approach is complementary to existing interventions. It is consistent with the recognized need for integrative modalities in addiction treatment. Neurofeedback itself is rarely employed as a stand-alone technique for addictions. Traditional addiction treatments feature gradual reduction of psychopharmacological agents along with psychotherapeutic support, including both psychodynamic and behavioral interventions. Successful neurofeedback may reduce or even eliminate the need for stimulants, antidepressants, mood stabilizers, antipsychotic medications, pain medications, and sleep aids. Neurofeedback training can also, over time, lead to greater insight, enhanced receptivity, and deeper engagement with the therapist. Throughout the process, a certain level of implicit trust is required for the trainee to "admit and permit" behavioral reinforcement; this makes the therapeutic context for this work critically important.

Model of brain function supporting EEG neurofeedback

The discovery during the "decade of the brain" that new neuronal growth does take place in the mature adult brain brings hope that even conditions previously considered intractable may be amenable to recovery. The discovery of neuronal growth in the adult human brain validated the notion of brain plasticity, even for those whose work was oriented entirely on structurally and neuroanatomically based models of chemical dependency. But brain plasticity does not depend upon new neuronal growth. It is an inherent property of neural systems.

Some reports document positive outcome rates of neurofeedback therapy that far exceed the typical 25–33% (1 year) sobriety rates achieved with other interventions. Addictive disease may be a constellation of learned behaviors that can be extinguished if and when the brain is given appropriate cues. Although addictive disease often has a heritable component, this should by no means serve as a justification for poor treatment response.

The following areas are critical to an understanding of neurofeedback's mechanism of action:

1. Architecture of neuronal networks
2. Organization of network functions
3. Dynamic management of states.

Architecture of neuronal networks

The human brain is perhaps one of the best examples of what has come to be known as a "small-world" model of networks. Both local and "global" connectivity characterize these networks. In the human brain, both local and global connectivity are quite extensive. Brain-based neurons that manage more distant communications are the pyramidal cells; these receive inputs locally through some 1000 to 10 000 dendritic connections. When dendritic inputs exceed threshold criteria, the neuron generates an action potential, a brief electrical transient capable of signal propagation. Action potentials progress the length of the axon; the axon itself ramifies many times and thus also distributes its signal to many nodes in the zone of the dendritic tree. In addition to this local network, each pyramidal cell also sends its axon to distal cortical regions via the white matter. Synaptic junctions can receive signals from any other synaptic junctions within typically as few as three synaptic links. We are wired in a way that marvelously maximizes and makes accessible all the global connectivity of which we are potentially capable. Cortical loci are "aware" of what is going on in any other part at any time.

Organization of network functions

A second key aspect of the "small-world" model of networks is that of hierarchical organization. In the brain, this hierarchy of control has several levels. At the top rung are the cortical neurons, numbering about ten billion. At the next level are the thalamus and the other subcortical nuclei (visible in medical brain imagery studies). The foundation or base of the hierarchy is the brainstem. Because the brainstem's role is so basic, its functions tend to be taken for granted, much like the heartbeat.

The implication for neurofeedback is this: any attempt to modify brain function communicates with the entire brain and with the entire regulatory hierarchy, all the way to the brainstem. *Neurofeedback reaches every brain level that is managed within this regulatory hierarchy.*

Central regulation of brain function is paramount here. EEG feedback accesses the organization of large-scale synaptic information transport. Fortunately, the rules are again very simple. A single excitatory post-synaptic potential is incapable of generating another action potential in the target neuron; there must be a co-conspirator that arrives within a very narrow time window. Therefore, the operation performed by the neuron, stated mathematically, is that of "coincidence detection." This process imposes very narrow timing constraints on all synaptic information transport since the "opportunity window" in this process is only about 10 milliseconds. The potential for functional deterioration of this transmission is obvious.

One role of the neuron is that of a correlation detector. Consider, however, that brain function cannot depend upon the functionality of each and every individual neuron. Information is instead encoded in neuronal assemblies. The brain gets the message through by utilizing many pathways, acting in unison. In other words, the brain is organized for massive parallel processing.

"Binding" – the necessity to discriminate which neuron is part of the dance and which is not – is therefore a major question in neuroscience. Time binding has been proposed as an explanation for how the brain elegantly solves this problem: simultaneity in firing defines the state of belonging to the ensemble. Firing coincidence at the individual neuronal level translates to simultaneity at the level of the neuronal ensemble.

When neurons fire in groups, the resulting signal is sufficiently large to be detectable at the scalp in the EEG. The EEG records continuing brain activity as it constructs and then deconstructs neuronal assemblies. The brain also arranges for repetition of *nearly* the same firing pattern at characteristic frequencies. The result is that the EEG depicts numerous packets of activity, each at its own characteristic frequency.

Neurologist Simon Farmer succinctly described this model (Farmer, 2002):

> We are beginning to understand that brain rhythms, their synchronization and de-synchronization, form an important and possibly fundamental part of the orchestration of perception, motor action and conscious experience and that disruption of oscillation and/or temporal synchronization may be a fundamental mechanism of neurological disease.

As a neurologist, Farmer restricts his discourse to neurological conditions, but these concepts clearly have wider application.

All these features of neuronal assemblies either are, or should be, under tight regulation by the brain. Gross malfunction shows up in cases of seizure disorder, dementia, and traumatic brain injury. Understanding EEG tracings that are characteristic of these disorders helps to illuminate EEG findings in subjects with addictive disorders.

Even the healthy brain provides electrophysiologic access to brain activity during operant conditioning or subtle stimulation. Neurofeedback works by a reciprocal process. On the one hand, neurofeedback "invites" the brain to alter its activity; on the other hand, the brain – an entity seeking to maintain its integrity and stability – acts to counter this interference. *The result of repeating this brain challenge is to strengthen the regulatory loops.*

Significantly, this process does not depend on the presence of EEG abnormalities. The process works to enhance regulatory control, not to bring it into existence de novo. Fortunately, this is the usual state of affairs – absent gross and incapacitating pathology. Thus, in treating addictions, the EEG "entering behavior" of almost all patients is sufficient to respond well to the treatment. This is because only minor increments in regulatory control are needed to make a life of abstinence a realistic possibility.

Dynamic management of states

In treating addiction, it is critical to take into account the importance of arousal states and affect regulation in treatment. The dynamics of brain function and regulation underpin addictive dysfunction. The relevance of the principles of brain dynamics in both functional and dysfunctional patterns makes effective intervention possible. The neuroscientist Walter Freeman expressed the concept succinctly (Freeman, 2000):

> Every neuron and every patch participates in every experience and behavior, even if its contribution is to silence its pulse train or stay dark in a brain image . . .

And, along similar lines, the following (ibid, p. 134):

> The . . . communities of modules in the two hemispheres, cooperating through the brainstem, the corpus callosum, and the other inter-hemispheric commissures, express a single, global, dynamic framework.

These comments support the observations made by many neurofeedback clinicians that a very limited number of training protocols are sufficient to move the brain globally to better function. Still, it matters a great deal which part of the cortex is trained and which parts of the whole domain of EEG frequencies are targeted in training. Again, some very simple rules apply. The lower EEG frequencies tend to organize more persistent states, whereas the higher EEG frequencies tend to underpin transient activity such as specific cognitive events. As for location on the scalp, knowledge about localization of function is clearly of relevance here. Alternatively, treatment of addicted patients typically does not target localized function, but instead targets very basic regulatory mechanisms that are broadly distributed and not localized at all.

It is best to think of this work, first, as addressing particular regulatory systems. The ebb and flow of the EEG at any one locale reflects the activation–relaxation dynamics of specific brain networks, and these are constituents of what are called phasic and tonic arousal. Scalp EEG tracings profile levels of arousal. The alcoholic brain often records a tonic high-arousal condition – for which neurofeedback offers a remedy. In fact, arousal regulation/dysregulation is the main clinical issue in the neurofeedback treatment of substance abusers.

Second, affect regulation is another target of neurofeedback training in an addicted population, as so many exhibit concurrent mood instabilities or mood-unstable personality disorders. One school of thought correlates personality disorders with disorders of attachment during early childhood. Through neurofeedback, the underlying circuitry governing

emotional attachment is directly trainable. Prevailing psychotherapies may address obstacles to emotional attachment, but they do not access the organic basis of these obstacles directly. Neurofeedback successfully targets both the symptoms and the root causes of persistent addiction because:

1. It trains the brain to modulate overarousal, a maladaptive dysphoric state that often triggers attempts to "self-medicate" the hyperarousal.
2. It addresses the underlying, unremediated disorders of attachment that often have developed into maladaptive behavior patterns, personalities, and lifestyles.
3. Neurofeedback training broadly targets executive function. Impulsivity and behavioral disinhibition are evidence of diminished executive function. Neurofeedback training moderates obsessive/compulsive tendencies and thrill-seeking behavior. This training also impacts satiety and reward systems, modulating drives ranging from appetite awareness to drug-seeking behavior. Concomitantly, neurofeedback leads to improvements in working memory and cognitive function. As the proper hierarchy of regulation is restored to neural networks, patients experience greater mastery across the neuropsychiatric spectrum, including gains in cognitive function.

Satiety, behavior, and the brain

Neurofeedback prepares the neural substrate for a drug-free existence. Drug-seeking behavior is often in response to a felt need. One possible remedy is to train the central nervous system (CNS) to function in the absence of that drug. Neurofeedback helps to alter brain reward circuitry so that the association between pleasure and satiety and the use of a specific drug is diminished. Neurofeedback does not provoke the extreme states of euphoria associated by users with many drugs. However, the enhanced capacity for feeling joy and pleasure (on a daily, consistent basis) that often results from effective neurofeedback training does allow the person to sustain and enjoy sobriety.

What about nicotine addiction? It is quite apparent to many smokers that their brains function better when they smoke. These people give up smoking at some considerable cost to themselves and perhaps to their relationships and work performance as well. The first intervention in smoking cessation is to train the brain that nicotine no longer offers performance increments. Then the cessation of smoking can take center stage.

The success of this strategy is most evident in work with marijuana smokers. In many cases, clients gave up marijuana quite unintentionally once they began EEG training. People routinely report, at some point in neurofeedback treatment, "I forgot to use!"

Patients are usually more surprised by this phenomenon than clinicians, who have observed it in many cases of treatment. The same has been reported for nicotine addiction.

The role and treatment of trauma

The discussion above hinges on the clinical process of neurophysiological normalization. Neurophysiological normalization may be a required component of stable, sustained abstinence (e.g. where marijuana use is driven by a felt need).

Addictive behavior coupled with a history of trauma makes treatment more complex, more challenging. Some addictions are difficult to treat unless the underlying trauma is somehow addressed as well.

Traumatic episodes are events in which the individual's survival was suddenly threatened, or when life-threatening events were observed in those near and dear. Traumatic events also include episodes in which the patient "merely" interprets or perceives that a given event may be life-threatening. Individuals are also traumatized by life events that don't necessarily kill or maim so much as bleed the spirit or vitality of a person to a grossly debilitating extent. Such individuals may seek out and/or benefit from "soul-work" – therapy for a person whose life force has been crushed in some way so that it cannot seek and find positive expression. Neurofeedback can be helpful here as well. By positive reinforcement – rewarding low EEG frequencies – treatment helps the person to encounter his "existential self." Under these conditions, traumas can be resolved, and healing and reconstitution of the self often occurs. People report these therapeutic experiences (often in retrospect) as life-altering. The process is another aspect of "self-repair," in that the role of the therapist is to facilitate and assist the healing that the patient invokes, using his own resources. The use of neurofeedback technology to facilitate this process is known as "alpha-theta training."

Alpha-theta training has three goals. First, it physiologically, psychologically, and perceptually distances the environment, which allows the person to focus inward calmly. Second, it quiets cortical function in general and the verbal "self-censor" in particular. This allows the core self to emerge into awareness by means of imagery. Alpha-theta sessions are often suffused with imagery that is dream-like, that is hypnagogic in quality. Third, the EEG becomes more coherent (wave forms become more similar) over larger brain regions: this enlarges the subjective boundary of self and helps draw others into one's affective embrace. Key historical relationships that had been problematic in the past can be quite suddenly restructured and perceived differently, in a more positive frame. Early childhood trauma may be defused and integrated. In some instances, the greatest perceived benefit of this training is identified by the patient with a particular session within the sequence of what is now called "deep-state" training. Observers unfamiliar with the process and its theoretical basis can find much that seems mysterious and unsystematic here. Healing from within is not confined to linear or methodologically rigid parameters.

Recovery from treatment-resistant addiction can require improved cerebral regulation as well as a "deeper" healing of injuries to the self. Ideally, the result is transformational, such that addiction no longer fills a need or, for that matter, has any place in the evolved life. In practice, results often fall short of the ideal. Nonetheless, neurofeedback has proven to be a valuable tool that allows some to maintain abstinence, recover function, and make progress in their lives.

The historical development of neurofeedback

A review of neurofeedback history is essential for three reasons: 1) it documents the depth and breadth of prior research; 2) it yields understanding of why neurofeedback still attracts sceptics, and 3) it provides a basis for current treatment approaches. Deep-state training began with Joe Kamiya, who first demonstrated successful reinforcement of alpha rhythms in 1962 (Kamiya, 1969; Kamiya & Noles, 1970). Kamiya then published a study demonstrating that alpha training was successful in moderating trait anxiety (Hardt & Kamiya, 1978). It was not long, however, before the alpha work caught public attention. Reports of idyllic experiences with altered states brought the technique into favor with the psychedelic crowd who wished simply to avoid the downside of the LSD experience. This development in turn disqualified the technique for formal academic research, and whatever minimal research that was done seemed destined to fail. Alpha training fell quite precipitously into disrepute, and this is largely attributed to one negative outcome study (Lynch *et al.*, 1974). Subsequently, only isolated clinicians and researchers carried the work forward, operating outside of the academic community and without benefit of grant funding.

M. Barry Sterman pioneered the movement involved in training physiological normalization. Sterman worked at the Sepulveda Veterans Administration Hospital in Los Angeles. Initially the work was thought to have limited application to seizure management, and later to the "neurobiological deficit" of attention deficit hyperactivity disorder (ADHD) in children. Proponents insisted at the time that they did not regard the technique as broadly applicable to psychological dysfunction. Even within the biofeedback community itself, the work did not gain much of a beachhead. The research was richly applauded, accepted, and, ironically, ignored. Who needed EEG feedback when there was peripheral biofeedback? In any event, biofeedback therapists weren't inclined to work with seizure disorders. The field of neurology, meanwhile, had no use for a behavioral technique for managing seizures. By 1985, funding for EEG feedback research at the NIH had run dry. Again, only isolated clinicians carried the torch.

Jim Hardt, a student of Joe Kamiya, was the first to work successfully with addictions using alpha training (Hardt, 2007). One of his early clinical successes is illustrative of the process. The case is described in Hardt's recent book, *The Art of Smart Thinking* (p.106):

In 1979, I had the opportunity to provide alpha training to a woman who I later discovered to be a multiple drug-user and a drug dealer. I did not know that she and her husband (also a dealer) were consuming almost an ounce of cocaine a day between them. She was drinking a fifth of hard liquor to take the edge off the cocaine, and she smoked tobacco daily, and took LSD, psilocybin, mescaline, and marijuana on a regular basis. She also took tranquilizers and stimulants to change her mind state whenever she wanted and in whatever direction she wished. Her personal motto was, "Excess is not enough!"

On the fifth day of her alpha training she described "falling into a pool of alpha," which forever changed her life. Although she had no intention of reducing or stopping her drug use when she started alpha training, and in spite of the fact that she liked her drug use lifestyle and thought her life was "working very well," her drug use began to fall away. Within six weeks of the end of her alpha training, she was not using any drugs. Even the tobacco smoking

had stopped. And now, she found that she could no longer live with her husband, who had not done the alpha training, and who continued to use and to deal drugs.

Hardt had a 9-year follow-up with this person, who continued her drug-free life, even to the point of spurning caffeine. This case violates all the expectations. There was not even the desire to quit drugs, and yet the training had a health-promoting and constructive effect. There had been no "hitting bottom" or other crisis to launch this person on the path to recovery. Moreover, there was ongoing benefit of the training even after its cessation. In this case, the entire training sequence was transformational in effect. Yet, there was no single transformative moment (as is sometimes the case).

Work with the theta band found favor in the research by Tom Budzynski on twilight learning. By holding people in a theta-dominant state just short of stage-one sleep with reinforcement techniques, Budzynski found that while in that state they were highly suggestible. The boundary of the self was more "permeable" (Budzynski, 1972). Soon thereafter, however, Budzynski's interest diverged to the peripheral biofeedback modalities that were of interest and were receiving grant funding at that time.

Elmer Green and his colleagues (with the active support of Karl Menninger) conducted the principal work with alpha-theta training (Green *et al.*, 1970; 1974). This research used alpha training mainly as an entry portal to states of theta dominance, with which the transformative experience was more directly associated. In this model, activity in both theta and alpha bands was reinforced. However, this research did not focus on or purport to address psychopathology in general or addictions in particular.

Lester Fehmi propelled a third initiative in studying alpha. Fehmi pioneered multi-channel alpha training to promote large-scale alpha coherence over the posterior cortex to still the sensory cortices and promote the capacity for more global, diffuse, and immersed states of attention to counter the Western bias toward narrowly focused attention (Fehmi, 1978; Fehmi and Robbins, 2007).

Neurofeedback in addictions treatment: what the research shows

The pivotal research of the biofeedback group at the Menninger Clinic resulted in the large-scale application of alpha-theta training to veteran alcoholics at the nearby Veterans Administration Hospital in Topeka,

Kansas (Goslinga, 1975). Twemlow and Bowen reported on trends in self-actualization scores with EEG feedback on 76 subjects (Twemlow & Bowen, 1976; 1977). Significantly, the only predictor of self-actualization scores that emerged with EEG training was religiosity. Perhaps patients with a high baseline religiosity score were more likely to experience "imagery with high religious impact, including experiences of white light, crucifixion, and other metaphors of death and rebirth" while in the theta-dominant state.

In 1977, Watson, Herder, and Passini published a study on 25 alcoholics who were given 10 hours of alpha training and then compared to matched controls (Passini *et al.*, 1977; Watson *et al.*, 1978). The study yielded evidence of improvement on state and trait anxiety, and 18-month follow-up yielded evidence of reduced alcohol consumption (Watson *et al.*, 1978). A third study, in which alpha training was done with 66 psychiatric patients and compared with no-treatment controls, yielded no significant differential changes (on 54 measures) outside of chance expectation. This negative outcome is not at all surprising given current understanding (vide infra).

Additional early studies

The study that revived interest in alpha-theta neurofeedback applications for addiction was undertaken by Eugene Peniston, a psychologist then employed at the Fort Lyon Veterans Administration (VA) facility to work with Vietnam veteran alcoholics. He also adapted the Menninger protocol for his work, having personally had an experience with the protocol at Menninger in the course of a training program. Ironically, he did not react well to the feedback session personally, and had to be strongly encouraged to try it again. Subsequent experiences were also wrenching, but they led him to undertake this research with some of his patients. Peniston also had a personal motivation: his brother had succumbed to alcoholism.

Following the basic Menninger protocol, the EEG training was preceded by eight 30-minute sessions of temperature biofeedback, which serves to give people a first experience with the concept of self-regulation training. Further, it calms an overactive sympathetic nervous system and brings people down from over-aroused states. The thermal biofeedback was augmented with exercises in paced, slow breathing to promote relaxation. The EEG training involved fifteen 30-minute sessions of alpha-theta training. The alpha band was set at 8–13 Hz, and the theta band at 4–8 Hz. Reward was a continuous tone for as long as threshold conditions were met. Guided imagery augmented the EEG training with verbal inductions given prior to entry into the training phase. The details of these aspects of the protocol are described in a later publication (Peniston & Kulkosky, 1999).

A total of 20 participants entered the program, with 10 receiving feedback in addition to the normal residential treatment program. Participants had to have a history of at least four prior treatment failures for alcoholism. The average was 5.4 treatment failures. They also had to have a confirmed history of alcoholism extending more than 20 years.

On follow-up, the control group stayed true to form. All had to be readmitted to another round of treatment within 18 months of completion. By contrast, all 10 of the experimental subjects were successful over the initial 18-month follow-up period, and, in fact, remained successful over the subsequent 10 years or more of informal follow-up. In this context, *successful* meant no more problem drinking. Interestingly, one of the 10 was able to return to social drinking without a problem. Two of the participants thought the EEG training was "for the birds," and immediately headed for the local bar upon release from the program. They both became ill at once and found that they had lost their tolerance for alcohol, a quite common outcome of alpha training. This alcohol-mediated illness has since become known as the "Peniston flu." Because of this early relapse, they were initially listed as treatment failures by Peniston. However, in view of their sustained sobriety after this initial episode, these two should be counted among the treatment successes. This meant 100% success where none would have been expected!

A firestorm met Peniston's work within the biofeedback community when it was presented at the 1990 annual meeting in Washington DC. The original Biofeedback Research Society had been organized in 1969 around the impetus of alpha training. When that became discredited in the mid-seventies, they sought refuge in biofeedback using peripheral modalities. Biofeedback therapists and researchers did not want to be reminded of the disgrace visited upon the organization by the early alpha training. They were convinced they had seen the last of alpha training.

Yet, Peniston had brought considerable supportive data to bear. First of all, there were clear changes in the percentage of time patients exceeded the threshold in alpha-theta training. Second, the experimental group demonstrated significant recovery on the Beck Depression Scale. Third, the control group showed increases in beta-endorphin levels over the course of the study. These were attributed to the stress of the therapy. Such an increase was not found in the experimental group.

Additionally, Peniston showed substantial normalization in subtest scores on the Millon Clinical Multiaxial Inventory (MCMI) and the Sixteen Personality Factor (16-PF) Questionnaire among the experimentals (Peniston & Kulkosky, 1990). Significant decreases occurred in MCMI scales labeled schizoid, avoidant, passive aggression, schizotypal, borderline, paranoid, anxiety, somatoform, dysthymia, alcohol abuse, psychotic thinking, psychotic depression, and psychotic delusion. Alcoholics receiving the standard medical treatment showed significant decreases only in two MCMI scales – avoidant and psychotic thinking – and an increase in one scale, the compulsive. On the 16-PF Questionnaire (Cattell *et al.*, 1970), the EEG training led to significant increases in warmth, abstract thinking, stability, conscientiousness, boldness, imaginativeness, and self-control. The training appeared to produce fundamental changes in personality variables that supported the observation of sustained sobriety.

By 1991, Peniston had published yet another study on the application of alpha-theta training to PTSD (Peniston & Kulkosky, 1991). A criticism directed at his earlier study was that he had not so much demonstrated remediation of alcoholism per se, but rather of PTSD, to which the alcoholism was secondary. Although this was a criticism that Peniston could accept, his next study formally focused on PTSD rather than on alcohol dependence. Because of the intimate association of PTSD and substance abuse, and because it supports the case for alpha-theta training, the study is an important part of the story.

A total of 29 Vietnam veterans was recruited into a study similar to that described above. This study administered 30 sessions of alpha-theta training, and then used the Minnesota Multiphasic Personality Inventory (MMPI) to track changes in personality variables. Favorable change occurred among the experimentals on nearly all the clinical subscales of the MMPI. The most substantial changes were in the depression, psychopathic deviate, paranoia, psychaesthenia, and schizophrenia subscales. The PTSD subscale of the MMPI improved by

a factor of two-thirds among the experimentals, while remaining unchanged among the controls.

On follow-up after 30 months, only three of the 15 experimentals reported having had any disturbing flashbacks. All three were given six booster sessions of neurofeedback, in the course of which one subject required rehospitalization. All of the 14 controls had to be admitted to Veteran's Administration treatment centers at least twice for additional PTSD-related treatment within the 30-month period.

Finally, in 1993, Peniston published yet another study in which recovery from PTSD was evaluated with four-channel EEG synchrony training to see if it offered any advantage over conventional single-channel alpha training (Peniston *et al.*, 1993). No comparison group was involved. The explicit synchrony training promotes a state of global coherence in the alpha and theta bands, which is more conducive to the often-sought disengaged, internally focused, state. However, outcomes were not dramatically different from prior feedback experience in such dual-diagnosis patients (PTSD and alcoholism). Follow-up among the 20 subjects at 26 months revealed four participants who showed recurrence of PTSD symptoms. Outcomes with respect to alcohol consumption were not reported.

The brusque rejection of Peniston's work upon first presentation to the biofeedback community relegated the continuation of research and replications to the select subset who were hardy and committed. Only a few of these studies have been published. In an outcome study, Saxby showed changes in personality variables similar to Peniston and documented sustained relapse prevention in 13 of 14 participants over a 21-month follow-up (Saxby & Peniston, 1995). Steve Fahrion, of the Menninger group, published a single case study that tracked EEG measures and personality factors (Fahrion *et al.*, 1992). Byers also documented normalization of personality measures (Byers, 1992). Kelley reported on a 3-year outcome study of alpha-theta neurofeedback training for problem-drinking among the Dine' (Navajo) people (Kelly, 1997). He took care to integrate the feedback work into the existing cultural paradigms. Kelley reported extinction of drinking behavior and reduced incidence of destructive behaviors in 16 of the 20 participants.

More recently, a European study applied a very different EEG training technique to the problem of alcohol dependency. The technique of transiently altering the slow cortical potential (low-frequency EEG), which was developed in application to seizure management, was employed with seven patients hospitalized for their alcoholism. In follow-up at 4 months after release from the hospital, six of the seven had retained sobriety, and these six were the ones who had demonstrated mastery of the skill of controlling their slow cortical potential (Schneider *et al.*, 1993).

Bodenhamer-Davis published follow-up results for the Peniston protocol with juvenile offenders (Bodenhamer-Davis & Callaway, 2004). Follow-up after 7–9 years found 80% maintenance of abstinence, and a rearrest rate down by half with respect to the comparison group. Burkett reported results mirroring those of Peniston for a tough clinical population, homeless crack addicts (Burkett *et al.*, 2004). Alpha-theta neurofeedback was added to a faith-based mission for the homeless in Houston. Substantial success was achieved according to multiple criteria: that the homeless person be housed, maintain work, and remain drug-free.

In addition to the published reports, various conference presentations attested to the successful insertion of alpha-theta training into real-world clinical practice. Tom Allen reported that it had become a central component of his treatment of juvenile substance abusers. Dr. Nancy White tracked MMPI data for 41 successive alcoholics in her private psychology practice and found consistent remediation on the depression scale. Fahrion employed alpha-theta training with parolees from the Kansas prison system. Whereas the results were generally positive in this case, they also showed a disappointingly high dropout rate.

More recently, Smith and Sams (2004) reported on a pilot study of neurotherapy in application to youthful offenders who were also substance abusers. The study was carried out in a therapeutic community where the youngsters typically stayed for 12 months. The median number of arrests for the treatment group (30 in number) had been two. Nearly all were of upper middle class in socioeconomic status, and nearly all were Caucasian.

Neurofeedback was also added to a 12-step-based program. Training was at a rate of four sessions per week; this program involved heart rate variability (HRV) training, which is thought to impact emotional responsivity. Significantly, the neurofeedback protocol falls into the category of physiological normalization. No alpha-theta training was done with this group, although it is possible that the HRV training served as a surrogate.

The outcomes reported for this pilot study mirrored the Peniston and CRI-Help data in nearly every respect: length of stay improved with the number of sessions; those who received a minimum of 24 sessions graduated from the program at a 100% rate. Even those who had only 12 sessions doubled their length of stay over controls who did without neurofeedback. Mean Beck Depression Inventory scores ($n = 30$) declined from 25.5 to 11.3. Psychiatric medications decreased among 50% of trainees, and increased in only one trainee, who also happened to be the one person to suffer relapse later. All group continuous performance test scores improved to normative levels, with all effect sizes exceeding one standard deviation. Average MMPI scores ($n = 30$) improved from 64.5 before training to 55.6 after training. If one disregards the masculine/feminine category where change was neither seen nor expected, the average change in the remaining nine categories was 10 points. Average changes of 10 or more points were observed for: depression (17), hysteria (15), hypochondriasis (12), schizophrenia (12), and paranoia (10). More than 90% achieved abstinence, and those who experienced brief relapse returned to recovery activity quickly. Only one relapsed irretrievably.

Two studies failed to corroborate Peniston's work. The first was a comparison of electromyography (EMG) biofeedback, transcendental meditation, and alpha-theta feedback with standard treatment of alcoholics (Taub *et al.*, 1994). Whereas enhanced clinical success was achieved within the EMG and transcendental meditation arms of the study, this success was not demonstrated in the alpha-theta arm. EEG advocates met this report with some suspicion because Taub was viewed as part of the biofeedback contingent that would just as soon see alpha-theta training disappear.

The second study was a university-based project that attempted to evaluate *pure feedback*, stripped of all the personal touches and concerned support that were part of the service provided by Peniston in the original work (Graap & Freides, 1997). Unsurprisingly, the study failed to support Peniston's findings, since therapeutic caring cannot be subtracted from the mix in the interest of pure science without sacrificing some treatment outcome variance.

By this time, Peniston's work had taken root among many clinicians – who pointed out that the training cannot be separated from its supportive context to stand on its own. Purifying and distilling the technique down to its essence for purposes of research was not a viable option. Some neurofeedback proponents insisted that narrow-minded academic researchers were once again impugning the work of sensitive and competent clinicians, just as had happened in the early days of the alpha work.

Somewhat piqued by criticism of their failed replication, Graap and Freides uncharitably pointed out that some of Peniston's data seemed to indicate that the populations in his two studies were not entirely independent. Peniston defended himself, but the controversy did not entirely subside. In any event, Graap and Freides never published the results of their study (Graap and Freides, 1998).

Another criticism directed at the Peniston study was that the numbers were too small to allow firm conclusions. This criticism was statistically unsound at best and, perhaps, even disingenuous. The number of subjects required is a function of effect size, and in this case the contrast between experimentals and controls was so radical that the number of subjects was quite adequate to rule out the null hypothesis.

Nevertheless, during the mid-90s a large-scale replication of Peniston's work was organized at EEG Spectrum, then headed by Siegfried Othmer, the co-author of this chapter. The principal modification was that EEG training would replace thermal training prior to the alpha-theta work. This research was done in collaboration with CRI-Help, a Residential Treatment Center in Los Angeles. The intent was to assess the role of neurofeedback in as life-like a situation as possible; hence staff at CRI-Help were trained to provide the service.

The study's intent was to focus on alcoholism, but there weren't enough cases to meet group size objectives in reasonable time. Subsequently, study subject criteria were expanded to include other drugs as well. Heroin, crack cocaine, and methamphetamine users represented 30% of the treatment population; 10% were alcoholics. Nearly all subjects were multi-drug users. Everyone received the standard Minnesota Model treatment, with the experimentals also receiving neurofeedback; controls received additional individual and group psychotherapy.

Executive function can be regarded as the highest echelon of motor planning. Training the circuitry of motor control at any point inevitably trains executive function as well. The placement at Fz (Fz and other sites refer to the standard International 1020 system of electrode placement) gets the frontal region explicitly

involved. Right hemisphere training was done with a parietal bias to calm down phasic arousal. For more extensive details of this protocol and for the clinical results that were obtained, see Othmer *et al.* (1999). The alpha-theta training used 8–11 Hz for the detection of alpha and 5–8 Hz for theta, with electrode placement at Pz (International 10-20 System). The neurofeedback consisted of a combination of SMR-beta training and alpha-theta training. SMR-beta training refers to the original procedure developed by Barry Sterman for seizure management, with a slight modification: the beta training, at 15–18 Hz, was used with the left hemisphere and the SMR-beta training, at 12–15 Hz, was used on the right. SMR refers to the sensorimotor rhythm first identified by Sterman. Electrode placement was C3-Fz for left hemisphere training, and C4-Pz for right hemisphere training. The principal objective of this protocol was improved regulation of arousal and enhanced executive function. Training to elevate amplitudes of the resting rhythm of the sensorimotor system moves the person to lower and more controlled states of tonic arousal. The slightly higher frequency training on the left side was often helpful for depression.

With 121 participants entering the program, group size was now adequate to withstand any potential statistical criticism, provided one could aggregate the data for the different drugs. When the results were later analyzed separately for the different drugs, this assumption was supported. The two groups were matched on the Addiction Severity Index. Those with a diagnosed psychotic or personality disorder or a seizure disorder were excluded from participation.

Results surfaced almost as soon as the training began. Even within the first couple of weeks of training (rate of two sessions per day), a statistically significant group effect in retention rate was demonstrated. This is shown in Fig. 19.1. During this period of time, only the SMR-beta training was done; this argues for a significant role for SMR-beta training in the overall protocol. The proximate goal in this training was to normalize the measures on a continuous performance test – the TOVA (test of variables of attention). Participants were re-tested after ten sessions. If TOVA scores had not normalized by that point, the subject was given ten additional sessions. The average number of sessions to TOVA normalization was 13, showing that the majority of subjects were able to normalize their TOVA scores within ten sessions (the median was ten).

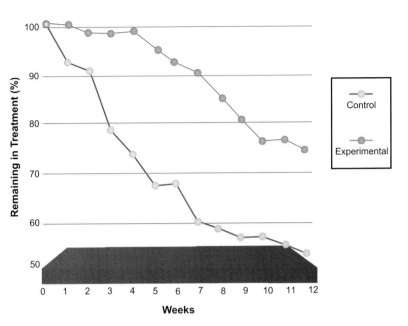

Figure 19.1 Retention in therapy for the experimental and control groups over the duration of the treatment program. Attrition rate for the controls was twice that of the experimentals. Significant differences appeared even during the SMR-beta phase of the EEG training.

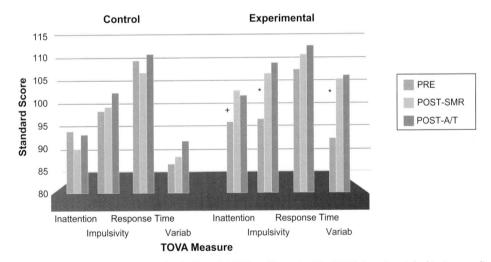

Figure 19.2 Pre-post standard scores are shown for the Test of Variables of Attention (the TOVA). Experimental subjects normalized all of their TOVA subtest scores with an average of 13 training sessions.

The average TOVA scores for the two cohorts are reproduced in Fig. 19.2. Remarkably, all post-training scores for the experimental group exceeded norms. This was somewhat surprising given the history of the participants. Many had been referred by Los Angeles County. Many were jobless. Some were homeless. About 30% had done prison time, and were likely to have had a history of psychological or physical trauma. CRI-Help estimates that their organization deals with the most challenging population that is engaged in regular addictions treatment anywhere.

A neurocognitive test battery was also given to all participants, but here the experimentals distinguished themselves from the controls significantly only on delayed recall testing. Though memory is one excellent measure of brain function, on the basis of the good continuous performance test data one might have expected a broader range of improvement. Gains were also observed on immediate recall and on the

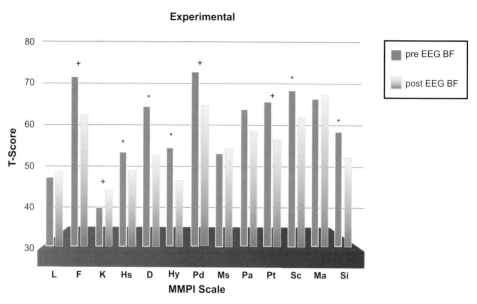

Figure 19.3 Pre-post MMPI data are shown for the experimentals. Substantial normalization of elevated scores is indicated. A star is used to indicate a significant treatment interaction, whereas a plus indicates significant change that nevertheless did not reach the level of significant treatment interaction.

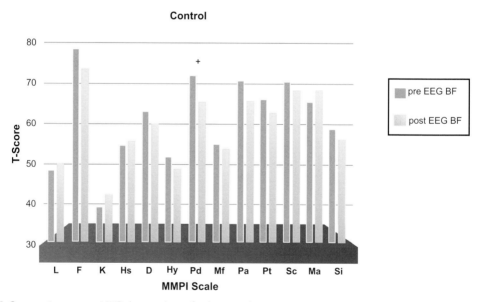

Figure 19.4 Comparative pre-post MMPI data are shown for the controls.

Tower Test, but there was no significant treatment interaction.

Following Peniston's method, the MMPI was also administered before and after the study, and the results mirrored his earlier data. The results are shown in Fig. 19.3 for the experimentals, and in Fig. 19.4 for the controls. A common thread running through all of these studies is the large change in the depression scale among experimental subjects. Additionally, the CRI-Help study confirmed Peniston's work with respect to significant changes in the hypochondriasis, conversion hysteria, and schizophrenia scales. The consistent direction of these changes over all studies indicates that this training clearly improved a

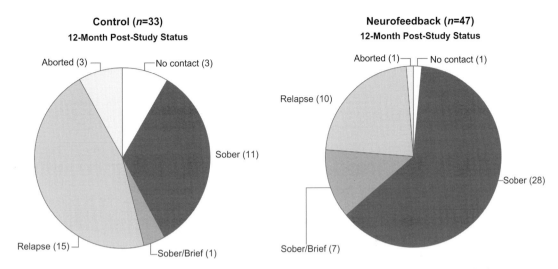

Figure 19.5 Relapse data are shown for the period 12 months post-graduation. Experimentals exhibit a three times higher success rate in maintaining abstinence if brief relapsers are included (35 versus 12).

number of aspects of the trainees' mental health status.

Relapse was tracked in these individuals over a 3-year period, but has been formally reported only for the first year. The data are shown in Fig. 19.5. In interpreting the data, one must consider that, at the end of the program, the graduating cohorts are no longer equivalent owing to the much higher attrition rate among controls.

A policy perspective would refer back to the point of entry into the program, where the groups are still matched. An arbitrary person inserted into the experimental program would have a three times higher likelihood of being relapse-free at the end of 1 year compared to someone who had received the standard treatment alone. This turns a success rate of nominally 20% into a success rate of more than 60%.

The current status

Given the novelty of the neurofeedback approach, it was difficult to get this work published. It finally appeared in the *American Journal of Drug and Alcohol Abuse* in August of 2005 (Scott *et al.*, 2005). The study had taken 4 years, and the subsequent path to publication had taken about 5 years. Since that time, numerous protocol enhancements have evolved through clinical application. Peniston reported a number of abreactions in the course of his training. The CRI-Help study had already changed to a reinforcement band of 5–8 Hz versus the prior 4–8 Hz, and the problem of abreactions essentially resolved. Apparently, this change could be

made with no loss in overall clinical efficiency. Further positive changes have also occurred since.

In the CRI-Help study, Principal Investigator William Scott found that a number of people reacted badly to alpha reinforcement. Often, these people would show high alpha amplitudes at inception. In these cases, it was beneficial first to train alpha down before administering the standard protocol later. One may think of this modification as additional training toward functional normalization, distinct from the alpha-theta sessions, where the primary purpose is experiential. Hence, there is no conflict in training alpha first down and then up in the same individual. The first phase takes place as part of the alert-state training, and the second takes place in a state of low arousal, or deep-state, training.

Subsequent evolution of the technique has taken two forms. First, it was found that if the alpha reward frequency was individualized to the client, the response to the reinforcement became more consistently favorable. This adjustment mostly falls in a narrow range between 10 and 11 Hz, but the fine-tuning turns out to be quite effective.

A second change arose from the work of Les Fehmi and Jim Hardt, who consistently rewarded alpha in a multi-channel configuration. The multi-channel set-up favors the emergence of a spatially distributed state of alpha synchrony, rather than merely promoting higher alpha amplitude in the raw EEG. Rewarding for alpha synchrony explicitly accelerates achievement of the real objective of this training. Simply rewarding higher alpha amplitudes could be contraindicated when the alpha band appears to be a zone of vulnerability, as it may be in cases of minor traumatic brain injury, fibromyalgia, and migraine. The more significant evolution occurred in the first stage of training, where the objective is enhanced physiological self-regulation. With the simple modification of allowing the reward frequency to be individually optimized, the training has become much more diverse, more effective, and also more targeted. Expanding the range of reward frequencies and shifting the reward frequency based on the person's response to the training has stretched the effectively reinforcible EEG spectrum up to 40 Hz and even down to 0.01 Hz (Othmer & Othmer, 2007). The traditional SMR-beta training most directly addresses activation of the motor system and what might be called cognitive arousal, the very quality that determines how well one handles a challenge like a continuous performance test. The expansion of the training window to both lower and higher frequencies showed that the vast majority of trainees have an even greater need for training at lower frequencies. The impact on affective states is much more immediate and compelling at low frequencies, with the additive benefit of greater impact on felt states, which in turn promotes engagement with the overall process. One might term this affective arousal, in that the training constructively addresses fear conditioning, trait anxiety, and affect disregulation.

Interconnection and normalization

With the option of training at low frequency along with the optimization strategy, trainees usually gravitate toward the training they most need at the particular time. This has produced a greater recognition of the role that psychological trauma, particularly early childhood trauma, plays in eliciting dysregulation, a condition that biofeedback strategies effectively remediates. A two-pronged strategy has evolved for addressing the trauma formations that underlie many treatment-resistant addictions. The first training, also referred to as "alert-state" training (formerly SMR-beta), addresses the physiological dysregulation, and the "deep-state" (alpha-theta) training tackles psychodynamic aspects.

The connections between treatment-resistant addictive disease and trauma, and their response to neurofeedback, offers the tantalizing possibility that neurofeedback may be applicable to other conditions as well. A history of trauma often accompanies severe chronic pain conditions, the major eating disorders, and intractable, severe, migraine. Such history is often found in treatment-resistant fibromyalgia, and chronic fatigue syndrome as well. Finally, there is a correlation of psychological trauma with disease mortality (Boscarino, 2008).

With addictive disease, the primary therapeutic effect of neurofeedback is its impact on the networks that perceive and process the trauma. Often the patient has experienced no physical injury. Psychological trauma starts as a "software" problem, which may then become progressively encoded in pathological central network relations. This paves the way, neuronally, for encoding and preferential firing of neuronal pathways resulting from subsequent trauma. In this fashion, the patient's vulnerability continues to increase. The accompanying syndromes then appear structurally based and even untreatable. The neurofeedback paradigm, however, approaches these clinical challenges as "software" problems, problems that are amenable to modification owing to the inherent plasticity of neural networks. The postulated pathological network relations have three principal features. First, the whole "system" becomes less stable; second, deviations appear in cortical–subcortical linkages; third, deviations appear in cortical connectivity. The instabilities are directly observable clinically in the variability of symptom severity over time, in the appearance of episodic conditions, and in fluctuating functionality. The subcortical dysfunctions are accessible by means of imaging technology such as SPECT and PET. From the standpoint of network theory, a hierarchical needs assessment shows that the first priority is to restore system stability. The second priority is to restore the (vertical) hierarchy of regulation, from brainstem to cortex; the third priority is to normalize the (horizontal) linkages between cortical regions where these may be anomalous.

Because neural networks are so tightly linked, any of the standard neurofeedback approaches will impact the system at all three levels. One can refine and optimize intervention, however, by taking advantage of *localization of function*. Executive function has a left frontal bias; emotional regulation has a right frontal bias; cerebral stability is optimized by targeting interhemispheric timing relationships, etc. There are also known frequency relationships. For example, cognitive function has a higher frequency bias; affect regulation has a lower frequency bias. The left hemisphere has a higher frequency bias than the right, and so on.

The two kinds of training that have emerged appeal to two fundamental aspects of the self: the first is the self in interaction with the outside world – this involves the usual gamut of concerns of the cognitive scientist from sensory processing to executive function to the organization of movement. The second involves the so-called *essential* self, the existential self that moves through time as a consistent psychic entity, maintaining a core character continuity throughout all the vicissitudes of life. In this self, the internal gyroscope is wound up, the moral compass is set, and the range and depth of emotional sentience are tuned. The addict requires attention and training in both domains, and these are directly accessible through interaction with the neuronal networks.

In addition to psychological trauma, there is also the problem of minor traumatic brain injury. These head injuries don't involve skull fracture or penetrating wounds, and, regrettably, may escape the careful attention of medical professionals. There is nothing minor, however, about the symptoms that are typically reported. Unfortunately, such symptom presentations are often unsupported by conventional CT imagery, and are thus largely discounted. Though dysfunction may last throughout life, the causal connection with the prior head injury is unlikely to be established. A recent evaluation of some 845 patients at New York addictions treatment centers found that 54% had suffered a minor traumatic brain injury (Gordon *et al.*, 2004). So, minor traumatic brain injury could be a significant etiological factor in intractable addiction. The lack of structural evidence of injury indicates that, as with psychological trauma, a major component of dysfunction lies within the domain of disturbed network relations. There is much evidence for this in functional imaging studies (Hoffman *et al.*, 1996; Thornton, 2005). Recoveries and other positive outcomes achieved through neurofeedback further support this functional model of minor traumatic brain injury (Walker *et al.*, 2002).

The stealth factor

One may consider both psychological trauma and minor brain injury as *stealth* conditions that may have gone largely unrecognized when patients present for addiction treatment. Each type of dysfunction is ultimately due to deficits in the brain's capacity to self-regulate. The remediation of these deficits is a necessary part of addiction treatment. Fortunately, neurofeedback training

substantially addresses these disregulations, but they must also be recognized and tracked throughout adjunctive therapies as well.

At this point we are perhaps in a better position to understand the poor outcomes of some of the earlier studies. Alpha reinforcement training is not likely to help people with unremediated traumatic brain injury, and may even be counterproductive. For many substance abuse patients, a narrow focus on the addiction status in treatment is unlikely to yield success. It is vital to address the psychological, psychopharmacological, social, spiritual, and neurophysiologic bases of the condition.

Eugene Peniston brought all the necessary elements of the recovery process together systematically, perhaps for the first time. Subsequent attempts to distil from this work the single "active ingredient" failed from the start. Many ingredients are involved in the task of restoring wholeness. Restoration of adequate self-regulatory status is, however, indispensable as a preparatory step for the journey toward self-actualization. Succeeding developments have only built upon and refined the Menninger/Peniston approach.

The transformative event

There is evidence that addictive behavior can be extinguished by the use of specific biofeedback techniques. Success is now possible for patient populations previously considered untreatable. Neurofeedback kindles a recovery process that the brain continues on its own. The process appears to be increasingly self-reinforcing as treatment progresses. Neurofeedback can be considered a *healthy kindling* process, where success means a transformed life, a life in which addiction no longer fits. This extension of healthy adaptation is a benefit that seems to evolve beyond (time-limited) neurofeedback treatment protocols.

Sometimes, the process of change is sudden and is attributed to a single transformative event (which typically occurs in the alpha-theta phase of the training). This kind of result is described by one therapist as follows:

> A 45-year-old male came to me for practicum work after his initial training as a neurofeedback therapist. He had never done any alpha-theta training on himself. After 15 minutes of training at Pz, he gasped, grabbed the arms of the chair, and began sobbing. At the end of the 30-minute training period, he was initially unable to describe his experience except to say that he was "overwhelmed by

the beauty." After lunch, he came back to the office and described the following scene: "I felt an odd sensation of floating. I was startled at first but then relaxed into the experience. I then floated up out of my chair and accelerated rapidly to a point high above the Earth where I remained suspended, watching the Earth and the stars. The visual experience was incredibly beautiful. I then knew that I was connected to everything in the universe and that I was nurtured and loved by it all. There was no experience of time. Then, I was gently drawn back to my chair where I was immersed in waves of pleasant emotion. " In a later recollection, he reported as follows: " For the next two days, I anguished over my inability to get back to that beauty during alpha-theta training. On the last day, I set the expectation that I would resolve the longing for the experience. After just a few minutes of training, I was back among the stars and all the beauty and sense of peace. After a while, I was drawn back to Earth."

The therapist commented that this man had worked for years in an adversarial environment involving oversight of government contracts. He had become, by his own admission, suspicious and guarded. He has since become warm, friendly, and engaging.

This type of experience is not uncommon in the alpha-theta training. Even more than with physiological normalization work, one has the sense that neurofeedback simply sets the stage for this kind of personal growth. Witnessing such healing in patients leaves the therapist more humble in regard to his own role in the process. With the client doing so much of the work, there is no need for the therapist to be intrusive. The *sine qua non* of this process is that there be a trusting relationship with the therapist. It is also critical that the therapist have his own traumas well resolved. Perhaps the circumstances for such a positive, supportive relationship were absent in the failed replication by Graap and Freides, where the objective was to test the intrinsic, uncontaminated alpha-theta procedure.

Early researchers trying to replicate the alpha training of Kamiya and Hardt made the mistake of thinking that alpha could be trained in isolation. In actual fact, the alpha amplitude remains intimately connected with and responsive to the state of the person. If conditions for the elevation in alpha amplitudes are lacking, no amount of reinforcement will make a difference. It would be akin to bird watching during a storm – the two activities are simply not compatible. This misunderstanding may also have contributed to the failed replications of the studies of Graap and Freides, and that of Taub.

In other words, treatment efficacy is complex. Indeed, all the early experiments by Les Fehmi in enhancing alpha in his own brain were complete failures. He could not get there by merely striving for it. Having discovered that a modest surrender to the process was necessary, he tried to practise that – but failed as well. It was necessary for him to *truly* surrender to the process, on every psychological level. So, merely subjecting someone to this procedure for a given length of time is not a predictor, let alone a guarantee, of a positive outcome. It is crucial to determine whether the given reinforcement results in state change. That in turn is likely to depend on variables such as trust, or sense of safety, or even, as was seen in Fehmi's own case, a complete absence of striving toward the goal. These uncodified yet nonetheless necessary contexts may not have been adequately provided in earlier research settings.

One of the present authors (S. O.) had an experience similar to Fehmi's – the alpha amplitudes would just not move! Yet, in a subsequent session involving verbal induction, the author yielded to the process readily. Fehmi utilizes verbal induction with all his clients along with (and independent of) his instrumental work. This availability of multiple pathways to success likewise puts the Taub study in a very different light. The success of the EMG and transcendental meditation arms in that study illustrates that different pathways may converge upon a common goal.

The transformative event is not unique to alpha-theta training (although, arguably, alpha-theta training is safer and more healthful than other paths). LSD, for example, was used in addiction treatment in the 1960s. One or two LSD sessions during an extended 6-month course of therapy made a large difference in outcomes that may only be attributed to these singular events. In three different universities, recovery at a 50% level was documented (Abrahamson, 1961). Recovery is sometimes achieved after the individual has a "peak experience." The affective component of the experience is what seems to matter. In one study, subjects were first given penicillamine; their LSD experiences were identical except for a dampening of affect. The opportunity for recovery, however, was thereby lost (Maslow, 1971).

Stanislov Grof routinely observed such transformative events in the course of his holotropic breathwork (Grof, 2000). In this approach, hyperventilation leads to a state of hypocapnia (reduced CO_2 levels in the brain), resulting in vasoconstriction that, in turn, alters the EEG toward theta- and delta-dominant states. Such states favor access to traumatic memories as well as to altered states. The peak experience, or transformative event, thus provoked gave subjects a rare glimpse of the "actualized" self, which in turn became the subjects' map for further inner work and growth.

The technique of eye movement desensitization and reprocessing similarly works by stimulating the low EEG frequencies where traumas are preferentially accessed. Hypnosis too typically moves subjects into states where low EEG frequencies are dominant. Indeed, one of the present authors refers to[1] alpha-theta deep-state training as "EEG hypnosis."

What differentiates modern alpha-theta training from these other techniques is the precision afforded by the use of EEG. What distinguishes the neurofeed-back approach in general is the fact that one tech-nique can address multiple aspects of the dysregulated brain – up to and including the brain in a state of addiction.

The transformative event, when it occurs, leaves little doubt regarding its significance. But it is not essential to the therapeutic process, and it should not be an explicit objective in treatment. When we asked participants with good outcomes to explain their sta-ble abstinence, all cited the twelve-step group experi-ence in which they were still involved. None named the neurofeedback. This was disappointing to us, of course, but hardly surprising. The effect of biofeed-back tends to be gradual, cumulative, and always ego-syntonic. Thus, it could conceivably hover somewhere beneath the person's radar. Because of the way this progress integrates with the developing self, accom-modations are subtly made so that the biofeedback contribution is subsumed in the increasingly autono-mous version of self that the person narrates.

Summary

This chapter provides evidence that addictive behav-iors may be conceptualized as *disorders of dysregula-tion*. Such disorders may have both a structural and a functional basis. Addressing the functional aspect of these disorders results in a surprising degree of recov-ery. Observing and modifying the EEG using neuro-feedback methodologies can change dysregulated

brain networks to regulated ones; this operant reinforce-ment strategy works toward the recovery of numerous domains of brain function. Neurofeedback is an entirely new treatment resource for conditions such as addiction that currently do not readily respond to pharmacologi-cal intervention or to cognitively based therapies. This approach is particularly successful in resolving trau-ma formations – both psychological and physical – that can impede clinical success in many other clinical domains. A comprehensive approach that addresses mul-tiple aspects of neuronal dysregulation manifestly enhanc-es success in addiction treatment. The data compel consideration of EEG neurofeedback for inclusion in contemporary treatment programs. Additionally, the efficacy of neurofeedback and the mechanisms by which it works may argue for adopting a more inclu-sive "systems-level" perspective on the problem of addiction.

Conclusion

Stable recovery from addiction may be more likely when modern neurophysiological and behavioral tech-nologies are combined with traditional medical and psychotherapeutic interventions. The model for these advances is the neural network encoding that makes the brain accessible to therapeutic intervention at the neuronal level. The technique of operant conditioning of EEG variables, combined with psychotherapy and pharmacological support, works to enhance clinical outcomes, even among the most challenging clinical populations.

Global remediation of mental functioning – rather than targeting addiction in isolation – is a compelling clinical strategy, given the high prevalence of comorbid conditions, including PTSD, minor traumatic brain injury, personality disorders, impulse control problems, behavioral disinhibition, anxiety, and mood disorders. These comorbidities, like addiction, feature deficits in neural network functioning, and these deficits may be treated by means of neurofeedback training.

Restoring the brain's regulatory and cognitive function by means of neurofeedback also heals psy-chological wounds by inducing and reinforcing par-ticular network states that favor trauma resolution, and subsequent progress toward self-actualization.

[1] Dr. Steinberg has used alpha-theta in his clinical neuropsy-chology practice for nearly two decades. He has also used EMDR and hypnosis, but prefers the clinical successes attained through neurofeedback and alpha-theta.

References

Abrahamson, H. (ed.) (1961). *The Use of LSD in Psychotherapy*. New York: Josiah Macy Foundation.

Bodenhamer-Davis, E. & Callaway, T. (2004). Extended follow-up results of Peniston protocol results with chemical dependency. *Journal of Neurotherapy*, **8**(2), 135.

Boscarino, J. A. (2008). Psychobiologic predictors of disease mortality after psychological trauma: implications for research and clinical surveillance. *Journal of Nervous & Mental Disease*, **196**(2), 100–7.

Budzynski, T. H. & Stoyva, J. M. (1972). Biofeedback techniques in behavior therapy. In *Behavior and Self-Control*, D. Shapiro, T. X. Barber, L. V. DiCara *et al.* (eds). Chicago: Aldine, pp. 437–59.

Burkett, V. S., Cummins, J. M., Dickson, R. M. & Skolnick, M. H. (2004). Treatment effects related to EEG biofeedback for crack cocaine dependency in a faith-based homeless mission. *Journal of Neurotherapy*, **8**(2), 138–40.

Byers, A. P. (1992). The normalization of a personality through neurofeedback therapy. *Subtle Energies*, **3**(1), 1–17.

Fahrion, S. L., Walters, E. D., Coyne, L. & Allen, T. (1992) Alterations in EEG amplitude, personality factors, and brain electrical mapping after alpha-theta brainwave training. *Alcoholism: Clinical and Experimental Research*, **16**, 547–52.

Farmer, S. F. (2002). Neural rhythms in Parkinson's disease. *Brain*, **125**, 1175–76.

Fehmi, L. G. (1978). EEG biofeedback, multi-channel synchrony training, and attention. In *Expanding Dimensions of Consciousness*, A. Sugarman & R. E. Tarter (eds). New York: Springer Publishing Company, pp. 152–82.

Gordon, W., Fenske, C., Perez, K. & Brandau, S. (2004). *Comorbidity between TBI and Substance Abuse*. Paper presented at: Strengthening Systems: Investing for Results. Alcoholism and Substance Abuse Providers of New York State 7th Annual Statewide Conference, New York, NY.

Goslinga, J. J. (1975). Biofeedback for chemical problem patients: a developmental process. *Journal of Biofeedback*, **2**, 17–27.

Graap, K. & Freides, D. (1998). Regarding the database for the Peniston alpha-theta EEG biofeedback protocol. *Applied Psychophysiology and Biofeedback*, **23**(4), 265–72.

Graap, K., Ready, D. J., Freides, D., Daniels, R., & Baltzell, D. (1997). EEG biofeedback treatment for Vietnam veterans suffering from post traumatic stress disorder. *Journal of Neurotherapy*, **2**, 65–66

Green, E. E., Green, A. M. & Walters, E. D. (1970). Voluntary control of internal states: psychological and physiological. *Journal of Transpersonal Psychology*, **2**, 1–26.

Green, E. E., Green, A. M. & Walters, E. D. (1974). Alpha-theta biofeedback training. *Journal of Biofeedback*, **2**, 7–13.

Grof, S. (2000). *Psychology of the Future*. New York: SUNY Press.

Hardt, J. V. (2007). *The Art of Smart Thinking*. Santa Clara: BioCybernaut Press.

Hardt, J. V. & Kamiya, J. (1978). Anxiety change through encephalographic alpha feedback seen only in high anxiety subjects. *Science*, **201**(4350), 79–81.

Hoffman, D., Stockdale, S. & van Egeren, L. (1996). EEG neurofeedback in the treatment of mild traumatic brain injury. *Clinical EEG*, **27**, 6.

Kamiya, J. (1969). Operant control of the EEG alpha rhythm and some of its reported effects on consciousness. In *Altered States of Consciousness*, C. T. Tart (ed.). New York: Wiley, pp. 519–29.

Kamiya, J. & Noles, D. (1970). The control of electroencephalographic alpha rhythms through auditory feedback and associated mental activity. *Psychophysiology*, **6**, 76.

Kelly, M. J. (1997). Native Americans, neurofeedback, and substance abuse theory: three year outcome of alpha/theta neurofeedback training in the treatment of problem drinking among Dine' (Navajo) People. *Journal of Neurotherapy*, **2**(3), 24–60.

Lynch, J. L., Paskewitz, D. & Orne, M. T. (1974). Some factors in the feedback control of the human alpha rhythm. *Psychosomatic Medicine*, **36**, 399–410.

Maslow, A. (1971). *The Farther Reaches of Human Nature*. New York: Viking Press, p. 108.

Othmer, S. F. & Othmer, S. (2007). Interhemispheric EEG training; clinical experience and conceptual models. In *Handbook of Neurofeedback: Dynamics and Clinical Applications*, J. R. Evans (ed.). New York: Haworth Medical Press, pp. 109–36.

Othmer, S., Othmer, S. F. & Kaiser, D. A. (1999). EEG biofeedback: an emerging model for its global efficacy. In *Introduction to Quantitative EEG and Neurofeedback*, J. R. Evans & A. Abarbanel (eds). San Diego: Academic Press, pp. 243–310.

Passini, F. T., Watson, C. B., Dehnel, L., Herder, J. & Watkins, B. (1977). Alpha wave biofeedback training therapy in alcoholics. *Journal of Clinical Psychology*, **33**, 292–9.

Peniston, E. G. & Kulkosky, P. J. (1989). Alpha-theta brainwave training and beta endorphin levels in alcoholics. *Alcoholism: Clinical and Experimental Results*, **13**(2), 271–9.

Peniston, E. G. & Kulkosky, P. J. (1990). Alcoholic personality and alpha-theta brainwave training. *Medical Psychotherapy: An International Journal*, **3**, 37–55.

Peniston, E. G. & Kulkosky, P. J. (1991). Alpha-theta brainwave neurofeedback therapy for Vietnam veterans with combat-related posttraumatic stress disorder. *Medical Psychotherapy: An International Journal*, **4**, 47–60.

Peniston, E. G., & Kulkosky, P. J. (1999). Neurofeedback in the treatment of addictive disorders. In *Introduction to Quantitative EEG and Neurofeedback*, J. R. Evans & A. Abarbanel (eds.). San Diego: Academic Press.

Peniston, E. G. Marrinan, D. A., Deming, W. A. & Kulkosky, P. J. (1993). EEG alpha-theta brainwave synchronization in Vietnam theater veteran with combat-related posttraumatic stress disorder and alcohol abuse. *Medical Psychotherapy: An International Journal*, **6**, 37–50.

Scott, W. C., Kaiser, D. A., Othmer, S. and Sideroff, S. I. (2005). Effects of an EEG biofeedback protocol on a mixed substance abusing population. *American Journal of Drug and Alcohol Abuse*, **31**(3), 455–69.

Schneider, F., Elbert, T., Heimann, H. *et al.* (1993). Self-regulation of slow cortical potentials in psychiatric patients: alcohol dependency. *Biofeedback Self Regulation*, **18**(1), 23–32.

Smith, P. N. & Sams, M. W. (2004). Neurofeedback with Youth Offenders. A pilot study in the use of analog/QEEG-based remedial neurofeedback training. Presentation at ISNR Annual Conference, August 8, 2004

Taub, E., Steiner, S. S., Smith, R. B., Weingarten, E. & Walton, K. G. (1994). Effectiveness of broad spectrum approaches to relapse prevention in severe alcoholism: a long-term, randomized, controlled trial of transcendental meditation, EMG biofeedback, and electronic neurotherapy. *Alcohol Treatment Quarterly*,

Thornton, K. (2005). EEG biofeedback for reading disabilities and traumatic brain injury. *Child and Adolescent Psychiatric Clinics of North America*, **14**(1), 137–62.

Twemlow, S. W. & Bowen, W. T. (1976). EEG biofeedback induced self-actualization in alcoholics. *Journal of Biofeedback*, **3**, 20–5.

Twemlow, S. W. & Bowen, W. T. (1977a). Sociocultural predictors of self actualization in EEG biofeedback treated alcoholics. *Psychological Reports*, **40**, 591–8.

Twemlow, S. W. & Bowen, W. T. (1977b). Biofeedback induced energy redistribution in the alcoholic EEG. *Journal of Biofeedback*, **3**, 14–19.

Walker, J. E., Norman, C. A. & Weber, R. (2002). Impact of QEEG-guided coherence training for patients with a mild traumatic brain injury. *Journal of Neurotherapy*, **6**, 31–43.

Watson, C. G., Herder, J. & Passini, E. T. (1978). Alpha biofeedback therapy in alcoholics. An 18-month follow-up. *Journal of Clinical Psychology*, **34**, 765–9.

20

The new pharmacotherapies for alcohol dependence

Barbara J. Mason & Marni Jacobs

Introduction

Alcohol dependence is a prevalent, chronic disorder with significant worldwide public health consequences. It is a disorder that affects the brain, spirit, and behavior, and yet the brain is often neglected in traditional interventions. The newer medications approved for alcohol dependence have been shown to safely and effectively augment the modest efficacy of existing behavioral treatments and self-help strategies for reducing the high risk of drinking relapse after an initial period of abstinence. Primary goals for alcoholism pharmacotherapy typically include maintaining abstinence, increasing the duration of an abstinent interval prior to a lapse, and reducing the intensity of drinking if a relapse occurs. Such drug effects may also serve to increase retention in behavioral treatment and self-help groups, thereby facilitating behavioral changes supportive of an alcohol-free lifestyle.

The medications in recent decades that have been found to be effective for the treatment of alcohol dependence in independent, placebo-controlled studies that have been replicated across continents are acamprosate (Campral) and naltrexone (ReVia, Vivitrol), although results are not uniformly positive. Both acamprosate and naltrexone are gaining increasing availability worldwide by prescription for the treatment of alcohol dependence, and there is scientific and clinical interest in examining these drugs in combination, given their high tolerability, moderate effect sizes, different pharmacological profiles, and potentially different effects on drinking outcomes.

Key similarities between acamprosate and naltrexone in the treatment of alcohol dependence

Acamprosate and naltrexone share many important features in the treatment of alcohol dependence. The two drugs both have good safety profiles and are generally acceptable to alcohol-dependent patients. Unlike disulfiram or sedative drugs, neither naltrexone nor acamprosate interacts with alcohol. Clinical investigations show no evidence of tolerance, dependence or the emergence of a withdrawal syndrome or rebound drinking when treatment is ceased (Mason, 2001). Additionally, although both drugs act in the brain, neither drug has any overt psychoactive, e.g. mood-altering or sedative, effects on the central nervous system (CNS).

Key differences between acamprosate and naltrexone in the treatment of alcohol dependence

An important difference between the two drugs relates to their mechanism of action. Naltrexone is an opioid receptor antagonist, which blocks the endogenous opioid reward system. It may thereby reduce the rewarding effect of alcohol. Acamprosate, on the other hand, is a taurine analog, and acts primarily by normalizing the dysregulation of NMDA-mediated glutamatergic neurotransmission that occurs during chronic alcohol consumption, withdrawal, and for an indeterminate period thereafter, thus attenuating one of the physiological mechanisms that may prompt relapse (Littleton, 2007). These different mechanisms of action may endow the two drugs with efficacy for different components of drinking behavior. In terms of the kinetics of their effects, naltrexone has a rapid onset of action, but its activity is not sustained following removal of the drug (Anton et al., 2001; O'Malley et al., 1996). In contrast, acamprosate has a slow onset of action, requiring around 1 week to reach steady-state levels in the nervous system (Saivin et al., 1998), but its effects on drinking behavior have been shown to persist for up to 1 year after the treatment is completed (e.g. Sass et al., 1996). Finally, the two drugs have different adverse event and overall tolerability profiles. An overview of the efficacy endpoints and

Table 20.1 Overview of published data on the efficacy and safety of acamprosate and naltrexone, alone and in combination, in the treatment of alcohol dependence

	Acamprosate	Naltrexone	Combination
Efficacy parameters			
Increases abstinence	Yes	Maybe	Maybe
Decreases heavy drinking	Maybe	Yes	Maybe
Long-term efficacy (≥ 1 year)	Yes	No	Unknown
Sustained efficacy post-treatment (≥ 6 months)	Yes	No	Unknown
Compliance	Good	Variable	Good
Contingent on a specific psychosocial intervention	Independent	Variable	Unknown
Safety parameters			
Interaction with alcohol	No	No	No
Intrinsic dependence potential	No	No	No
Overall safety profile	Good	Good	Good
Hepatic impact	No	Yes	Yes
Clinically relevant drug interactions	No	Yes	Yes
Use in opioid users, methadone patients	Suitable	Unsuitable	Unsuitable

safety of acamprosate and naltrexone, alone and in combination, is presented in Table 20.1.

Acamprosate

Summary of acamprosate efficacy for the treatment of alcohol dependence

Acamprosate was initially studied in Europe, and more recently, in Brazil, Korea, Australia, and the US. The acamprosate published double-blind, placebo-controlled clinical trial database includes over 6500 outpatients from 15 countries and is reported in 23 published studies that are summarized in Tables 20.2 and 20.4. Twenty-one of these trials (i.e. all but Lhuintre *et al.*, 1990 and Mason *et al.*, 2006) used relatively equivalent methodology in terms of entry criteria, treatments, handling of dropouts, outcome measures and assessment of compliance. Additionally, one study found support for acamprosate's efficacy in an adolescent population as opposed to an adult population (Niederhofer & Staffen, 2003). Patients received the psychosocial intervention typical of their treatment setting. Treatment duration ranged from 2 to 12 months with 13 trials 6 months or longer in duration. Patients were generally recently detoxified and typically had been abstinent for about 5 days at entry into the trials. In these studies, the principal efficacy measure was abstinence, which was assessed as the rate of

patients completing the trial with no consumption of alcohol at all, the cumulative proportion of the study duration when the patients remained abstinent, and/or the time to first drink.

The results have been consistent in the majority of published studies, and generally show a significant beneficial effect of acamprosate on abstinence outcomes relative to placebo (Table 20.2). A factor of two in the difference in the proportion of patients achieving stable abstinence was observed in approximately one-third of studies. A beneficial effect on the time to first drink was also frequently observed.

Overall, the published placebo-controlled studies demonstrate the efficacy of acamprosate for supporting abstinence over a broad range of patients in association with a variety of different psychosocial interventions. A number of these studies assessed the persistence of a treatment benefit after the study medication was stopped, and found acamprosate efficacy was maintained for up to 12 months post-treatment relative to placebo.

The Tempesta *et al.* (2000) study also assessed the frequency and amount of alcohol consumed per day in those patients who had a relapse, in addition to the primary abstinence outcomes described above. During active treatment, acamprosate subjects had significantly less frequent drinking episodes and consumed less alcohol during relapses than patients on placebo, although these effects on drinking were not sustained

Table 20.2 Summary of published, randomized, double-blind, placebo-controlled trials of acamprosate treatment of alcohol dependence

	n	Months of study	Days to relapse Acamprosate	Placebo	Rate of total abstinence (%) Acamprosate	Placebo	Cumulative abstinence duration Acamprosate	Placebo	Rate of heavy drinking Acamprosate	Placebo	Completion of double-blind treatment (%) Acamprosate	Placebo	Reference
Short-term efficacy studies	85	3			61[a]	32					47	37	Lhuintre et al., 1985
	569	3									61	62	Lhuintre et al., 1990[d]
	127	3			29	33					31	29	Roussaux et al., 1996
	142	2	14	8	37	32	81%	70%	60	61	74	69	Namkoong et al., 2003
	75	3			43[a]	20							Baltieri & De Andrade 2004
	169	3	34	33	20	18	66 days	57 days			75	66	Morley et al., 2006
	26	3			54[a]	15	80 days[a]	33 days					Niederhofer & Staffen 2003*
Intermediate duration efficacy studies	102	6			24[a]	4	60 days[a]	49 days[a]			66[a]	21	Pelc et al., 1992
	61	6			38[b]	17	43%[a]	24%					Ladewig et al., 1993
	302	6	111[a]	55	39[a]	26	49%[a]	36%			57	55	Barrias et al., 1997
	262	6	45[a]	15	20[a]	10	34 days[a]	24 days			41[a]	31	Geerlings et al., 1997
	246	6	151[a]	61	43[a]	30	72%[a]	59%			53[a]	38	Poldrugo, 1997

	n	Months										Reference
	581	6	37	40	34	39	77 days	81 days		35	35	Chick et al., 2000b
	330	6	158[a]	58	58[a]	45	66%[a]	54%	A < P[a]	76	74	Tempesta et al., 2000
	288	6			35[b]	26	93 days[a]	74 days		65	61	Gual & Lehert, 2001
Long-term efficacy studies	272	12	165[a]	112	45[a]	25	62%[a]	45%		58[a]	40	Sass et al., 1996
	448	12	55[a]	43	18[a]	7	139 days[a]	104 days		42	37	Whitworth et al., 1996
Dose-ranging studies	538	12	153[a] (2 g)	102	19 (2 g)	11	223 days[a] (2 g)	173 days		55[a] (2 g)	36	Paille et al., 1995
			136[a] (1.3 g)		18 (1.3 g)		198 days[a] (1.3 g)			47[a] (1.3 g)		
	188	3	56[a] (2 g)	15	51[a] (2 g)	26	63%[a] (2 g)	38%		68[a] (2 g)	52	Pelc et al., 1997
			56 (1.3 g)		44[a] (1.3 g)		59%[a] (1.3 g)			70[a] (1.3 g)		
	601	6					58%[a] (2 g)	52%		41[a] (2 g)	55	Mason et al., 2006**
							63%[a] (3 g)			51 (3 g)		
Combined efficacy of acamprosate and disulfiram	110	12			25[a]	5	40%[a], 55% (+disulfiram)[c]	21%, 31% (+disulfiram)		35[a]	35	Besson et al., 1998

A, acamprosate; P, placebo; <,> indicate the direction of any significant effects reported when the actual values are not reported. [a]Difference between acamprosate and placebo groups, P <0.05. [b]Difference between acamprosate and placebo groups, P < 0.1 and P > 0.05. [c]Difference between acamprosate and disulfiram subgroup versus other subgroups, P <0.05; P<0.05. [d]Difference between acamprosate and placebo groups. [d]γ-glutamyltransferase level was the primary outcome measure in this study and was significantly lower in acamprosate patients than in placebo patients (1.4 ± 1.56 versus 2.0 ± 3.19¥ upper limit of normal, P = 0.016). The only study that has been done in adolescents, aged 16–19 years. **Covariate-adjusted intention-to-treat population.

191

at post-treatment follow-up. Similar effects were noted in a 2003 study that combined data from 15 placebo-controlled treatment studies to assess whether patients who had taken one or more drinks since the previous study visit reported a fewer number of drinking days, lower average number of drinks per day, and consumed less alcohol in total with acamprosate versus placebo (Chick *et al.*, 2003). The authors reported that among relapsers, acamprosate was significantly associated with less quantity and frequency of drinking compared to placebo. The increased control over drinking when relapse occurred suggests that continuing acamprosate treatment during a relapse may have clinical benefits.

A multi-center, double-blind, placebo-controlled clinical trial of acamprosate was conducted in the US in support of FDA approval, which was granted on July 29, 2004. This trial differed from the European clinical trials in several ways (summarized in Mason & Ownby, 2000): patients were generally not medically detoxified (only 10%) and many were actively drinking at inclusion. Patients with a history of use of other drugs of abuse were not excluded so that the safety of acamprosate could be evaluated in patients with a history of polysubstance abuse, and these constituted 75% of the study population. Both these factors are generally considered negative determinants on alcoholism treatment outcome. Additionally, double-blind treatment was augmented with a manual-guided counseling program for all participants, in keeping with US clinical trial conventions (www.alcoholfree.info; Mason & Goodman, 1997). Cumulative abstinence duration did not differ across groups in the intention-to-treat population, although there were trends in the hypothesized direction. However, a significant difference between acamprosate and placebo treatment groups was found in cumulative abstinence duration and in measures of drinking consumption in the intention-to-treat population after adjusting for relevant baseline variables (e.g. severity of polysubstance abuse) and treatment exposure. Benefits of acamprosate were especially robust in patients who had a clearly identified goal of abstinence at the start of treatment; such motivation may have offset the lack of detoxification or initial abstinence for many in this sample. In addition, this American trial compared a higher dose of 3 g per day with the standard dose of 2 g per day used in Europe, and generated outcome data consistent with a linear dose–response relationship, again applying the above co-variates. There were no deaths, serious

adverse drug-related events, or group differences in the rate of drug discontinuation, thus supporting acamprosate's excellent safety profile in this heterogeneous US sample (Mason *et al.*, 2006).

In two studies that failed to detect a difference between acamprosate and placebo (Chick *et al.*, 2000b; Namkoong *et al.*, 2003), a large proportion of patients (30% and 68%, respectively) were drinking in the days immediately prior to randomization, as in the US trial discussed above (Mason *et al.*, 2006). This may have affected the result, as the pharmacological target of acamprosate is present following abstinence initiation in patients with current alcohol dependence. However, a multi-center trial that initiated double-blind treatment concurrent with inpatient detoxification obtained positive results with acamprosate relative to placebo during 6 months of subsequent outpatient treatment (Gual & Lehert, 2001). An advantage to this strategy is that acamprosate steady state is achieved during abstinence on an inpatient unit and prior to hospital discharge. In another inconclusive study, which was much smaller, many patients had less severe alcohol-related problems (corresponding to the DSM-III/IV definitions of alcohol abuse; American Psychiatric Association, 1987) and did not fulfil the criteria for alcohol dependence with the associated CNS changes that acamprosate targets (Roussaux *et al.*, 1996). More recently, in an Australian study that failed to detect any differences between acamprosate and placebo, the authors reported that patients in the study had extremely high levels of emotional distress and moderate levels of disability in mental function. Participants were also given the option of manualized compliance therapy, and it is not clear whether or not participation in this therapy had an effect on treatment groups (Morley *et al.*, 2006). A large ($n = 1289$) open-label multinational acamprosate study in Europe found equivalent benefits of acamprosate across a variety of concomitant behavioral treatments (Pelc *et al.*, 2002). Recent open-label experience with acamprosate in Australia confirmed the efficacy of acamprosate in conjunction with cognitive behavioral therapy (CBT) over CBT alone (Feeney *et al.*, 2002), and the equivalent efficacy of acamprosate alone and in conjunction with brief intervention or CBT (de Wildt *et al.*, 2002) for abstinence as well as drinking intensity outcomes.

In support of FDA approval for acamprosate, data were re-analyzed from three European double-blind placebo-controlled trials (13, 48, and 52 weeks in length), in which complete abstinence was the primary outcome measure (Paille *et al.*, 1995; Sass *et al.*, 1996; Pelc *et al.*, 1997). A total of 998 alcohol-dependent patients were included in these studies, with the majority abstinent at randomization. In contrast to the original analyses, patients with missing data or with unknown status, as well as patients with a positive assessment of drinking on any study variable evaluated at each visit, were considered "not abstinent," resulting in a more stringent definition of abstinence. Re-analysis of the rate of complete abstinence, percentage of days abstinent, and the time to first drink confirmed the original findings for the efficacy of acamprosate versus placebo (Kranzler & Gage, 2008).

Safety and tolerability of acamprosate in patients with alcohol dependence

The safety profile of acamprosate appears favorable (Rosenthal *et al.*, 2008). The only adverse event consistently reported across trials more frequently in acamprosate-treated patients with respect to placebo-treated patients was mild and transient diarrhea. Across clinical trials, the rate of early terminations owing to drug-related adverse events did not differ between acamprosate- and placebo-treated patients. Pharmacovigilance subsequent to the commercialization of acamprosate in 1989 has not identified any health risk associated with acamprosate use in over 1.5 million patients. Re-analysis of safety data by the FDA noted an increase in suicidal ideation but not completed suicides in patients treated with acamprosate. All patients with alcohol dependence should be monitored for suicidality owing to the increased risk associated with the disorder. Acamprosate is renally excreted and treatment of patients with severely compromised renal functioning is contraindicated (see package insert for guidance).

Clinical predictors of acamprosate efficacy

In an large-scale effort to ascertain whether acamprosate is more efficacious in certain populations, a pooled analysis on seven European trials was performed. This investigation assessed a number of potential predictors of efficacy, including physiological dependence at baseline, family history of alcoholism, age of onset of alcohol dependence, anxiety symptomatology at baseline, craving at baseline, and gender. The pooled analysis evaluated data on over 1450 patients; however, acamprosate efficacy was not associated with any of the identified predictor variables (Verheul *et al.*, 2005).

Compliance with acamprosate

Compliance with acamprosate in the double-blind, placebo-controlled trials was typically >85%, and not different from placebo; this is important for a drug that has to be given twice or three times daily owing to low bioavailability. Patients who are not participants in a clinical trial may be less motivated to be medication-compliant. However, strategies to increase compliance with dosing in this population may include: 1) suggesting that patients reaffirm their commitment to their recovery with every dose; 2) prescribing the drug in blister cards rather than bottles as the cost is the same but blister cards show the day and time each dose is to be taken; 3) request that patients bring their blister cards to their follow-up appointments so that it can be determined if a dose at a particular time of day is being missed that can be linked with an activity of daily living, like a meal or brushing teeth, as a dose reminder; and 4) using the blister card as "prime real estate" on which patients may write inspirational messages to support their recovery.

Use of acamprosate in patients with comorbid psychiatric disorders

A number of Axis I disorders frequently co-occur with alcohol dependence; however, until recently, their effect on alcohol use outcomes in the context of pharmacotherapy has been under-studied. One significant feature of acamprosate is that it normalizes alcohol-related changes in sleep architecture, which may have beneficial effects in the treatment of both alcoholism and comorbid disorders characterized by sleep disturbance (Koob *et al.*, 2002; Staner *et al.*, 2006). Furthermore, unlike naltrexone, acamprosate is not metabolized in the liver, and therefore there are no known or suspected drug interactions. Drug interaction studies have found acamprosate to be safe for use in patients being treated with antidepressants, anxiolytics, antipsychotics, naltrexone, and disulfiram (Besson *et al.*, 1998; Saivin *et al.*, 1998; Mason *et al.*, 2002; Johnson *et al.*, 2003).

Naltrexone

Summary of naltrexone efficacy for the treatment of alcohol dependence

The clinical database for naltrexone is considerably more heterogeneous methodologically than that of acamprosate, reflecting the fact that the drug was readily available for an earlier indication (opiate dependence) and early trials were therefore investigator-driven, with different investigators choosing different methodologies. This situation has the advantage that the drug has been evaluated under a wide range of conditions, but also the limitation that studies are difficult to compare with one another. Until recently, most of the studies have been small, single-center studies with a treatment duration of 3 months and involved oral medication (50 mg/day). Recently, multi-center trials of long-acting injectable forms of naltrexone have been reported (Kranzler *et al.*, 2004; Garbutt *et al.*, 2005). The most commonly reported endpoint of the naltrexone trials has been relapse to heavy drinking (typically defined as > five drinks/day in males and > four drinks/day in females), and it is on this measure that efficacy has been most consistently demonstrated (Table 20.3).

However, the demonstration of a decrease in relapse has not been observed in all studies, including the largest to date (Krystal *et al.*, 2001; *n* = 627). There are a number of factors that could explain this. For example, since the effect of naltrexone may be to reduce consumption when drinking, potential treatment effects in the clinical trials may be diluted by patients who remain abstinent throughout. If the analysis is restricted to patients who resume drinking during the trials, then the size of the treatment effect may be increased (Volpicelli *et al.*, 1992; Morris *et al.*, 2001), or, in one study, an effect revealed where none existed before (Oslin *et al.*, 1997). Similarly, re-analysis of two negative clinical trials examined drinking trajectories and found that naltrexone doubled the odds of following the abstainer trajectory as opposed to the constant drinking trajectory, suggesting that naltrexone may have a clinically meaningful effect for certain patients even in studies where it failed to show efficacy in planned analyses (Gueorguieva *et al.*, 2007).

The effect of naltrexone on relapse may be to some extent dependent on associated psychotherapy, especially in non-abstinent patients. In a 3-month trial by O'Malley *et al.* (1992), patients were stratified into those that received CBT and those that received supportive therapy. Among non-abstinent patients, only those receiving CBT showed a benefit from naltrexone on relapse. Two trials of 6 months' (Balldin *et al.*, 2003) and 8 months' (Heinälä *et al.*, 2001) duration replicated the interaction with CBT originally noted by O'Malley *et al.* (1992), in which groups receiving concomitant CBT, but not supportive therapy, showed naltrexone effects on relapse relative to placebo. Similar

results were described in a study comparing treatment with naltrexone or placebo combined with either CBT or motivational enhancement therapy (MET) (Anton *et al.*, 2005). Researchers found that naltrexone, independent of therapy assignment, increased time to first relapse, and that the CBT/naltrexone group did better than any other groups on a variety of outcome measures, including the MET/naltrexone group. Conversely, in a recent multi-center trial, naltrexone combined with CBT techniques and medication management had worse outcomes than naltrexone and medication management alone (Anton *et al.*, 2006). Unlike the majority of acamprosate trials, controlled trials of naltrexone given in conjunction with non-standardized (treatment as usual) behavioral treatment have not been reported.

There are few data to support a beneficial long-term treatment effect with naltrexone. The single 1-year study to have been performed failed to reveal any difference between naltrexone and placebo on any outcome measure (Krystal *et al.*, 2001). In addition, follow-up of the O'Malley and Anton study samples revealed no significant drug effects within a few months after medication was discontinued (O'Malley *et al.*, 1996; Anton *et al.*, 2001). The absence of enduring post-treatment drug effects may be a function of the brief half-life of naltrexone (4 hours) and its active metabolite, 6-beta-naltrexol (15 hours), and the fact that antagonism of endogenous opioid receptors by naltrexone does not induce neurochemical changes that persist following drug elimination.

More recently, a study focused on long-term treatment with naltrexone suggested that naltrexone's suppressant effects on drinking are limited to the first 3 months of treatment (Davidson *et al.*, 2007). Researchers found no significant differences in percentage of days abstinent or percentage of heavy drinking days between patients who received 24 weeks of treatment with naltrexone as compared with patients who received 12 weeks of treatment with naltrexone followed by 12 weeks of placebo. Medication compliance was found to be low in the final 12 weeks of the study in both groups, which also may have had an effect on drinking outcomes.

Safety and tolerability of naltrexone in patients with alcohol dependence

Although the overall safety profile of naltrexone is good, poorly tolerated adverse events, principally

Table 20.3 Summary of published, randomized, double-blind, placebo-controlled trials of naltrexone treatment of alcohol dependence

	n	Months of study	Days to relapse		Rate of total abstinence (%)		Cumulative abstinence duration		Rate of heavy drinking (%)		Completion of double-blind treatment (%)		Reference
			Naltrexone	Placebo	Naltrexone	Placebo	Naltrexone	Placebo	Naltrexone	Placebo	Naltrexone	Placebo	
Short-term efficacy studies	104	3	N+CBT=NR[a]	P+CBT=25	N+CBT=28[a]	P+CBT=21	N+CBT=96%[a]	P+CBT=90	N+CBT=43[a]	P+CBT=NR	N+CBT=34	P+CBT=40	O'Malley et al., 1992
			N+ST=NR[a]	P+ST=35	N+ST=61[c]	P+ST=19	N+ST=96%[a]	P+ST=91%	N+ST=34[a]	P+ST=NR	N+ST=22	P+ST=41	
	70	3	N>P[a]		54	43	N>P[a]		23[a]	54	69	60	Volpicelli et al., 1992
	44	3	N=P		N=P		N=P		14	35	N=P		Oslin et al., 1997
	97	3			44	35			35[b]	53	73	73	Volpicelli et al., 1997
	131	3			47	33	90%[a]	82%	38[a]	60	87	78	Anton et al., 1999
	175	3	N=P		18	19			N=P		41	42	Chick et al., 2000a
	183	3	50	56	30	35	79%	84%	12	8	59[a]	79	Kranzler et al., 2000
	183	3	Nefazodone=50		Nefazodone=32		Nefazodone=83%		Nefazodone=11		Nefazodone=73		Monterosso et al.,
	128	3	N<P[a]		N=P				5[a]	9	N=P		Monti et al., 2001
	111	3	18	17	54	51			N<P[a]		69	57	Morris et al., 2001
	171	3	N=P				N=P		N=P		67	62	Gastpar et al., 2002
	202	3	30	29	73	65	65%	63%	8[b]	19	60	58	Guardia et al., 2002
	107	3	90[a]	42			N=P		34[a]	53	59	67	Latt et al., 2002
	145	3	N=P				N=P		N=P		76	67	Killeen et al., 2004
	40	3.5					N=P		N=P		55	65	Huang et al., 2005

(Continued)

Table 20.3 (Cont.)

n	Months of study	Days to relapse Naltrexone	Days to relapse Placebo	Rate of total abstinence (%) Naltrexone	Rate of total abstinence (%) Placebo	Cumulative abstinence duration Naltrexone	Cumulative abstinence duration Placebo	Rate of heavy drinking (%) Naltrexone	Rate of heavy drinking (%) Placebo	Completion of double-blind treatment (%) Naltrexone	Completion of double-blind treatment (%) Placebo	Reference
160	3	N > P[a]						N+CBT=38[a] N+MET=44[a]	P+CBT=60 P+MET=56	N+CBT=79 N+MET=80	P+CBT=88 P+MET=77	Anton et al., 2005
169	3	39	33	9	11	58 days	57 days	39	43	67	65	Morley et al., 2006
103	3	N = P		N = P				N = P		77	76	O'Malley et al., 2007
Intermediate duration efficacy studies												
121	8							N+CBT=73[a,b]	P+CBT=97	69 Overall		Heinala et al., 2001
118	6	N+CBT=57[c] N+ST=20	P+CBT=22 P+ST=18			N+CBT=68 days N+ST=56 days	P+CBT=53 days P+ST=50 days	N+ST=93 N+CBT=21[a] N+ST=34	P+ST=88 P+CBT=38 P+ST=39	N = P	N = P	Balldin et al., 2003
120	6	N = P		N = P		N = P		N = P		N = P	N = P	Oslin et al., 2008
116	8							55[a]	74	45[a]	26	Ahmadi et al., 2004
Long-term efficacy studies												
627	12	72	62			3-month outcomes: 89% 12-month outcome: 85%	86% 82%	38	44	73 Overall		Krystal et al., 2001
Long-acting injectable naltrexone studies												
315	3	11	6	18[a]	10	53[a]	46	77	84	80	75	Kranzler et al., 2004
627	6					380 mg: N=P 190 mg: N=P		380 mg: N<P[a] 190 mg: N<P[b]		380 mg:60 190 mg:60	61	Garbutt et al., 2005

N, naltrexone; P, placebo; NR, actual values not reported in the original study; CBT, cognitive behavioral therapy; ST, supportive therapy; MET, motivational enhancement therapy; <,> indicate the direction of any significant effects reported when the actual values are not reported. [a]Difference between naltrexone and placebo groups, $P < 0.05$. [b]Difference between naltrexone and placebo groups, $P < 0.10$ and $P > 0.05$; [c]Medication × therapy interaction, $P < 0.05$.

nausea and headache, resulted in 15% of patients discontinuing treatment in an open-label usage study of naltrexone (Croop *et al.*, 1997). Additionally, care has to be taken in prescribing the drug to certain patient populations. Naltrexone shows a dose-dependent hepatotoxicity (see the package insert), and is thus contraindicated in patients with significant hepatic impairment, which is frequently encountered in alcohol-dependent populations. Thus, liver function tests (LFTs) should be obtained prior to treatment initiation and repeated periodically during naltrexone treatment. The clinical trials of naltrexone have typically been conducted in patients without significant impairment in hepatic function (LFTs < 3 × ULN (upper limit of normal)). Another consequence of the hepatic impact of naltrexone is the possibility of drug–drug interactions. A potentially clinically significant interaction has recently been reported between naltrexone and non-steroidal anti-inflammatory drugs (Kim *et al.*, 2001). This study found elevated LFTs in study participants receiving both medications, although the doses of naltrexone used were higher than the typical 50 mg daily dose. Importantly, naltrexone is contraindicated for use in patients taking prescribed or illicit opioid drugs. Antagonism of the effects of these drugs at opiate receptors will generally precipitate an opiate withdrawal syndrome. Hence, naltrexone would be contraindicated for methadone-maintained patients with alcohol dependence, or those with needs for narcotic analgesics.

Clinical predictors of naltrexone efficacy

Some studies suggest naltrexone treatment may be more beneficial in some alcohol-dependent patients than others. Scientists have suggested these moderating effects may be because of either genetic differences or particular patient characteristics, which may or may not be related. One early study explored the hypothesis that patients could be matched to both psychopharmacological and psychotherapy treatments based on certain pre-treatment characteristics. The treatment matching variables investigated included craving, alcohol dependence severity, and cognitive measures of learning and memory. Results suggested that patients experiencing higher levels of craving and poorer cognitive functioning derive the most benefit from naltrexone versus placebo, supporting the hypothesis that therapeutic treatment supplemented with naltrexone may help to reduce some of the negative prognosis associated with high craving and poor learning and memory ability (Jaffe *et al.*, 1996).

A number of traits have been addressed in multiple studies, such as age of drinking onset and family history of alcohol abuse. An open-label controlled trial looking at treatment with naltrexone plus psychotherapy versus treatment with psychotherapy alone found that a family history of alcoholism, early age at onset of drinking problems, and comorbid use of other drugs of abuse were predictive of a positive response to naltrexone (Rubio *et al.*, 2005). In a more recent study, naltrexone decreased urge levels in participants with younger age of alcoholism onset, increased time in between drinks in participants who had more relatives with alcohol problems, and reduced the stimulating effects of alcohol in women (Tidey *et al.*, 2008).

The relationship between family history of alcoholism was also shown in a human laboratory study that found the number of drinks consumed during a drinking period was significantly decreased by the 100 mg dose of naltrexone in drinkers with a family history of alcoholism. Secondary analysis among male drinkers alone revealed that 100 mg of naltrexone significantly decreased drinking in participants with a family history of alcoholism, but increased drinking in those without (Krishnan-Sarin *et al.*, 2007). Similar effects were seen in a 12-week naltrexone treatment study where, although a dichotomized measure of family history of alcohol problems was not shown to have any interaction with medication efficacy, naltrexone resulted in lower drinking rates among patients with a higher percentage of relatives with a drinking problem (Rohsenow *et al.*, 2007). The above studies indicate that certain patients may benefit more from naltrexone treatment than others, based on a variety of clinical factors. In addition, the relationship between family history of alcohol abuse and naltrexone treatment efficacy provides support for an interaction between genetic factors and response to treatment.

Scientists have looked at polymorphisms in the D4 dopamine receptor (*DRD4*) gene and the mu-opioid receptor (*MOR*) genes as potential moderators of the effectiveness of naltrexone in heavy drinkers. Polymorphisms on the *DRD4* gene have not been as well studied as those on the *MOR* gene, and the few existing studies have produced mixed results as to whether or not any gene *x* medication interaction exists (McGeary *et al.*, 2006; Tidey *et al.*, 2008). However, a number of human and animal studies have suggested that the mu-*MOR* modulates alcohol intake through its effects on reward and stress responsivity. More specifically, the A118G polymorphism of the *OPRM1* gene has been shown to confer functional differences to mu-opioid receptors, in that the G variant binds beta-endorphin three times more strongly than the A variant (Ray & Hutchinson, 2004; 2007).

A functional polymorphism of the opioid receptor gene *OPRM1* that has been studied with regard to individual response to treatment with naltrexone is Asn40Asp. Genetic studies have shown that individuals with one or two copies of the Asp40 allele treated with naltrexone have significantly lower rates of relapse and a longer time to return to heavy drinking than those homozygous for the Asn40 allele (Oslin *et al.*, 2003; Anton *et al.*, 2008). Contradictory studies have found no significant interactions between any individual single nucleotide polymorphism (SNP) studied and naltrexone treatment response (Gelernter *et al.*, 2007). These results suggest that the Asp40 allele of the *OPRM1* gene may predict the clinical treatment response to naltrexone in alcoholic individuals, although this relationship may be obscured by other efficacious concomitant treatments, such as behavioral intervention.

Compliance with naltrexone

Strategies to support medication compliance may need to be emphasized to optimize therapeutic outcome with naltrexone. In four trials that did not show efficacy in intent-to-treat analyses, treatment effects were revealed when a subgroup of compliant patients were analyzed separately (Oslin *et al.*, 1997; Volpicelli *et al.*, 1997; Chick *et al.*, 2000a; Monti *et al.*, 2001). Even in the context of CBT, treatment effect sizes approximately doubled in a placebo-controlled trial of naltrexone when only the most compliant individuals were considered (Baros *et al.*, 2007). These findings suggest that monitoring compliance may optimize treatment response, and the techniques described above with regard to maximizing treatment compliance with acamprosate may apply equally. Furthermore, in response to the compliance issues noted with daily oral administration of naltrexone, an intramuscular formulation has been approved that releases naltrexone for 1 month following injection into the buttock. One multi-center dose-ranging trial has been reported with this formulation in alcohol dependence that found significant effects on heavy drinking in the higher dose condition, with a 14.1%

rate of discontinuation owing to adverse events, primarily nausea, injection site reaction, and headache (Garbutt *et al.*, 2005). Patients who were males and abstinent at treatment initiation derived the most beneficial effects from active treatment.

Use of naltrexone in patients with comorbid psychiatric disorders

Although naltrexone has been approved by the FDA for the treatment of alcohol dependence, no medications have been approved for individuals with alcohol dependence and comorbid psychiatric disorders. Emerging studies have begun to investigate the use of naltrexone in these patients, in order to evaluate the drug's safety and efficacy in patients with such comorbidities. One of the most common disorders occurring with alcoholism is depression. Naltrexone works by blocking mu-receptors, an important reward pathway in the brain, and data from case reports and a controlled trial have found an exacerbation of depressive symptoms in patients with alcohol dependence being treated with naltrexone (Farren & O'Malley, 1999; Latt *et al.*, 2002; Schurks *et al.*, 2005). In contrast, Petrakis *et al.* (2007) found no relationship between the diagnosis of depression and naltrexone treatment on alcohol use outcomes, psychiatric symptoms, or reporting of side-effects, suggesting that naltrexone is safe for use in alcohol-dependent individuals dually diagnosed with depression. Naltrexone has also been studied for safety and efficacy in combination with antidepressants. Studies show conflicting results on whether there is an added benefit of giving naltrexone in combination with antidepressants with regard to drinking outcomes; however, it is worthwhile to note that no adverse effects were noted in combining its use with treatment for depression (Oslin, 2005, Krystal *et al.*, 2008). Studies looking at patients dually diagnosed and undergoing pharmacological treatment for other psychiatric disorders such as schizophrenia-spectrum disorders, bipolar disorder, PTSD, and personality disorders suggest that naltrexone is safe for use in these patients and may be associated with better drinking-related outcomes (Petrakis *et al.*, 2005; 2006a; 2006b; Brown *et al.*, 2006; Batki *et al.*, 2007; Ralevski *et al.*, 2007). However, it is important that patients with a history of psychiatric disorders, primarily depression, be monitored for depressive symptoms while being treated with naltrexone.

Meta-analyses of acamprosate and naltrexone

Another level of review of acamprosate and naltrexone efficacy in alcohol dependence is meta-analysis. Since meta-analyses combine data from multiple studies for re-analysis, the sample size available for analysis is thereby increased, strengthening the ability to detect treatment effects. In recent years, meta-analyses have been performed for both acamprosate and naltrexone, yielding consistent results. Whereas some studies have focused on the treatment effects of the individual drugs, others have looked at the drugs by comparison to determine which treatment is more efficacious in alcohol-dependent individuals.

A 2004 meta-analysis looked at the effect of acamprosate on the maintenance of abstinence from alcohol and included data from 17 randomized, placebo-controlled trials (RCTs) that were considered to be of good quality and were reasonably comparable. Analyses involved 4087 alcohol-dependent individuals and showed that continuous abstinence rates at 6 months were significantly higher in patients treated with acamprosate as compared with placebo (Mann et al., 2004). Meta-analyses focused on the efficacy of naltrexone have also been positive. A systematic review and meta-analysis of seven RCTs published between 1976 and January 2001 indicated that subjects treated with naltrexone experienced significantly fewer episodes of relapse when compared to subjects on placebo (Streeton & Whelan, 2001). A larger meta-analysis of 24 RCTs presented in 32 papers that included 2861 individuals found that naltrexone significantly decreased relapse in short-term treatment (Srisurapanont and Jarusuraisin, 2005).

Meta-analytic principles assume random assignment to treatments. Nevertheless, treatment with acamprosate and naltrexone has also been compared in two meta-analyses that combined RCTs of both drugs, although the subjects did not have an equal chance of randomization to naltrexone if they were participants in an acamprosate trial, and vice versa. One such study extracted data from all placebo-controlled studies of both drugs to calculate a mean effect size. Both drugs were found to have modest but significant effects on treatment retention and drinking outcomes, and researchers concluded that, based on limited comparisons of the two medications, there appeared to be no statistical difference in their efficacy in treating alcohol-dependent patients (Kranzler &

Van Kirk, 2001). Another meta-analysis sought to examine the efficacy profiles of acamprosate and naltrexone, as well as compare them with one another, and found acamprosate to be more effective in preventing a lapse, and naltrexone to be more effective at preventing a lapse from becoming a relapse to heavy drinking (Rosner et al., 2008). Although the outcome measures varied between studies, the above meta-analyses concluded that both acamprosate and naltrexone had significant effects on drinking outcomes in alcohol-dependent individuals. These approved pharmacotherapies should be considered for use in patients seeking treatment for alcohol dependence, with choice of medication reflecting the safety considerations discussed above, as well as patient goals and preferences.

Acamprosate and naltrexone in combination

Pharmacokinetic and pharmacodynamic safety studies of acamprosate and naltrexone, alone and in combination

The safety of administering acamprosate and naltrexone, in combination, relative to administering each drug independently, was evaluated in two well controlled pharmacokinetic (PK) and pharmacodynamic (PD) inpatient studies (Mason et al., 2002; Johnson et al., 2003). Initially, a double-blind, multiple dose, within subjects, randomized three-way crossover drug interaction study was conducted in 24 healthy volunteers with the aim of examining the safety of the standard therapeutic doses of acamprosate (2 g/day) and naltrexone (50 mg/day), given alone and in combination (Mason et al., 2002). A complete absence of negative interactions on measures of safety, tolerability, and cognitive function supported the absence of a contraindication to coadministration of acamprosate and naltrexone in clinical practice. Unexpectedly, coadministration of acamprosate with naltrexone significantly increased the rate and extent of absorption of acamprosate, as indicated by an average 33% increase in acamprosate maximum plasma concentration, 33% reduction in time to maximum plasma concentration, and 25% increase in area under the plasma concentration–time curve. These findings suggested that combination treatment may make acamprosate more available systemically, with no decrease in tolerability, which may have clinical advantages.

These PK and PD findings were replicated and expanded upon in a clinical sample of 23 non-treatment-seeking volunteers with alcohol dependence (Johnson *et al.*, 2003). Subjects were assessed in a double-blind, placebo-controlled, multiple dose, within subjects, randomized four-way crossover dose-ranging PD/PK study of naltrexone (50 mg/day versus 100 mg/day) and acamprosate (2 g/day versus 3 g/day), given alone and in combination. Naltrexone administration significantly increased plasma acamprosate levels, in a dose-dependent relationship. Unlike the earlier study, more side-effects were noted with the combination of medications than with either medication alone. However, adverse events overall tended to be infrequent, of mild to moderate intensity, and were resolved with reassurance and symptomatic treatment. The absence of a contraindication to coadministration of acamprosate and naltrexone in clinical practice was again supported, although the authors suggest additional clinical monitoring with combined treatment. The authors also proposed further clinical study to evaluate whether the increased levels of acamprosate in plasma obtained with naltrexone coadministration produced any advantage for dosing above the standard therapeutic doses of acamprosate (2 g/day) and naltrexone (50 mg/day).

Efficacy of acamprosate and naltrexone in combination

The clinical utility of combination treatment has recently been demonstrated in two single-site placebo-controlled clinical trials in Germany and Australia (Kiefer *et al.*, 2003; Feeney *et al.*, 2006). In the earlier investigation, following detoxification, 160 volunteers with alcohol dependence participated in 12 weekly CBT group sessions and were randomized to receive double-blind acamprosate (2 g/day) or naltrexone (50 mg/day), alone or in combination, or placebo. Time to first drink, time to relapse, and cumulative abstinence time were the primary outcome measures; however, patients who relapsed were removed from the study. This precluded the traditional assessment of cumulative abstinence time over the complete study duration and contributed to a high rate of study discontinuation. Overall, all active medication groups had better outcomes than placebo. The combined medication group had significantly lower relapse rates than acamprosate and placebo but not naltrexone. Naltrexone showed a greater effect on relapse than

acamprosate. Group differences on cumulative abstinence time were not reported. No serious adverse drug experiences were observed, although diarrhea and nausea occurred with higher frequency in the combination treatment groups.

In the Australian investigation, 236 patients were matched across gender, age group, prior alcohol detoxification, and dependence severity, and assigned to one of three medication groups: CBT + acamprosate, CBT + naltrexone, or CBT + combined medication (Table 20.4). Outcome measures included program attendance, abstinence, and, for those who relapsed, cumulative abstinence duration and days to first drink. Across medication groups, CBT + combined medication produced the greatest improvement across all outcome measures, although the differences did not reach clinical significance. CBT + naltrexone was found to be as effective as combined medication, although the trend seemed to favor combined medication. Withdrawal owing to adverse medication effects was minimal, and the investigators concluded that the medication combination was well tolerated, and that the addition of both medications resulted in measurable benefit.

The COMBINE Study, a large collaborative effort sponsored by the National Institute on Alcohol Abuse and Alcoholism, was recently undertaken to evaluate the utility of combined acamprosate (3 g/day) and naltrexone (100 mg/day) treatment for alcohol dependence. This RCT, conducted between January 2001 and January 2004, evaluated 1383 recently abstinent, alcohol-dependent participants from 11 academic sites around the US. Patients received medical management (MM) with 16 weeks of treatment with naltrexone, acamprosate, combined naltrexone and acamprosate, or placebo, with or without combined behavioral intervention (CBI), resulting in eight treatment groups. A ninth group received CBI only. Researchers found no advantage for combined medications and patients receiving MM with naltrexone, CBI, or both fared better on drinking outcomes although differences were slight as all groups improved significantly from baseline. However, a higher rate of adverse events was noted in the combined medication groups, including 11 patients treated with naltrexone experiencing elevations in LFTs ≥ 5 ULN. Acamprosate, on the other hand, showed no evidence of efficacy, with or without CBI, and no combination produced better efficacy than naltrexone or CBI alone in the presence of MM (Anton *et al.*, 2006).

Table 20.4 Summary of published trials of acamprosate and naltrexone in combination

	n	Months of study	Days to relapse	Rate of total abstinence (%)	Cumulative abstinence duration	Rate of heavy drinking	Completion of double-blind treatment (%)	Reference
			Acamprosate, naltrexone, combination, or placebo	Acamprosate, naltrexone, combination, or placebo	Acamprosate, naltrexone, combination, or placebo		Acamprosate, naltrexone, combination, or placebo	
Short-term efficacy studies	160	3	N > P[a]	N > P[a]				Kiefer et al., 2003
			A > P[a]	A > P[b]				
			C > P[a]	C > P[a]				
			C > A[c], C = N, N = A	C > A[a], C = N, N = A				
	236	3	CBT + A = 27 days	CBT + A = 51	CBT + A = 45 days		CBT + A = 66[c]	Feeney et al., 2006*
			CBT + N = 27 days	CBT + N = 66	CBT + N = 50 days		CBT + N = 80	
			CBT + C = 37 days	CBT + C = 68	CBT + C = 54 days		CBT + C = 83	
	1383	4			MM + N = 80%	MM + N = 68%	MM + N = 57	Anton et al., 2006**
					MM + A = 76%	MM + A = 71%	MM + A = 63	
					MM + C = 81%	MM + C = 65%	MM + C = 61	
					MM + P = 74%	MM + P = 76%	MM + P = 70	
					CBI + MM + N = 76%	CBI + MM + N = 67%	CBI + MM + N = 67	
					CBI + MM + A = 78%	CBI + MM + A = 68%	CBI + MM + A = 67	
					CBI + MM + C = 78%	CBI + MM + C = 74%	CBI + MM + C = 58	
					CBI + MM + P = 80%	CBI + MM + P = 71%	CBI + MM + P = 73	

A, acamprosate; N, naltrexone; C, combined acamprosate & naltrexone; P, placebo; CBT, cognitive behavioral therapy; CBI, cognitive behavioral intervention; MM, medical management. [a]Difference between treatment and placebo groups, $P < 0.05$. [b]Difference between treatment and placebo groups, $P < 0.1$ and $P > 0.05$. [c]Difference between acamprosate or naltrexone alone and combination treatment groups, $P < 0.5$. *Sequential, non-randomized study. No placebo group used. **Cell × cell comparisons not reported. N + MM > N + MM + CBI for % abstinent days; N < P for heavy drinking in factorial model.

Conclusions

Acamprosate and naltrexone both appear to be of use in the treatment of alcohol dependence above and beyond the effects of counseling alone. The two drugs have each demonstrated efficacy relative to placebo in patients receiving concomitant counseling, but they also differ in a number of important ways. A key difference between the two drugs relates to their mechanism of action. Naltrexone is an opioid receptor anatagonist which blocks the endogenous opioid reward system. It may thereby reduce the rewarding effect of alcohol. Acamprosate, on the other hand, normalizes the dysregulation of NMDA-mediated glutamatergic neurotransmission that occurs during chronic alcohol consumption and withdrawal, and thus attenuates one of the physiological mechanisms that may prompt relapse. These different mechanisms of action may endow the two drugs with efficacy for different components of drinking behavior, with naltrexone primarily reducing heavy drinking and acamprosate primarily maintaining abstinence. In terms of the kinetics of their effects, naltrexone has a rapid onset of action, but its activity is not sustained following elimination of the drug. In contrast, acamprosate has a slower onset of action, requiring around 1 week to reach steady-state levels in the nervous system, but its effects on drinking behavior typically persist after the treatment is completed. The two drugs also have different adverse event and overall tolerability profiles.

While studies of drug efficacy in alcohol-dependent patients are generally favorable, some conflicting findings have been presented. Differences in treatment benefits have been suggested, primarily with naltrexone, with regard to specific types of concomitant psychotherapies or patient characteristics that may moderate its effects. Clinical studies and post-marketing experience indicate that these drugs are typically safe when used as approved by the FDA in alcohol-dependent patients, including those dually diagnosed with psychiatric disorders. However, as noted above, naltrexone is contraindicated in those patients using prescribed or illicit opiates, and baseline and follow-up liver function tests in patients treated with naltrexone are warranted, given its potential hepatotoxicity. Support for enhanced efficacy of combination treatment relative to acamprosate alone was provided by two single-site placebo-controlled combination treatment clinical trials; however, this finding was not replicated in a multi-center study which also found higher rates of adverse events associated with combination treatment. The majority of RCTs of either acamprosate or naltrexone given in conjunction with counseling show significantly improved alcoholism treatment outcome relative to counseling administered with placebo. This evidence base suggests both acamprosate and naltrexone should be routinely considered by medical professionals for patients entering alcoholism treatment, taking into account the patient's goals and preferences as well as the safety considerations outlined above.

Acknowledgments

Support for this work was provided by R01AA012602 and R37AA014028. Appreciation is expressed to Karyn Coveney for her assistance in the preparation of this manuscript. This manuscript is a revision of earlier articles (Mason, 2003; 2005), portions of which are reprinted with permission from *European Neuropsychopharmacology*, **13**(6), Mason, B. J. (2003). Acamprosate and naltrexone treatment for alcohol dependence: an evidence-based risk-benefits assessment, 2003, pages 469–75, with permission from Elsevier; and reprinted with permission from *Journal of Studies on Alcohol*, Suppl. 15, 148–56, 2005, copyright by Alcohol Research Documentation, Inc., Rutgers Center of Alcohol Studies, Piscataway, NJ 08854, USA.

Disclosure

Dr. Mason has served as a consultant and/or received research support from DuPont Pharma and Alkermes / Cephalon, the manufacturers of naltrexone; Lipha Pharmaceuticals, Inc., a subsidiary of Merck Sante s.b.s. and Forest Laboratories, Inc., the manufacturers of acamprosate.

References

Ahmadi, J., Babaeebeigi, M., Maany, I. *et al.* (2004). Naltrexone for alcohol-dependent patients. *Irish Journal of Medical Sciences*, **173**, 34–7.

American Psychiatric Association. (1987). *Diagnostic and Statistical Manual of Mental Disorders*, 3rd edn revised. Washington DC: American Psychiatric Press.

Anton, R. F., Moak, D. H., Waid, L. R. *et al.* (1999). Naltrexone and cognitive behavioral therapy for the treatment of outpatient alcoholics: results of a placebo-controlled trial. *American Journal of Psychiatry*, **156**, 1758–64.

Anton, R. F., Moak, D. H., Latham, P. K. *et al.* (2001). Posttreatment results of combining naltrexone with cognitive-behavior therapy for the treatment of alcoholism. *Journal of Clinical Psychopharmacology*, **21**, 72–7.

Anton, R. F., Moak, D. H., Latham, P. *et al.* (2005). Naltrexone combined with either cognitive behavioral or motivational enhancement therapy for alcohol dependence. *Journal of Clinical Psychopharmacology*, **25**, 349–57.

Anton, R. F., O'Malley, S. S., Ciraulo, D. A., COMBINE Study Research Group *et al.* (2006). Combined pharmacotherapies and behavioral interventions for alcohol dependence: the COMBINE study: a randomized controlled trial. *Journal of the American Medical Association*, **295**, 2003–17.

Anton, R. F., Oroszi, G., O'Malley, S. *et al.* (2008). An evaluation of mu-opioid receptor (OPRM1) as a predictor of naltrexone response in the treatment of alcohol dependence: results from the Combined Pharmacotherapies and Behavioral Interventions for Alcohol Dependence (COMBINE) study. *Archives of General Psychiatry*, **65**, 135–44.

Balldin, J., Berglund, M., Borg, S. *et al.* (2003). A 6-month controlled naltrexone study: combined effect with cognitive behavioral therapy in outpatient treatment of alcohol dependence. *Alcoholism Clinical and Experimental Research*, **27**, 1142–9.

Baltieri, D. A. & De Andrade, A. G. (2004). Acamprosate in alcohol dependence: a randomized controlled efficacy study in a standard clinical setting. *Journal of Studies on Alcohol*, **65**, 136–9.

Baros, A. M., Latham, P. K., Moak, D. H., Voronin, K. & Anton, R. F. (2007). What role does measuring medication compliance play in evaluating the efficacy of naltrexone? *Alcoholism: Clinical and Experimental Research*, **31**, 596–603.

Barrias, J. A., Chabac, S., Ferreira, L. *et al.* (1997). Acamprosate: multicenter Portuguese efficacy and tolerance evaluation study. *Psiquiatria Clinica*, **18**, 149–60.

Batki, S. L., Dimmock, J. A., Wade, M. *et al.* (2007). Monitored naltrexone without counseling for alcohol abuse/dependence in schizophrenia-spectrum disorders. *American Journal on Addictions*, **16**, 253–9.

Besson, J., Aeby, F., Kasas, A., Lehert, P. & Potgieter, A. (1998). Combined efficacy of acamprosate and disulfiram in the treatment of alcoholism: a controlled study. *Alcoholism: Clinical and Experimental Research*, **22**, 573–9.

Brown, E. S., Beard, L., Dobbs, L. & Rush, A. J. (2006). Naltrexone in patients with bipolar disorder and alcohol dependence. *Depression and Anxiety*, **23**, 492–5.

Campral® (acamprosate calcium) [package insert]. St. Louis, MO: Forest Pharmaceuticals, Inc., 2005.

Chick, J., Anton, R., Checinski, K. *et al.* (2000a). A multicentre, randomized, double-blind, placebo-controlled trial of naltrexone in the treatment of alcohol dependence or abuse. *Alcohol and Alcoholism*, **35**, 587–93.

Chick, J., Howlett, H., Morgan, M. Y. & Ritson, B. (2000b). United Kingdom Multicentre Acamprosate Study (UKMAS): a 6-month prospective study of acamprosate versus placebo in preventing relapse after withdrawal from alcohol. *Alcohol and Alcoholism*, **35**, 176–87.

Chick, J., Lehert, P. & Landron, F. (2003). Does acamprosate improve reduction of drinking as well as aiding abstinence? *Journal of Psychopharmacology*, **17**, 397–402.

Croop, R. S., Faulkner, E. B. & Labriola, D. F. (1997). The safety profile of naltrexone in the treatment of alcoholism. Results from a multicenter usage study. The Naltrexone Usage Study Group. *Archives of General Psychiatry*, **54**, 1130–5.

Davidson, D., Wirtz, P. W., Gulliver, S. B. & Longabaugh, R. (2007). Naltrexone's suppressant effects on drinking are limited to the first 3 months of treatment. *Psychopharmacology*, **194**, 1–10.

De Wildt, W. A., Schippers, G. M., Van Den Brink, W. *et al.* (2002). Does psychosocial treatment enhance the efficacy of acamprosate in patients with alcohol problems? *Alcohol and Alcoholism*, **37**, 375–82.

Farren, C. K. & O'Malley, S. S. (1999). Occurrence and management of depression in the context of naltrexone treatment in alcoholism. *American Journal of Psychiatry*, **156**, 1258–62.

Feeney, G. F., Young, R. M., Connor, J. P., Tucker, J. & McPherson, A. (2002). Cognitive behavioural therapy combined with the relapse-prevention medication acamprosate: are short-term treatment outcomes for alcohol dependence improved? *Australian and New Zealand Journal of Psychiatry*, **36**, 622–8.

Feeney, G. F., Connor, J. P., Young, R. M., Tucker, J. & McPherson, A. (2006). Combined acamprosate and naltrexone with cognitive behavioural therapy is superior to either medication alone for alcohol abstinence: a single centre's experience with pharmacotherapy. *Alcohol and Alcoholism*, **41**, 321–7.

Garbutt, J. C., Kranzler, H. R., O'Malley, S. S. *et al.* (2005). Efficacy and tolerability of long-acting injectable naltrexone for alcohol dependence: a randomized controlled trial. *Journal of the American Medical Association*, **293**, 1617–25.

Gastpar, M., Bonnet, U., Boning, J. *et al.* (2002). Lack of efficacy of naltrexone in the prevention of alcohol relapse: results from a German multicenter study. *Journal of Clinical Psychopharmacology*, **22**, 592–8.

Geerlings, P. J., Ansoms, C. & Van Den Brink, W. (1997). Acamprosate and prevention of relapse in alcoholics. *European Addiction Research*, **3**, 129–37.

Gelernter, J., Gueorguieva, R., Kranzler, H. R., VA Cooperative Study #425 Study Group *et al.* (2007). Opioid receptor gene (OPRM1, OPRK1, and OPRD1) variants and response to naltrexone treatment for alcohol dependence: results from the VA Cooperative Study. *Alcoholism: Clinical and Experimental Research*, **31**, 555–63.

Gual, A. & Lehert, P. (2001). Acamprosate during and after acute alcohol withdrawal: a double-blind placebo-controlled study in Spain. *Alcohol and Alcoholism*, **36**, 413–18.

Guardia, J., Caso, C., Arias, F. *et al.* (2002). A double-blind, placebo-controlled study of naltrexone in the treatment of alcohol-dependence disorder: results from a multicenter clinical trial. *Alcoholism: Clinical and Experimental Research*, **26**, 1381–7.

Gueorguieva, R., Wu, R., Pittman, B. *et al.* (2007). New insights into the efficacy of naltrexone based on trajectory-based reanalyses of two negative clinical trials. *Biological Psychiatry*, **61**, 1290–5.

Heinala, P., Alho, H., Kiianmaa, K. *et al.* (2001). Targeted use of naltrexone without prior detoxification in the treatment of alcohol dependence: a factorial double-blind, placebo-controlled trial. *Journal of Clinical Psychopharmacology*, **21**, 287–92.

Huang, M. C., Chen, C. H., Yu, J. M. & Chen, C. C. (2005). A double-blind, placebo-controlled study of naltrexone in the treatment of alcohol dependence in Taiwan. *Addiction Biology*, **10**, 289–92.

Jaffe, A. J., Rounsaville, B., Chang, G. *et al.* (1996). Naltrexone, relapse prevention, and supportive therapy with alcoholics: an analysis of patient treatment matching. *Journal of Consulting and Clinical Psychology*, **64**, 1044–53.

Johnson, B. A., O'Malley, S. S., Ciraulo, D. A. *et al.* (2003). Dose-ranging kinetics and behavioral pharmacology of naltrexone and acamprosate, both alone and combined, in alcohol-dependent subjects. *Journal of Clinical Psychopharmacology*, **23**, 281–93.

Kiefer, F., Jahn, H., Tarnaske, T. *et al.* (2003). Comparing and combining naltrexone and acamprosate in relapse prevention of alcoholism: a double-blind, placebo-controlled study. *Archives of General Psychiatry*, **60**, 92–9.

Killeen, T. K., Brady, K. T., Gold, P. B. *et al.* (2004). Effectiveness of naltrexone in a community treatment program. *Alcoholism: Clinical and Experimental Research*, **28**, 1710–17.

Kim, S. W., Grant, J. E., Adson, D. E. & Remmel, R. P. (2001). A preliminary report on possible naltrexone and nonsteroidal analgesic interactions. *Journal of Clinical Psychopharmacology*, **21**, 632–4.

Koob, G. F., Mason, B. J., De Witte, P., Littleton, J. & Siggins, G. R. (2002). Potential neuroprotective effects of acamprosate. *Alcoholism: Clinical and Experimental Research*, **26**, 586–92.

Kranzler, H. R. & Van Kirk, J. (2001). Efficacy of naltrexone and acamprosate for alcoholism treatment: a meta-analysis. *Alcoholism: Clinical and Experimental Research*, **25**, 1335–41.

Kranzler, H. R. & Gage, A. (2008). Acamprosate efficacy in alcohol-dependent patients: summary of results from three pivotal trials. *American Journal on Addictions*, **17**, 70–6.

Kranzler, H. R., Modesto-Lowe, V. & Van Kirk, J. (2000). Naltrexone vs. nefazodone for treatment of alcohol dependence. A placebo-controlled trial. *Neuropsychopharmacology*, **22**, 493–503.

Kranzler, H. R., Wesson, D. R., Billot, L., Drug Abuse Sciences Naltrexone Depot Study Group. (2004). Naltrexone depot for treatment of alcohol dependence: a multicenter, randomized, placebo-

controlled clinical trial. *Alcoholism: Clinical and Experimental Research*, **27**, 533–9.

Krishnan-Sarin, S., Krystal, J. H., Shi, J., Pittman, B. & O'Malley, S. S. (2007). Family history of alcoholism influences naltrexone-induced reduction in alcohol drinking. *Biological Psychiatry*, **62**, 694–7.

Krystal, J. H., Cramer, J. A., Krol, W. F., Kirk, G. F. & Rosenheck, R. A. (2001). Veterans Affairs Naltrexone Cooperative Study 425 Group. Naltrexone in the treatment of alcohol dependence. *New England Journal of Medicine*, **345**, 1734–9.

Krystal, J. H., Gueorguieva, R., Cramer, J., Collins, J. & Rosenheck, R; VA CSP No. 425 Study Team. (2008). Naltrexone is associated with reduced drinking by alcohol dependent patients receiving antidepressants for mood and anxiety symptoms: results from VA Cooperative Study No. 425, "Naltrexone in the treatment of alcoholism". *Alcoholism: Clinical and Experimental Research*, **32**, 85–91.

Ladewig, D., Knecht, T., Leher, P. & Fendl, A. (1993). Acamprosate – a stabilizing factor in long-term withdrawal of alcoholic patients. *Ther Umsch*, **50**, 182–8.

Latt, N. C., Jurd, S., Houseman, J. & Wutzke, S. E. (2002). Naltrexone in alcohol dependence: a randomised controlled trial of effectiveness in a standard clinical setting. *Medical Journal of Australia*, **176**, 530–4.

Lhuintre, J. P., Daoust, M., Moore, N. D. *et al.* (1985). Ability of calcium bis acetyl homotaurine, a GABA agonist, to prevent relapse in weaned alcoholics. *Lancet*, i:1014–16.

Lhuintre, J. P., Moore N., Tran, G. *et al.* (1990). Acamprosate appears to decrease alcohol intake in weaned alcoholics. *Alcohol and Alcoholism*, **25**, 613–22.

Littleton, J. M. (2007). Acamprosate in alcohol dependence: implications of a unique mechanism of action. *Journal of Addiction Medicine*, **1**(3), 115–25.

Mann, K., Lehert, P. & Morgan, M. Y. (2004). The efficacy of acamprosate in the maintenance of abstinence in alcohol-dependent individuals: results of a meta-analysis. *Alcoholism: Clinical and Experimental Research*, **28**, 51–63.

Mason, B. J. (2001). Treatment of alcohol-dependent outpatients with acamprosate: a clinical review. *Journal of Clinical Psychiatry*, **62**(Suppl. 20), 42–8.

Mason, B. J. (2003). Acamprosate and naltrexone treatment for alcohol dependence: an evidence-based risk-benefits assessment. *European Neuropsychopharmacology*, **13**, 469–75.

Mason, B. J. (2005). Rationale for combining acamprosate and naltrexone for treating alcohol dependence. *Journal of Studies on Alcohol Supplement*, **15**, 148–56.

Mason, B. J. & Goodman, A. M. (1997). *Brief Intervention and Medication Compliance Procedures Therapist's Manual*. New York, NY: Lipha Pharmaceuticals, Inc.

Mason, B. J. & Ownby, R. L. (2000). Acamprosate for the treatment of alcohol dependence: a review of double-blind, placebo-controlled trials. *CNS Spectrums*, **5**, 58–69.

Mason, B. J., Goodman, A. M., Dixon, R. M. *et al* (2002). A pharmacokinetic and pharmacodynamic drug interaction study of acamprosate and naltrexone. *Neuropsychopharmacology*, **27**, 596–606.

Mason, B. J., Goodman, A. M., Chabac, S. & Lehert, P. (2006). Effect of oral acamprosate on abstinence in patients with alcohol dependence in a double-blind, placebo-controlled trial: the role of patient motivation. *Journal of Psychiatric Research*, **40**, 383–93.

McGeary, J. E., Monti, P. M., Rohsenow, D. J. *et al.* (2006). Genetic moderators of naltrexone's effects on alcohol cue reactivity. *Alcoholism: Clinical and Experimental Research*, **30**, 1288–96.

Monterosso, J. R., Flannery, B. A., Pettinati, H. M. *et al.* (2001). Predicting treatment response to naltrexone: the influence of craving and family history. *American Journal on Addictions*, **10**, 258–68.

Monti, P. M., Rohsenow, D. J., Swift, R. M. *et al.* (2001). Naltrexone and cue exposure with coping and communication skills training for alcoholics: treatment process and 1-year outcomes. *Alcoholism: Clinical and Experimental Research*, **25**, 1634–47.

Morley, K. C., Teesson, M., Reid, S. C. *et al.* (2006). Naltrexone versus acamprosate in the treatment of alcohol dependence: a multi-centre, randomized, double-blind, placebo-controlled trial. *Addiction*, **101**, 1451–62.

Morris, P. L., Hopwood, M., Whelan, G., Gardiner, J. & Drummond, E. (2001). Naltrexone for alcohol dependence: a randomized controlled trial. *Addiction*, **96**, 1565–73.

Naltrexone hydrochloride [package insert]. St. Louis, MO: Mallinckrodt, Inc., revised September 2003.

Namkoong, K., Lee, B. O., Lee, P. G., Choi, M. J., Lee, E; Korean Acamprosate Clinical Trial Investigators (2003). Acamprosate in Korean alcohol-dependent patients: a multi-centre, randomized, double-blind, placebo-controlled study. *Alcohol and Alcoholism*, **38**, 135–41.

Niederhofer, H. & Staffen, W. (2003). Acamprosate and its efficacy in treating alcohol dependent adolescents. *European Child and Adolescent Psychiatry*, **12**, 144–8.

O'Malley, S. S., Jaffe, A. J., Chang, G. *et al.* (1992). Naltrexone and coping skills therapy for alcohol dependence: a controlled study. *Archives of General Psychiatry*, **49**, 881–7.

O'Malley, S. S., Jaffe, A. J., Chang, G. *et al.* (1996). Six-month follow-up of naltrexone and psychotherapy for alcohol dependence. *Archives of General Psychiatry*, **53**, 217–24.

O'Malley, S. S., Sinha, R., Grilo, C.M. *et al.* (2007). Naltrexone and cognitive behavioral coping skills therapy for the treatment of alcohol drinking and eating disorder features in alcohol-dependent women: a randomized controlled trial. *Alcoholism: Clinical and Experimental Research*, **31**, 625–34.

Oslin, D. W. (2005). Treatment of late-life depression complicated by alcohol dependence. *American Journal of Geriatric Psychiatry*, **13**, 491–500.

Oslin, D., Liberto, J. G., O'Brien, J., Krois, S. & Norbeck, J. (1997). Naltrexone as an adjunctive treatment for older patients with alcohol dependence. *American Journal of Geriatric Psychiatry*, **5**, 324–32.

Oslin, D. W., Berrettini, W., Kranzler, H. R. *et al.* (2003). A functional polymorphism of the mu-opioid receptor gene is associated with naltrexone response in alcohol-dependent patients. *Neuropsychopharmacology*, **28**, 1546–52.

Oslin, D. W., Lynch, K.G., Pettinati, H. M. *et al.* (2008). A placebo-controlled randomized clinical trial of naltrexone in the context of different levels of psychosocial intervention. *Alcoholism: Clinical and Experimental Research*, **32**, 1299–308.

Paille, F. M., Guelfi, J. D., Perkins, A. C. *et al.* (1995). Double-blind randomized multicentre trial of acamprosate in maintaining abstinence from alcohol. *Alcohol and Alcoholism*, **30**, 239–47.

Pelc, I., LeBon, O., Verbanck, P., Lehert, P. H. & Opsomer, L. (1992). Calcium acetyl homotaurinate for maintaining abstinence in weaned alcoholic patients: a placebo controlled double-blind multi-centre study. In *Novel Pharmacological Interventions for Alcoholism*, eds. C. Naranjo & E. Sellers. New York: Springer, pp. 348–52.

Pelc, I., Verbanck, P., Le Bon, O. *et al.* (1997). Efficacy and safety of acamprosate in the treatment of detoxified alcohol-dependent patients. A 90-day placebo-controlled dose-finding study. *British Journal of Psychiatry*, **171**, 73–7.

Pelc, I., Ansoms, C., Lehert, P. *et al.* (2002). The European NEAT program: an integrated approach using acamprosate and psychosocial support for the prevention of relapse in alcohol-dependent patients with a statistical modeling of therapy success prediction. *Alcoholism: Clinical and Experimental Research*, **26**, 1529–38.

Petrakis, I. L., Poling, J., Levinson, C., VA New England VISN I MIRECC Study Group (2005). Naltrexone and disulfiram in patients with alcohol dependence and comorbid psychiatric disorders. *Biological Psychiatry*, **57**, 1128–37.

Petrakis, I. L., Poling, J., Levinson, C. *et al.* (2006a) Naltrexone and disulfiram in patients with alcohol dependence and comorbid post-traumatic stress disorder. *Biological Psychiatry*, **60**, 777–83.

Petrakis, I. L., Nich, C. & Ralevski, E. (2006b). Psychotic spectrum disorders and alcohol abuse: a review of pharmacotherapeutic strategies and a report on the effectiveness of naltrexone and disulfiram. *Schizophrenia Bulletin*, **32**, 616–17.

Petrakis, I., Ralevski, E., Nich, C., VA VISN I MIRECC Study Group (2007). Naltrexone and disulfiram in patients with alcohol dependence and current depression. *Journal of Clinical Psychopharmacology*, **27**, 160–5.

Poldrugo, F. (1997). Acamprosate treatment in a long-term community-based alcohol rehabilitation programme. *Addiction*, **92**, 1537–46.

Ralevski, E., Ball, S., Nich, C., Limoncelli, D. & Petrakis, I. (2007). The impact of personality disorders on alcohol-use outcomes in a pharmacotherapy trial for alcohol dependence and comorbid Axis I disorders. *American Journal on Addictions*, **16**, 443–9.

Ray, L. A. & Hutchison, K. E. (2004). A polymorphism of the mu-opioid receptor gene (OPRM1) and sensitivity to the effects of alcohol in humans. *Alcoholism: Clinical and Experimental Research*, **28**, 1789–95.

Ray, L. A. & Hutchison, K. E. (2007). Effects of naltrexone on alcohol sensitivity and genetic moderators of medication response: a double-blind placebo-controlled study. *Archives of General Psychiatry*, **64**, 1069–77.

Rohsenow, D. J., Miranda, R. Jr., McGeary, J. E. & Monti, P. M. (2007). Family history and antisocial traits moderate naltrexone's effects on heavy drinking in alcoholics. *Experimental and Clinical Psychopharmacology*, **15**, 272–81.

Rosenthal, R. N., Gage, A., Perhach, J. L., Goodman, A. M. (2008). Acamprosate: safety and tolerability in the treatment of alcohol dependence. *Journal of Addiction Medicine*, **2**, 40–50.

Rösner, S., Leucht, S., Lehert, P. & Soyka, M. (2008). Acamprosate supports abstinence, naltrexone prevents excessive drinking: evidence from a meta-analysis with unreported outcomes. *Journal of Psychopharmacology*, **22**, 11–23.

Roussaux, J. P., Hers, D. & Ferauge, M. (1996). Does acamprosate diminish the appetite for alcohol in weaned alcoholics. *Journal de Pharmacie de Belgique*, **51**, 65–8.

Rubio, G., Ponce, G., Rodriguez-Jiménez, R. *et al.* (2005). Clinical predictors of response to naltrexone in alcoholic patients: who benefits most from treatment with naltrexone? *Alcohol and Alcoholism*, **40**, 227–33.

Saivin, S., Hulot, T., Chabac, S. *et al.* (1998). Clinical pharmacokinetics of acamprosate. *Clinical Pharmacokinetics*, **35**, 331–45.

Sass, H., Soyka, M., Mann, K. and Zieglgänsberger, W. (1996). Relapse prevention by acamprosate. Results from a placebo controlled study on alcohol dependence. *Archives of General Psychiatry*, **53**, 673–80.

Schurks, M., Overlack, M. & Bonnet, U. (2005). Naltrexone treatment of combined alcohol and opioid dependence: deterioration of co-morbid major depression. *Pharmacopsychiatry*, **38**, 100–2.

Srisurapanont, M. & Jarusuraisin, N. (2005). Naltrexone for the treatment of alcoholism: a meta-analysis of randomized controlled trials. *International Journal of Neuropsychopharmacology*, **8**, 267–80.

Staner, L., Boeijinga, P., Danel, T. *et al.* (2006). Effects of acamprosate on sleep during alcohol withdrawal: a double-blind placebo-controlled polysomnographic study in alcohol-dependent subjects. *Alcoholism: Clinical and Experimental Research*, **30**, 1492–9.

Streeton, C. & Whelan, G. (2001). Naltrexone, a relapse prevention maintenance treatment of alcohol dependence: a meta-analysis of randomized controlled trials. *Alcohol and Alcoholism*, **36**, 544–52.

Tempesta, E., Janiri, L., Bignamini, A., Chabac, S. & Potgieter, A. (2000). Acamprosate and relapse prevention in the treatment of alcohol dependence: a placebo-controlled study. *Alcohol and Alcoholism*, **35**, 202–9.

Tidey, J. W., Monti, P. M., Rohsenow, D. J. *et al.* (2008). Moderators of naltrexone's effects on drinking, urge, and alcohol effects in non-treatment-seeking heavy drinkers in the natural environment. *Alcoholism: Clinical and Experimental Research*, **32**, 58–66.

Verheul, R., Lehert, P., Geerlings, P. J., Koeter, M. W. & van den Brink, W. (2005). Predictors of acamprosate efficacy: results from a pooled analysis of seven European trials including 1485 alcohol-dependent patients. *Psychopharmacology*, **178**, 167–73.

Volpicelli, J. R., Alterman, A. I., Hayashida, M. & O'Brien, C. P. (1992). Naltrexone in the treatment of alcohol dependence. *Archives of General Psychiatry*, **49**, 876–80.

Volpicelli, J. R., Rhines, K. C., Rhines, J. S. *et al.* (1997). Naltrexone and alcohol dependence. Role of subject compliance. *Archives of General Psychiatry*, **54**, 737–42.

Whitworth, A. B., Fischer, F., Lesch, O. M. *et al.* (1996). Comparison of acamprosate and placebo in long-term treatment of alcohol dependence. *Lancet*, **347**, 1438–42.Table 20.3 (Cont.)

Dialectical behavior therapy adapted to the treatment of concurrent borderline personality disorder and substance use disorders

Lisa Burckell & Shelley McMain

There is a high rate of co-occurrence of borderline personality disorder (BPD) and substance use disorders (SUDs). A recent review found that an estimated 57% of BPD individuals met the criteria for an SUD, while close to one-third of those with SUDs met the diagnostic criteria for BPD (Trull *et al.*, 2000). Individuals with both these disorders typically experience problems in many spheres of their lives, including higher levels of psychopathology (Darke *et al.*, 2004; Skodol *et al.*, 1999), higher rates of suicidal and non-suicidal self-injurious behaviors (Darke *et al.*, 2004; Links *et al.*, 1995; van den Bosch *et al.*, 2001; Stone *et al.*, 1987), a more severe substance use profile (e.g. earlier age of onset, higher rates of polydrug abuse, greater use of illicit substances (Darke *et al.*, 2004; Brooner *et al.*, 1997; Nace *et al.*, 1991), higher rates of sexual promiscuity and prostitution (Miller *et al.*, 1993), and higher rates of unemployment, compared to individuals with one of these diagnoses alone.

In light of these findings, it is not surprising that the treatment of concurrent BPD and SUDs presents a significant challenge. One of the few specialized treatments available is dialectical behavior therapy (DBT), originally developed by Marsha Linehan for the treatment of suicidal patients diagnosed with BPD (Linehan, 1993b). DBT-S is an adaptation of the original DBT protocol, designed for the treatment of individuals with concurrent BPD and SUDs (Linehan & Dimeff, 1997; McMain *et al.*, 2007).

This chapter provides an overview of DBT-S, beginning with a case presentation that highlights the clinical challenges associated with the treatment of SUD/BPD patients; this case is referred to throughout the chapter to illustrate how DBT-S strategies address these challenges. Next, we explain the co-occurrence of BPD and SUDs using DBT's biosocial theory, and then we highlight similarities and differences between DBT-S and other addiction treatments. The remainder of the chapter addresses the core strategies of DBT,

the modifications to the standard protocol for the treatment of co-occurring BPD and SUDs, and training opportunities in DBT-S.

Case example

"Marie" was a 35-year-old woman who met the criteria for BPD, alcohol dependence, and opiate abuse. She had a history of two suicide attempts, plus an accidental, near-fatal heroin overdose in the year preceding treatment. Marie was self-referred to our DBT program and agreed to participate in 1 year of treatment. Her goals were to eliminate suicidal behavior, abstain from heroin, and stop engaging in sexually promiscuous behavior. Initially she remained ambivalent about abstaining from alcohol but did agree to work to reduce her drinking.

Marie's family background included an extensive history of mental health and substance abuse problems. She described her mother as an emotionally volatile and sexually promiscuous alcoholic who was rarely at home and who frequently left her unsupervised. Her father was a workaholic who was emotionally distant. She recalled being sexually abused by an older cousin on repeated occasions between the ages of 5 and 12. Her parents divorced when she was 10, and after the divorce she lived with her father, who often criticized her for behaving like her mother.

Marie reported that she first tried alcohol at age 7, and during early adolescence began experimenting with various illicit substances. This experimentation had a rebellious flavor to it; she claimed that it was a way of saying "fuck you" to her father. Moreover, she found it easier to interact with people, particularly men, when she was intoxicated. Over the past 10 years, Marie was intimately involved with abusive men and she repeatedly engaged in casual sexual encounters with strangers. She frequented "seedy" bars in an effort to meet the only kind of men whom she thought would be interested in her. In these situations, she often minimized concerns for her personal safety (i.e. minimizing the risks involved in having unprotected sex with strangers).

Understanding the overlap of BPD and SUDs: DBT's biosocial theory

The biosocial theory of DBT not only offers an explanation for the co-occurrence of BPD and SUDs, but provides a coherent prescription for treatment. The model maintains that the core deficit among individuals with BPD is emotion dysregulation, and posits that BPD is the result of a breakdown in the emotion regulation system (Linehan, 1993b). Emotion dysregulation develops over time following repeated encounters between a constitutionally vulnerable individual and multiple invalidating environmental experiences (such as punishment, abuse, and criticism.) Substance abuse, like other impulsive behaviors – suicide attempts, promiscuity, and recklessness, for example – develops and is maintained either because it functions to regulate emotions and/or because it is a byproduct of dysregulated emotion.

There is growing empirical evidence that both BPD and SUDs are partially caused by constitutional irregularities in affect. For example, individuals with BPD report greater emotional intensity, faster reactivity, and delayed return to emotional baseline in response to emotion cues (e.g. Stiglmayr *et al.*, 2005). Among substance abusers, there is mixed support for the presence of a constitutional emotional vulnerability. Some studies (Elkins *et al.*, 2006; Jackson & Sher, 2003) support a strong association between alcohol use disorders and negative emotionality, a constitutional trait reflecting problematic emotion regulation. The relationship between illicit substance abuse and negative emotionality, however, has been shown to be less robust than the link to other temperamental traits such as impulsivity (Elkins *et al.*, 2006).

The role of invalidation in the development of both BPD and SUDs is supported as well. As many as 44% of individuals with BPD are estimated to have experienced sexual abuse (Battle *et al.*, 2004), which is regarded as a risk factor for the development of this disorder (for a review, see Paris, 1997). Less overtly pathogenic experiences such as parental criticism and emotional neglect are other forms of invalidation that contribute to emotional dysregulation. For example, evidence suggests that suicidal adolescents who have significant interpersonal problems (suicidality and high interpersonal conflict being two symptoms of BPD), are more likely than peers without these difficulties to have experienced parental neglect, emotional under-involvement, and criticism during childhood (Johnson *et al.*, 2002). Other research supports a link between self-injurious thoughts and behaviors and parental criticism among adolescents (Wedig & Nock, 2002). In related findings, partner criticism is associated with alcoholism (O'Farrell *et al.*, 1998) and SUD relapse (Fals-Stewart *et al.*, 2001).

The biosocial theory stresses reciprocity between emotional vulnerability and invalidating environmental experiences. Specifically, emotionally sensitive individuals often place unreasonable demands on others, which increases the likelihood that others will respond with invalidation. Conversely, contact with pervasively invalidating environments generates emotional sensitivity even among individuals who are less vulnerable. The consequence is a failure to learn how to modulate emotions effectively. In the absence of adaptive coping strategies to regulate emotion, these individuals use maladaptive ones, such as substance abuse, suicidal behavior, and impulsive sexual acts. While these maladaptive behaviors have negative long-term consequences, they are often highly reinforcing in the short-term because they effectively regulate emotions in the moment. For example, heroin numbs intense emotional pain, cocaine heightens euphoria, and self-injurious behaviors can relieve feelings of emptiness or elicit concern from others.

The biosocial theory can account for the development of Marie's problems. Marie had apparently been a colicky infant and a sensitive child; she remembered crying uncontrollably when she was dropped off at preschool, and she recalled that she needed a lot of soothing from the teachers. Her parents expressed irritation with this behavior and could not understand why she was unable to act like other children. During later childhood, Marie voiced fears about being left at home unsupervised, to which her parents usually responded by telling her to "grow up and stop acting like a baby." Marie claimed that her parents would only attend to her needs if she had a temper tantrum or exhibited other dramatic displays of emotion. She first tried alcohol at age 7, and recalled that she immediately enjoyed its taste. Later, during adolescence, she increasingly relied on alcohol and other illicit substances to numb her chronic pain, anger, and feelings of shame. The more she relied on alcohol, the more she craved it; this was due at least in part to physiological withdrawal. Her father generally ignored Marie unless she got into trouble at school, or arrived home intoxicated, or had angry outbursts.

Treatment overview

DBT-S is an adaptation of the original DBT protocol developed for suicidal patients with BPD. While it shares the same elements as standard DBT, it also incorporates some unique features. This section reviews the elements of standard DBT and the unique elements of DBT-S, and compares DBT-S with leading addiction treatment models.

DBT is a comprehensive, broad-based cognitive behavioral treatment whose overarching goal is to enhance behavioral stability to improve patients' overall quality of life. In the past two decades, it has been extended beyond treatment of BPD exclusively and has been adapted to other patient populations who experience significant behavioral dyscontrol problems (see Dimeff & Koerner, 2007 for a review). Theoretically, DBT is rooted in dialectics, learning theory, and Zen – three philosophies that inform case conceptualization and intervention strategies in DBT.

Dialectical theory stresses a systemic perspective. Behavior is understood within the larger context in which it develops and is maintained. Consistent with this perspective, DBT therapists focus on how the environment facilitates or inhibits change, and they help patients structure their environments to support positive change. In this regard, DBT-S, like twelve-step approaches (Alcoholics Anonymous, 1981), highlights the importance of developing a community that overtly supports sobriety. Another assumption in dialectical philosophy is that reality is complex, non-dualistic, and comprises multiple perspectives and natural tensions. Change is realized through the synthesis of opposing perspectives. This aspect is most evident in DBT's integration of learning theory and Zen philosophy.

In DBT, the primary dialectical synthesis involves balancing a focus on change with a focus on acceptance. Change strategies are informed by learning theory, which stresses that behavior develops according to learning principles (e.g. operant conditioning, classical conditioning, and modeling). The influence of learning theory is evident in DBT's emphasis on analyzing the factors that control the development and maintenance of behaviors. Like most cognitive behavioral treatments, DBT stresses the importance of clearly defining behavioral treatment targets and behavioral monitoring (e.g. through the use of diary cards). Using behavior analytic techniques, problematic behaviors are assessed, and controlling factors are isolated so that solutions can be generated. Other standard behavioral strategies are employed as well, such as contingency management, exposure, behavioral activation, and skills training.

The focus on acceptance is informed by Zen philosophy, which stresses that suffering stems from the failure to accept reality as it is. This approach emphasizes validation and attempts to help patients accept reality without judgment. The dialectical synthesis of acceptance and change emerges in session through the simultaneous use of both strategies: the therapist strategically shifts between pushing the patient to block dysfunctional behaviors and promote functional ones, while communicating acceptance of the functional intention underlying the patient's dysfunctional behavior. In DBT-S, the standard biosocial theory for BPD is expanded to include an explanation for the development of concurrent BPD and SUDs. DBT-S uses an integrated approach so that clinicians within the same program address addiction and mental health problems to provide a coherent and comprehensive approach to treatment. DBT-S uses a modified treatment target hierarchy and diary cards that have been adapted to accommodate SUD behaviors. Specific substance use goals are viewed from the context of a dialectical philosophy that balances a focus on abstinence and relapse prevention. In light of the evidence that individuals with co-occurring BPD and SUDs have higher rates of treatment dropout than do those with DBT alone, DBT-S also incorporates strategies to enhance treatment engagement. Finally, while DBT-S contains the standard DBT skills modules, it also includes skills that are particularly relevant to those with concurrent alcohol and other drug use.

Addictive behaviors, including the management of cravings, urges, and relapse

DBT-S shares many features with leading addiction treatment models. Similar to motivational interviewing (Miller & Rollnick, 2002), it incorporates specific interventions designed to build attachment to the therapist and treatment team, and utilizes techniques such as "devil's advocate" and "freedom to choose" to enhance motivation and commitment to change. It is also like structured relapse prevention (Marlatt & Donovan, 2005), in that it combines acceptance and change strategies to promote abstinence. And like twelve-step approaches, it is grounded in spirituality, drawing upon Buddhist philosophy just as twelve-step approaches emphasize Christian principles. Both treatments stress the importance of changing what is possible and accepting those things that cannot be changed, a key message in the twelve-step serenity prayer. Both DBT-S and twelve-step approaches emphasize the importance of the environment in supporting change.

Despite these similarities, DBT-S differs from many addiction treatment models in some fundamental ways. Whereas in motivational interviewing motivation is defined as an internal construct that is strengthened once ambivalence is resolved, DBT-S is viewed as a function of the reinforcers in the environment (Linehan & Dimeff, 1997). In contrast to structured relapse prevention, which focuses solely on maintaining abstinence, DBT-S is also designed to help patients achieve abstinence. Twelve-step approaches view addiction as a disease, whereas DBT-S conceptualizes addiction as a learned behavior that is often maintained because drinking and drugging function to regulate affect. Finally, twelve-step approaches view the support and fellowship of the community as the essential mechanism of change, whereas in DBT-S, the mechanism of change entails the development of functional behaviors within the patient.

Treatment and session structure

The standard DBT approach outlined by Linehan (1993b) takes into account the level of severity of substance abuse, psychiatric illness, and level of psychosocial functioning. Treatment is organized into different stages that therapeutically relate to the patient's severity of dysfunction. Stage 1 treatment is for patients with significant behavioral dyscontrol such as suicidal behaviors, substance abuse, and other behaviors that compromise treatment engagement (i.e. missing appointments or presenting to session in an intoxicated state), and often compromise quality of life. The goal of stage 1 treatment is to help patients develop control over their behavior. Once control is achieved, subsequent stages of treatment that address less severe problems may be initiated.

Stage 2 involves enhancing emotional experiencing or the reprocessing of trauma. Stage 3 is all about

achieving happiness, while stage 4 focuses on increasing the patient's capacity to sustain joy.

DBT-S is a stage 1 approach, and has widely been implemented in a 1-year time frame with good results, although the length of time needed to achieve behavioral control varies according to the severity of dysfunction. Treatment is organized into four distinct treatment modes: weekly individual sessions, a skills training group, phone consultation, and work with a consultation team. Skills training facilitates the acquisition of new behaviors; the four skills training modules are described in greater detail later in this chapter. Between-session phone contact with therapists is used to encourage patients to handle situations between sessions and to ensure skill generalization. The therapist consultation team is a community of DBT therapists that is used to motivate and support therapists in implementing effective treatment. This is especially important considering that clinicians can easily become demoralized by feelings of anger, hopelessness, and burnout when treating patients who often have multiple high-risk behaviors and frequent episodes of relapse.

The individual sessions address specific problems, and focus on improving motivation to change. Sessions are structured according to a treatment hierarchy. In order of priority, the focus is on: 1) life-threatening behaviors (risk of harm to self or others); 2) treatment sabotage behaviors (including those of both patient and therapist); and 3) substance use and other behaviors that deeply compromise quality of life. If substance use behaviors involve life-threatening behaviors (e.g. intentionally injecting heroin with HIV-infected syringes), they are identified as such and take higher precedence. Substance abuse behaviors are further divided into behavioral elements capable of both attaining and achieving abstinence. These targets are organized by a "Path to Clear Mind" target hierarchy (McMain et al., 2007). In sequence, the "Path to Clear Mind" involves: 1) decreasing substance abuse, whether involving the use of illegal drugs, the abuse of legally prescribed drugs, or using legally prescribed drugs not as prescribed; 2) decreasing urges and cravings to use drugs; 3) decreasing "apparently irrelevant behaviors" (e.g. walking by a liquor store if alcohol is a problem, socializing with drug users or dealers, keeping drug paraphernalia); and 4) decreasing clients' decisions to keep "at least for now" options to use drugs open. (This "option" often involves lying about drug use; keeping drug dealers' phone numbers, and behavioral flirting with a lifestyle they are working hard to leave behind.)

The primary therapist oversees the care of the patient, including the development of an overall treatment plan that is guided by a case formulation. The therapist manages suicide risk, facilitates the generalization of skills, helps the patient stay motivated and engaged in treatment, and focuses on ensuring that the patient completes out-of-session homework assignments.

> Patients use daily diary cards to monitor all relevant functional and problematic behaviors, such as urges to use drugs, actual drug use, prescription drug use, over-the-counter drug use, impulses to self-injure, suicide urges, emotions, and urges to quit therapy. Diary cards are reviewed at the start of each session, and a session agenda is collaboratively developed to ensure that the most critical behaviors are addressed.

Determining the session focus is illustrated by the case of Marie. One week, Marie arrived to session without having completed her diary cards and after missing the previous session. The session began with the therapist asking her to complete her diary card based on whatever she could remember. There had been no life-interfering behaviors since the last session, so the next highest priority behaviors were targeted: her therapy-interfering behavior (i.e. her failure to complete diary cards, her missed sessions) and her extensive alcohol consumption. Marie was initially reluctant to address these behaviors, explaining that she did not have the money to get to the session…and had run out of diary cards. When she and her therapist analyzed the factors contributing to this behavior, it became apparent that Marie's heavy alcohol use was the main reason she lacked funds for transportation to sessions. Though Marie was ambivalent about abstaining from alcohol at treatment outset, drinking was now interfering with treatment. Confronting her with this increased her willingness to work on her alcohol problems.

Orientation to treatment and establishing treatment goals

Before the formal treatment process is initiated, patients undergo an orientation phase, typically conducted during the period of the initial four meetings, whose main goal is to enhance motivation. DBT's emphasis on establishing a clear treatment framework is characteristic of most treatment models for BPD.

During the orientation phase, tasks include clarifying expectations, discussing the task of therapy, establishing the treatment time frame, collaboratively identifying treatment goals, and obtaining an explicit commitment from the patient to engage in treatment. Patients are educated about the characteristics, etiology, and prognosis of BPD and its relationship to substance abuse. To counter negative expectations about change, they are informed that both BPD and SUDs are treatable disorders. Patients are taught that their problems are learned, and can be understood and changed through the principles of learning theory. Therapists stress that treatment engagement is critical to success. Information is provided to patients about the empirical base of DBT to educate them about its potential benefits and to counter feelings of discouragement and hopelessness. An essential aspect of orientation involves identifying specific treatment goals and obtaining the patient's commitment to address these goals. At a minimum, before treatment is initiated, patients must agree to eliminate life-threatening behaviors and to remain in treatment.

Although abstinence from substance abuse is not mandatory for treatment participation, a commitment to achieve it is sought. A premise of DBT-S is that patients with BPD need to abstain to achieve stability, as substance abuse contributes to emotional instability, behavioral dysregulation, crisis behavior, and pain. Individuals with BPD are even more vulnerable than most people to the effects of substance abuse owing to their emotional sensitivity. Many patients see a commitment to permanent abstinence as an impossible and unrealistic goal; these same feelings often discourage them from attempting to quit alcohol and drugs. Furthermore, slips or relapses are a normal part of the recovery process, but patients often feel defeated and demoralized when relapse does occur after they have committed to abstain. At these moments of failure, they are more likely to abandon their goal of abstinence. At times like these patients are encouraged to balance their focus on abstinence with an equally weighted focus on harm reduction. This synthesis, referred to as "dialectical abstinence," involves simultaneously focusing on abstinence and on minimizing damage if a slip or relapse occurs. Patients are encouraged to stop using substances; however, rather than ruling it out forever, they are encouraged to focus on more manageable periods of time, such as minutes, hours, or days. When patients commit to abstain, they are directed to turn their minds fully towards abstinence, and are helped to identify and problem-solve any obstacles to their sobriety. The cognitive strategy of mentally "closing the door" on substance abuse is balanced with a focus on helping patients skilfully manage slips and relapses so that total damage is minimized. This dual focus maximizes the benefits of abstinence approaches and relapse prevention, since the length between periods of use is increased during abstinence and the frequency and intensity of use are reduced when slips occur (McMain *et al.*, 2007).

The process of obtaining a commitment to abstain is illustrated in the case of Marie. During her orientation phase, Marie readily committed to abstaining from heroin use; however, she was at first extremely ambivalent about stopping drinking, insisting that she drank no more than anyone else and that her drinking was not a problem because she did not do it every day. The therapist remained non-judgmental, but provided her with information about recommended drinking guidelines in an effort to increase her motivation. At the same time, the therapist emphasized that Marie was free to choose her goals. It became evident that the primary obstacle to Marie agreeing to abstain was her fear of not being able to follow through on this commitment. For example, she did not believe that she could be sober for more than a couple of days before she would "lose it." She thought it would be easier for her to reduce her use. However, the therapist strongly advised against this, stating that alcohol dependence had likely altered her brain in ways that would make it impossible for her to drink in moderation. Marie eventually agreed to commit to staying sober, and she felt that her focus on only one period of time (at a time) made abstinence seem more in her reach. She defined a specific length of time during which she felt she could commit to abstinence with almost absolute certainty. Once the end of this time period was reached, she was advised to re-commit to a new period of sober time.

Attachment strategies

The treatment of concurrent BPD and SUDs is complicated by poor treatment retention rates. Treatment dropout rates for substance-abusing BPD patients are estimated to be as high as 73% (Linehan *et al.*, 1999). Substance abuse heightens chaos and impulsivity in BPD patients, and contributes to employment difficulties, financial problems, legal issues, inadequate housing, medical complications, sexual promiscuity,

and increased exposure to abusive environments. Linehan and Dimeff (1997) characterize patients with co-occurring BPD and SUDs as "butterflies" who drift in and out of treatment and frequently fail to form a strong attachment to the therapist and to treatment. It is important for therapists to appreciate that these patients may not be motivated to fully engage in treatment – interventions are needed to enhance compliance.

In DBT-S, several specific attachment strategies are used to address treatment compliance problems. For example, during the orientation phase, patients are educated about the "butterfly" phenomenon. By anticipating the nature of the attachment problem for a specific patient, the therapist can troubleshoot obstacles to treatment engagement. The therapist and patient actively collaborate to develop a crisis plan, identifying people that can be contacted if the patient gets "lost" from treatment. Extra contact with patients is encouraged early in treatment, to forge and maintain a strong therapeutic bond. In DBT, the development of a strong attachment to the therapist and treatment program is regarded as a critical component of effective treatment, and nurturing a strong therapy relationship is emphasized throughout the course of treatment. At times, therapists may need to utilize active outreach strategies (e.g. home visits, holding sessions outside the office) to engage patients who are at risk of premature dropout from treatment.

The case of Marie illustrates how the "butterfly" problem can be addressed. During orientation, Marie informed her therapist that she had prematurely terminated treatment on several previous occasions because she lost interest or because she didn't like the therapist. Her therapist oriented Marie to the consequences of a "butterfly" attachment style, and helped increase her motivation to address this problem. Together, they identified several ways to increase Marie's commitment to treatment. For example, Marie and her therapist identified possible warning signs of Marie's dissatisfaction and withdrawal (e.g. late arrival to session, lack of completion of homework, and lack of communication with the therapist). They also developed a crisis plan that included identification of people whom the therapist could contact to help locate Marie if she failed to show to sessions.

Skills training

Standard DBT skills training includes four modules, designed to address one or more of the problems that individuals with BPD experience. *Mindfulness skills* focus on the ability to develop awareness of the moment, to allow patients to gain greater control over their attentional processes. Mindfulness is a critical skill, because awareness is a prerequisite for making changes in one's behavior, thinking, and emotional experience. *Emotion regulation skills* focus on developing one's ability to name and regulate emotional experience. *Distress tolerance skills* focus on learning ways to navigate crises without making them worse, through specific activities such as distraction and acceptance of present situations. Finally, *interpersonal effectiveness skills* are designed to help individuals with BPD assert their needs without damaging relationships or self-worth.

DBT-S supplements the standard DBT skills training with three new mindfulness skills ("Clear Mind," "urge surfing," and "alternate rebellion"), and two new distress tolerance skills ("adaptive denial" and "burning bridges"), all of which serve to promote abstinence from drugs.

Standard DBT describes three states of mind: reasonable mind, emotion mind, and wise mind (Linehan, 1993a). "Reasonable mind" is characterized by logic devoid of the influence of emotion, while "emotion mind" is characterized by emotion without the benefit of logic. Individuals with BPD often spend much of their lives acting from emotion mind and/or alternating between emotion mind and reasonable mind. The dialectical synthesis of these opposing states is "wise mind;" wise minds can access both emotional experience and reason, and can acknowledge what feels "right" in the moment. Learning how to access wise mind is critical for individuals who wish to make skilful choices, such as choosing personal skills rather than psychotropic substances to cope with emotional pain. In DBT-S, the emphasis on attaining and maintaining sobriety is designed to help the patient attain "clear mind," which individuals with co-occurring BPD and SUDs need to enter before they can access wise mind. Clear mind, like wise mind, is a dialectical synthesis of two opposing states of mind – clean mind and addict mind (Linehan & Dimeff, 1997). Individuals enter treatment in "addict mind" where their actions are controlled by urges to use. Once they have initially achieved and maintained sobriety, they enter "clean mind," a state characterized by denial that they can succumb to drug use. This sense of invincibility leads them to disregard planning for relapse or/and to ignore signs of vulnerability to

relapse. In clear mind, patients appreciate their sobriety and recognize the need to work actively to maintain sobriety. "Urge surfing" is based on the concept that urges do not persist indefinitely; urges rise and they inevitably fall. Individuals are encouraged to "surf" or ride out the urge by simply observing it, knowing that the urge will eventually subside.

"Alternate rebellion" is based on the mindfulness "how" skill of being effective. Effectiveness emphasizes doing what works to achieve goals and to avoid making things worse. Alternate rebellion is an important strategy for patients who may rely on substance use as a way to rebel or to express their individuality. Specifically, this strategy encourages patients to identify effective ways of expressing their individuality without compromising their sobriety or other goals.

Within the distress tolerance module, "adaptive denial" is used to help patients avoid thinking about unbearable and distressing thoughts (e.g. "I can never use again") and persuading themselves that they are committed to adaptive behaviors that serve a similar (if not better) function. For example, individuals with SUDs often find the idea of never being able to drink or take drugs incredibly distressing. Using adaptive denial would include blocking out this fact, and helping oneself to tune the thought out by going to a movie rather than by using drugs. "Burning bridges" focuses on teaching patients to remove all access to drugs to increase the likelihood that they will remain abstinent when the urges inevitably arise.

These new mindfulness skills were particularly helpful for Marie. After she initially became sober, she dismissed the importance of remaining vigilant to signs of relapse. Only after cycling through sobriety and relapse several times more did she appreciate the importance of the continued effort needed to remain abstinent. She also mentioned that urge surfing allowed her to have the patience to wait for urges to subside. Marie was a self-described "rebel" whose substance use reflected her fierce individuality. Over time, she recognized that she could express her individuality through tattoos and piercings rather than through compromise of her sobriety. For "bridge burning," she deleted her dealer's phone numbers and stopped socializing at bars.

Case management

Individuals with co-occurring BPD and SUDs often experience difficulties with basic needs, including housing, employment, and food. DBT-S treatment emphasizes coaching patients to manage their own difficulties rather than having therapists or others intervene for them, as is common with other case management approaches. In contrast to viewing patients as fragile and incapable of solving their own life problems, DBT-S is grounded in the assumption that patients are capable of managing crises if the therapist provides coaching. Teaching crisis management is critically important: patients learn to use skills that can make the difference between sobriety and relapse when future crises occur. Finally, DBT-S therapists assume a more active role in providing case management if and when a patient cannot readily access these services in the community.

At the start of treatment, Marie was unemployed and was thousands of dollars in debt. The therapist coached her to meet with both an employment counselor and a debt manager. Ultimately, Marie was able to secure a position and negotiate a long-term solution for her debt. She reported feeling like "a real person" because she was able to address these seemingly impossible problems.

Pharmacotherapy

The vast majority of substance abusing patients with BPD use prescribed medications (Zanarini *et al.*, 2004); therefore, management of pharmacotherapeutic treatment is an additional important consideration. Because inadequate management and poor compliance with medication regimens can compromise treatment, it is helpful to include pharmacotherapists on DBT treatment consultation teams (Linehan & Dimeff, 1997) – particularly addiction psychiatrists or other physicians with expertise in the treatment of addictions and psychiatric disorders. Pharmacotherapists may prescribe, monitor, and taper patients from psychotropic medications as indicated; they may also oversee the medical aspects of addictive behaviors such as medically assisted detoxification and opioid substitution therapy. In contrast to some other addiction models, such as twelve-step approaches, DBT-S does not proscribe the use of medications, especially since there is some empirical evidence supporting the pharmacological treatment of BPD (Bellino *et al.*, 2008). However, DBT emphasizes a "skills for pills" approach that focuses on overall reduction of medication as an important treatment goal, especially for patients whose use of medications

(e.g. benzodiazepines) is problematic. Pharmacotherapists can reinforce patients' use of skills rather than pills when appropriate. In sum, the participation of a pharmacotherapist on the treatment team can help to ensure better treatment coordination and continuity of care.

Empirical support for DBT-S

DBT-S has received more attention in the empirical literature than any other approach for the treatment of comorbid BPD and SUDs. Four randomized controlled trials have evaluated its clinical effectiveness. The first study evaluated the effectiveness of a 1-year trial of DBT-S for the treatment of BPD and substance dependence. Results showed that, compared to a treatment-as-usual condition, participants receiving DBT-S had greater reductions in drug use and better treatment retention rates (Linehan *et al.*, 1999). Another study (Linehan *et al.*, 2002) found that opiate-dependent women with BPD who received 1 year of DBT-S had significantly greater reductions in drug use over the course of treatment than did those receiving comprehensive validation therapy (CVT) and attending twelve-step meetings. At 1-year follow-up, only the DBT-S group maintained their gains, whereas the CVT group increased their drug use. Despite DBT's superiority on drug use outcomes, participants in the CVT had better rates of treatment retention. Results from the other two studies (McMain *et al.*, 2004; Verheul *et al.*, 2003) also support the use of DBT for BPD/SUDs.

There have been no clinical trials evaluating the use of DBT-S for individuals with a diagnosis of SUD only, i.e. without BPD. Although many patients may benefit from its therapeutic components, several factors should be considered when applying DBT-S to such individuals (McMain *et al.*, 2007). Several patient characteristics would support its use: 1) the substance abuse is related to emotional dysregulation (not the case for all individuals with SUDs); 2) the patients meet criteria for other Axis I and II disorders, i.e. have complex diagnostic presentations; and 3) the patients have repeated unsuccessful prior treatment episodes. However, in the absence of specific psychosocial supports, such treatment may be unwarranted as a first-line intervention. DBT-S is designed to treat the severe behavior dyscontrol associated with BPD/SUDs, and some individuals with SUDs alone can benefit from existing interventions without requiring such comprehensive treatment.

Training

Specialized training is required to implement DBT effectively. Training courses in DBT are widely available in many countries (e.g. US, Canada, England, and Germany). Currently the most extensive array is offered by the Behavioral Technology Company based in Seattle. Most courses focus on the development of conceptualization and interventional skills sophisticated enough to address the treatment of multi-disordered patients. Trainees learn the following:

- How to view patients with co-occurring BPD and SUDs through a non-pejorative lens. DBT's biosocial theory helps to explain how psychopathology develops and is maintained.
- How to structure treatment competently; how to use DBT's target hierarchy to prioritize treatment and session targets; and how to make optimal use of concrete intervention strategies.
- How to apply learning theory to help patients modify their behaviors (through the principles of learning). For example, clinicians are instructed in the use of therapeutic tools such as behavioral analysis, exposure, problem definition, contingency management, reinforcement, and behavioral monitoring.
- How to validate and communicate acceptance. Many clinicians enter training assuming that validation merely involves expressions of warmth and support, a perspective reinforced by counseling training programs. While validation can involve this stance, it does not require it. Clinicians are taught to be empathic while helping their patients make sense of their own behaviors. They learn that validation involves being radically genuine, engaging in the therapy relationship in an authentic and direct manner, using a style that neither condescends nor makes the patient feel even more fragile. For example, openly disclosing feelings of frustration or disappointment is a means of supporting the patient's ability to tolerate feedback.
- To master the flexible and strategic use of interventions, and to achieve a dialectical balance between acceptance and change strategies.

Ultimately, training in conceptualization and intervention increases clinicians' confidence and skill in managing patients who present with multiple problems. It remains to be established how much training is necessary to apply DBT-S effectively. Based on our experience, a solid background in cognitive behavioral approaches and personal flexibility are assets to learning this approach.

Summary

DBT-S is a therapeutic modality that has been designed to treat the specific issues common to individuals with co-occurring BPD/SUDs, including emotional and behavioral dyscontrol, multiple concurrent psychiatric disorders, and treatment-resistant behaviors. Although it has not been evaluated for the treatment of patients without comorbid substance use disorders, it may be a promising treatment option for individuals whose substance abuse is linked to emotion dysregulation and/or those for whom other treatment programs have not been effective.

References

Alcoholics Anonymous. (1981). *Twelve Steps and Twelve Traditions*. New York: Alcoholics Anonymous World Services.

Battle, C., Shea, T., Johnson, D. *et al.* (2004). Childhood maltreatment associated with adult personality disorders: findings from the collaborative longitudinal personality disorders study. *Journal of Personality Disorders*, **18**, 193–211.

Bellino, S., Paradiso, E. & Bogetto, F. (2008). Efficacy and tolerability of pharmacotherapies for borderline personality disorder. *CNS Drugs*, **22**, 671–92.

Brooner, R. K., King, V. L., Kidorf, M. *et al.* (1997). Psychiatric and substance use comorbidity among treatment-seeking opioid abusers. *Archives of General Psychiatry*, **54**, 71–80.

Darke, S., Williamson, A., Ross, J., Teesson, M. &Lynskey, M. (2004). Borderline personality disorder, antisocial personality disorder and risk-taking among heroin users: findings from the Australian Treatment Outcome Study (ATOS). *Drug and Alcohol Dependence*, **74**, 77–83.

Dimeff, L. A. & Koerner, K. (2007). *Dialectical Behaviour Therapy in Clinical Practice*. New York: Guilford Press.

Elkins, I. J., King, S. M., McGue, M. & Iacono, W. G. (2006). Personality traits and the development of nicotine, alcohol, and illicit drug disorders: prospective links from adolescence to young adulthood. *Journal of Abnormal Psychology*, **115**, 26–39.

Fals-Stewart, W., O'Farrell, T. & Hooley, J. (2001). Relapse among married or cohabitating substance-abusing patients: the role of perceived criticism. *Behaviour Therapy*, **32**, 787–801.

Inman, D. J., Bascue, L. O. & Skoloda, T. (1985). Identification of borderline personality disorder among substance abuse inpatients. *Journal of Substance Abuse Treatment*, **2**, 229–32.

Jackson, K. & Sher, K. (2003). Alcohol use disorders and psychological distress: a prospective state–trait analysis. *Journal of Abnormal Psychology*, **112**, 599–613.

Johnson, J. G., Cohen, P., Gould, M. *et al.* (2002). Childhood adversities, interpersonal difficulties, and risk for suicide attempts during later adolescence and early adulthood. *Archives of General Psychiatry*, **59**, 741–9.

Kosten, T. A., Kosten, T. R. & Rounsaville, B. J. (1989). Personality disorders in opiate addicts show prognostic specificity. *Journal of Substance Abuse Treatment*, **6**, 163–8.

Linehan, M. M. (1993a). Dialectical behavior therapy for the treatment of borderline personality disorder: implications for the treatment of substance abuse. In: *Research Monograph Series: Behaviour Treatments for Drug Abuse and Dependence*, L. Onken, J. Blaine & J. Boren. eds. Rockville, MD: National Institute of Health, 201–15.

Linehan, M. M. (1993b). *Cognitive Behavioural Treatment of Borderline Personality Disorder.* New York: Guilford Press.

Linehan, M. M. & Dimeff, L. A. (1997). *Dialectical Behavior Therapy Manual of Treatment Interventions for Drug Abusers with Borderline Personality Disorder.* Seattle, WA: University of Washington (unpublished work).

Linehan, M. M., Schmidt, H., Dimeff, L. A. *et al.* (1999). Dialectical behavior therapy for patients with borderline personality disorder and drug-dependence. *American Journal on Addictions*, **8**, 279–92.

Linehan, M. M., Dimeff, L. A., Reynolds, S. K. *et al.* (2002). Dialectical behavior therapy versus comprehensive validation therapy plus 12-step for the treatment of opioid dependent women meeting criteria for borderline personality disorder. *Drug & Alcohol Dependence*, **67**, 13–26.

Links, P. S., Heslegrave, R. J., Ronald, J. *et al.* (1995). Borderline personality disorder and substance abuse: consequences of comorbidity. *Canadian Journal of Psychiatry*, **40**, 9–14.

Marlatt, G. A. & Donovan, D. M. (2005). *Relapse Prevention: Maintenance Strategies in the Treatment of Addictive Behaviors*, 2nd edn. New York: Guilford Press.

McMain, S., Korman, L., Blak, T. *et al.* (2004). *Dialectical Behaviour Therapy for Substance Users with Borderline Personality Disorder: A Randomized Controlled Trial in Canada.* New Orleans: Association for the Advancement of Behavior Therapy Annual Meeting.

McMain, S., Sayrs, J., Dimeff, L. & Linehan, M. (2007). *Dialectical Behavior Therapy for Individuals with BPD and Substance Dependence.* New York: Guilford Press.

Miller, W. R. & Rollnick, S. (2002). *Motivational Interviewing: Preparing People for Change*, 2nd edn. New York: Guilford Press.

Miller, F. T., Abrams, T., Dulit, R. & Minna, F. (1993). Substance abuse in borderline personality disorder. *American Journal of Drug and Alcohol Abuse*, **19**, 491–7.

Nace, E. P. & Davis, C. W. (1993). Treatment outcome in substance-abusing patients with a personality disorder. *The American Journal on Addictions*, **2**, 26–33.

Nace, E. P., Davis, C. W. & Gaspari, J. P. (1991). Axis II comorbidity in substance abusers. *American Journal of Psychiatry*, **148**, 120.

O'Farrell, T., Hooley, J., Fals-Stewart, W. & Cutter, H. (1998). Expressed emotion and relapse in alcoholic patients. *Journal of Consulting & Clinical Psychology*, **66**, 744–52.

Paris, J. (1997). Antisocial and borderline personality disorders: two separate diagnoses or two aspects of the same psychopathology? *Comprehensive Psychiatry*, **38**, 237–42.

Skodol, A. E., Oldham, J. M. & Gallaher, P. E. (1999). Axis II. Comorbidity of substance use disorders among patients referred for treatment of personality disorders. *American Journal of Psychiatry*, **156**, 733–8.

Stiglmayr, C., Grathwol, T., Linehan, M. *et al.* (2005). Aversive tension in patients with borderline personality disorder: a computer-based field study. *Acta Psychiatrica Scandinavica*, **111**, 372–9.

Stone, M. H., Hurt, W. S. & Stone, D. K. (1987). The PI 500: long-term follow-up of borderline inpatients meeting DSM-III criteria. I. Global outcome. *Journal of Personality Disorders*, **1**, 291–8.

Trull, T. T., Sher, K. J., Minks-Brown, C., Durbin, J. & Burr, R. (2000). Borderline personality disorder and substance use disorders: a review and integration. *Clinical Psychology Review*, **20**, 235–53.

van den Bosch, L. M. C., Verheul, R. & van den Brink, W. (2001). Substance abuse in borderline personality disorder: clinical and etiological correlates. *Journal of Personality Disorders*, **15**, 416–24.

Verheul, R., van den Bosch, L. M. C., Koeter, M. W. J. *et al.* (2003). Dialectical behaviour therapy for women with borderline personality disorder: 12-month, randomised clinical trial in The Netherlands. *British Journal of Psychiatry*, **182**, 135–40.

Wedig, M. & Nock, M. (2007). Parental expressed emotion and adolescent self-injury. *Journal of the American Academy of Child and Adolescent Psychiatry*, **46**, 1171–8.

Zanarini, M. C., Frankenburg, F. R., Hennen, J., Reich, D. B. & Silk, K. R. (2004). Axis I comorbidity in patients with borderline personality disorder: 6-year follow-up and prediction of time to remission. *American Journal of Psychiatry*, **161**, 2108–14.

Addiction and emergency psychiatry

Richard Gallagher, Gregory Fernandez & Edward Lulo

The common prevalence of alcoholism and other substance-related addictive disorders, with their secondary medical consequences, warrants their characterization as the chief public health problem in our country. An obvious corollary is the great extent to which hospital and clinic settings must deal with such cases on a daily basis. Nowhere is the magnitude of this task more pressing than in our hospital emergency rooms (ER).

Medical emergency departments (EDs) are now the first choice option for acute, new onset patients and the last resort, as well, for any "medically unstable" individuals. This term is an elastic one, given the paucity of other practical options in our burdened healthcare system.

Emergency facilities are, moreover, the only medical settings mandated by law to treat all comers. The onus on emergency services is receiving increasing attention at a time when healthcare policy and economics are back in the forefront of the American political debate. A recent report by the American College of Emergency Physicians in Chicago highlighted the serious issue of overcrowding in EDs throughout the nation (Viccellio, 2008). In this climate, emergency services are challenged to deal swiftly and knowledgeably with the wide range of difficulties presented by the enormous population of substance abusers.

General statistics of emergency care and substance-abusing patients

Emergency departments carry a massive burden of caring for acute patients and in recent years many who are chronically ill as well. In the year 2005, 115.3 million people visited EDs in the US, an increase of about 20 million from 10 years earlier (Nawar et al., 2007). Despite the common utilization of EDs by the indigent for more chronic conditions, rates of admission from emergency services are rising, a clear indication of the serious, not trivial, nature of these presentations.

"Throughput" time is also increasing; the average wait time in one state system has risen to 163 minutes in a recent year, 5.4% higher than 2 years earlier (Illinois Hospital Association, 2005). Because of the expense and regulatory demands to treat a broader range of problems with the most up-to-date equipment and methodology, during this same interval the number of certified emergency departments has actually decreased from 4176 to 3795 (Nawar et al., 2007). EDs face pressure to treat more and sicker patients in less time, and so it is increasingly problematic to include in work-ups careful alcohol and substance abuse, as well as psychiatric, histories.

Data on the number of patients seen in medical EDs without appreciation of the extent of such concomitant disorders are hard to come by, but it is estimated that patients discharged without a full accounting of their substance abuse represent a significant percentage of the total. Our own freestanding psychiatric ED (which works closely with our medical ER, vide infra), together with our crisis team, treats approximately 6000 cases per year. Nearly 30% have active substance abuse problems and another 18% report past misuse. These findings are only elicited by skilled history-taking. Recognizing the complexity of extrapolating statistics from one hospital to another and being cautious about over-generalization on the basis of a population screened for psychiatric issues, we, nevertheless, believe such high rates of substance abuse in an ER setting reflect the magnitude of the national problem. Emergency services that do not inquire carefully and routinely of these histories are clearly missing the bulk of such cases. One may compare rates of substance abuse diagnosed in ERs with rates in the general population. Statistics purporting to show lower rates of substance abuse diagnoses in some ER settings in comparison to accepted, substantial rates in epidemiologic samples, suggest strongly that estimates are often grossly under-reported in many official surveys of ED patients.

Integrated emergency services: ideal organization and otherwise

Notwithstanding pressures to reduce waiting time, an ideal emergency service should be able to manage with expertise psychiatric patients, substance abusing ones, and the combination. Patients with co-occurring substance abuse and psychiatric disorders are common (Substance Abuse and Mental Health Services Administration, 2002). The dually diagnosed in particular have been shown to have significantly higher rates of ER utilization (Curran *et al.*, 2008).

Proper management of these cases in ERs ultimately results in cost savings, it has been argued (Curran *et al.*, 2008). Sensible planning is key. Emergency medical and psychiatric services are organized in one of two ways. The more standard emergency room facility involves a combined medical and psychiatric emergency area where patients are evaluated in the same general space within a single hospital building. This arrangement has the advantage of concentrating resources within a limited amount of space. It ensures rapid communication and quick transfer of individuals among the different "medical services" in charge of the patients' respective problems. The drawbacks frequently involve overcrowding, "turf issues," and serious time demands.

Typical dilemmas arise: who sees the patient first or who is required to see the patient at all? How much time can be devoted to discussing at length and in depth the patients' full histories, most especially a careful probe of the use of alcohol or other drugs? (This need is especially important with a busy service precisely when the history of such use is not immediately obvious or initially minimized or denied; both scenarios are more the rule than the exception.) Other questions follow: whose service and management needs are prioritized as the case unfolds? If a patient is waiting for a surgical or other complex consultation, who decides when to interrupt or whether to call a "substance abuse" consult at all? How long does one wait for the consultation? Who deals with the inevitable, complex, "disposition" problems, with the constant, perceived need to have patients exit from busy ERs as expeditiously as possible?

With sensible organization and good faith on the part of staff, ERs may find practical and sensibly routinized ways to deal with conflicting agendas. Many emergency settings, however, face considerable turmoil and staff tensions over such concerns. There must

be clear expectations and guidelines as to the disciplines chiefly responsible for the heterogeneous patients and the prioritizing of the multiple evaluations. Frequently, clinicians who deal with even a major substance abuse problem feel rushed or treated as "second class" staff in a busy, single emergency room.

We think it preferable to have a separate, freestanding psychiatric (and substance abuse) emergency service, when feasible. This method of care is not inexpensive, but is of great appeal to more strictly medical ERs for its assistance to their overall burden. This setting should be assigned the primary responsibility for both psychiatric and substance abusing patients and the "dually diagnosed." This "psych. ER" is optimally part of a larger hospital campus with its own, physically separate, medical/surgical emergency room. Such is our experience, for instance, at the Westchester Medical Center in the northern suburbs of metropolitan New York City.

The Westchester Medical Center is affiliated with a major academic training program at the New York Medical College. It has a separate emergency facility for psychiatric and substance abuse evaluations in a building detached from the main hospital. The medical center also encompasses a broad range of other services, including outpatient clinics and a 700-bed acute general hospital. The psychiatric facility on campus (known as the Behavioral Health Center – hereafter BHC) has around 100 psychiatric beds. The ED at BHC serves as its own admission service, obviating duplication, conflicts, and the expense of a separate admission department. Good communication and cooperation between the non-contiguous "medical ER" and the "psych. ER" are critical and not without potential conflicts. The physical separateness of the services, however, allows each its own pace, routine, and comfort level. Each is responsible for the patients their respective staff is most experienced in handling.

This arrangement allows the work to proceed at its own speed without concern for the medical clearance, which is completed before the patient is sent to the BHC. The service can concentrate on developing a staff highly knowledgeable in this specialized area and aware of disposition options and interim solutions to these vexing concerns. Ideally the service should have close ties to a full range of psychiatric inpatient beds, detoxification facilities, rehab services, outpatient resources of all varieties, and a reasonably functioning shelter or "respite" system. Ongoing networking with area services allows an ER to control its critical "back door."

An ideal psychiatric ER must exist within a supportive, overall treatment system aimed at disposing of patients with a minimum of bottlenecks. All care systems struggle at times for resources and aftercare options. It is important, however, that local planners and responsible government agencies adequately fund emergency resources, including ensuring suitable dispositions from our overcrowded system.

Another argument for conducting substance abuse evaluations within a separate, psychiatric, ER is the need for maximal experience with behaviorally out of control and otherwise disruptive patients. Medical ERs may have this ability, too. Nevertheless, a distinct area set aside for these inevitable tasks is preferable. Staff in psych. ERs are accustomed to handling psychotic and otherwise highly agitated individuals and so bring a level of confidence and efficiency to this task seldom found in non-psychiatric personnel. (Psychiatric or other specially trained staff may, of course, be "on call" to a medical ER.) Space considerations are sometimes involved. Space in standard ERs is often at a premium. Even with recent expansions – not infrequent in the past few years, given present needs – the general workload and updated equipment seem always to fill the additional space. While psychiatric settings may become overcrowded, too, primary consideration has usually been paid to ensuring room for control procedures as well as the expertise in monitoring agitated patients and their subsequent placement. Medical ERs often find such clinical situations taxing and annoying; there is often expressed concern from medical personnel that the patient will perturb other patients or their families. There may be a consequent rush to refer such patients precipitously or to make hasty dispositions before options have been fully explored. (Some medical ERs have separate areas designated for emergency placement of the acutely out-of-control individual; our experience suggests this arrangement is workable, but still less than ideal.)

EDs often differ widely, as well, in the length of stay permitted. It is desirable to have "crisis beds" located directly in the ER. At the BHC these are called "EOB" (for "emergency observation beds") and our local laws allow us to house patients for up to 72 hours, involuntarily if need be. These beds are invaluable in allowing completion of sometimes complex assessments and mobilization of outside help. They assure at least brief continuity of care for those patients in need. As required by state law, the modal patient is the dually diagnosed, although it is fair to note that most acutely unstable substance abusers have an acute, psychological impairment, if only in the nature of an "adjustment disorder."

Collaboration with a community psychiatric outreach service is also preferable. Mobile services were cited in a recent task force on emergency care to represent the ideal in titrating admissions and promoting utilization of services to the most available facilities. In Westchester and in New York State generally, geographical locales ("catchment" areas) are served by a government subsidized "mobile crisis team," part of an integrated "CPEP" or "comprehensive psychiatric emergency program." This collaboration allows emergency services critical control of their "front door," too. The outreach team can visit appropriate cases in the community or deal with an immediate crisis via telephone. We foster close working relationships with the local police departments, who highly value such assistance with their frequent substance abusing "EDPs" (the police term for behaviorally problematic and often substance abusing "emotionally disturbed persons"). We keep daily records of services available throughout the county and can shuttle patients to available facilities without overloading any one ER.

Systems of care around the world, of course, may lack the resources or organization to implement an ideal flow of patient care to appropriate assessment centers and on to suitable follow-up facilities. Promotion of such systems when the economic or political climate allows is important. Knowing the "ideal" always makes planning easier, even if compromises are inevitable. Private facilities are often accessible by the more affluent. A public safety net, nevertheless, often proves life-saving for all, regardless of socioeconomic status, and is especially critical to the indigent.

These preconditions have been treated at length in recognition of the chief obstacle to quality ED care, as almost universally noted in various surveys, i.e. care that is overly rushed. Position papers for emergency services of late have questioned whether waiting for urine toxicology screens is even practical nowadays. Generally, ED staffs are capable and caring, but few ER directors disagree that excessive demands and time issues frequently make the delivery of service less than optimal. Secondary medical problems can sometimes be missed when the focus is on the life-threatening ones. The same may be said a fortiori of substance abuse and psychiatric assessments in general in emergency settings. Frequently ERs are pressed even to complete suicidal evaluations, with the recent result that US regulatory agencies have had to mandate them as an ER priority. Substance abuse, either alone or complicating psychiatric conditions, increase rates of self-destructiveness greatly. It is fair to say that it is the single major risk factor accompanying dysphoric states of mind. Careful retrospective reviews of emergency cases with poor and sometimes tragic outcomes confirm that improved care required more time latitude. A recent survey at New York University showed conclusively that those who leave emergency rooms prior to completing a satisfactory evaluation are at high risk for subsequent worsening of their clinical condition and overt self-harm (American Psychiatry News, 2008).

Steps of emergency care

It cannot be emphasized too strongly that sufficient resources and time empower the ED staff for the work of which they are well capable, but often find impractical in real world settings. The next need is to ensure procedures for the actual care itself. It is useful to divide ER interventions into a diagnostic/assessment and acute response phase and into a "general" treatment recommendation stage, although these twin tasks are generally intertwined.

Assessment/acute treatment response

Because of the complexity, heterogeneity, and acuity of cases involving substance abusers in EDs, care of such individuals often proves challenging to ED staffs from a technical point of view. The initial inquiry should encompass all drugs taken, illicit and licit, to include tobacco, caffeine, and herbal medication. Patients should be quizzed about what is "in their medicine cabinet," and what they take to alleviate pain, help with tension or sleep, or enhance their mood.

Frequently, ERs, almost as a matter of course, attempt to shorten the process of their evaluations, once alcohol or drug use is suspected as the primary problem. We advise caution in this regard. Even with patients well known to the emergency service (the "frequent fliers," in ER parlance), careful, standard work-ups are generally indicated. Short-cuts should be avoided. Despite the initial impressions of staff, underlying medical or psychiatric issues may be emerging. Given unhealthy and destructive lifestyles,

patients are prone to new onset medical issues, even if previously in reasonable physical health.

The medical work-up should include all standard exams and laboratory tests. A thorough physical exam should encompass an especially careful assessment of the liver, nose, heart, and dermatological abnormalities (e.g. scars, bruises, needle tracks). This exam should be combined with a good neurological screening assessment and a full mental status exam. Laboratory testing should include a CBC and basic metabolic panel (with liver function tests), and should be alert for the abnormalities found most frequently in alcoholic or substance abusing individuals. We order EKGs, Rapid Plasma Reagin (a test for syphilis), amylase, hepatitis antigens (at least HepB surface Ag), blood iron, B-12, and confidential HIV testing, when indicated. These patients are often depressed secondary to acute or chronic substance abuse. We generally order a TSH and further thyroid testing, as needed. For individuals whose physical health is seriously impaired by their drug use and/or whose mental alertness is acutely compromised, more specialized testing such as X-rays, PPD (Purified Protein Derivative for TB screening), and neuroimaging studies, may be ordered. All patients receive a urine toxicology screen and occasional blood toxicology for suspected, unusual ingestions. While not all substance abuse is routinely picked up on either testing (*vide infra*), screening often prompts the patient to admit substance abuse issues otherwise not disclosed. Strong resistance to urine testing is almost pathognomonic of substance abuse.

With addicted patients, special skill and patience is often required to sort out neurological from psychiatric deficits, especially if the patient is intoxicated or in withdrawal. The latter states may be surprisingly prolonged, especially with sedative hypnotic abuse (and particularly the longer acting diazepam or clonazepam). A few individuals each year present to our ED as diagnostic dilemmas and are found to have late onset or unusually prolonged benzodiazepine withdrawal. Similarly complicated to assess are patients with pre-existing cognitive limitations, including the traumatic brain-injured, the developmentally disabled, and the elderly. Those with highly prolonged abuse histories, especially of alcohol, frequently need a CT scan or MRI. Ready consultation by neurology may be indicated in many of these cases.

Caution should be given to interpretation of the laboratory and toxicology results. Urine and blood tests are accurate and available only for certain ingested substances. False negatives are the primary concern in ERs. Emergency services must also be aware of the potential for false positives. Non-steroidal anti-inflammatory drugs, such as ibuprofen and naprosyn, for instance, can result in a positive identification for cannabis.

Marijuana itself is rarely a primary concern in emergency evaluations but is appropriately screened routinely. More often marijuana use accompanies other acute substance abuse ER presentations. Without adopting an alarmist tone with those experimenting with marijuana or those who smoke it intermittently, we, nevertheless, warn ER patients of its illegal and "gateway" status and do not minimize its longer term risks. With more chronic users we emphasize the potential for multiple target organ damage – especially to the lungs, reproductive system, and the brain. We point out the frequency with which we see memory difficulties and development of an amotivational inclination with long-term use.

Far more problematic to ERs are abusers of alcohol, by a large margin the most common substance use population seen in our emergency facilities. If ethanol is suspected or reported, a breathalyzer can be confirmatory; we screen all patients routinely with this device. Figures in themselves are estimates; individual tolerance varies so considerably that the actual figure may be less important than the clinical state. Without constant recalibration, moreover, breathalyzers are often set too high or too low and much of the final reading depends on the depth of inspiration. It has been demonstrated that breath tests generally report lower figures than blood samples (Currier *et al.*, 2006).

Routines of ER care for alcoholics should include orders for folate, vitamins, and thiamine. The recommended dose of folic acid is 1 mg to aid in reversal of polyneuropathy and to prevent thrombocytopenia. Multivitamins (with folic acid often included) are indicated given the frequent overall poor nutrition of alcoholics. Thiamine 100 mg IM qd for 3 days followed by 100 mg PO qd is most advisable; the benefits of thiamine administration far outweigh the potentially dire consequences of delayed therapy. In more severe cases, maintenance of fluid and electrolyte imbalance may be indicated, since these patients are susceptible to low levels of potassium, glucose, and magnesium. Fluid losses are not uncommon from the tendency to vomit and, in cases of more serious withdrawal, from fever or diaphoresis.

Many ERs, especially those with training programs, employ fixed assessment and treatment protocols, although we prefer to rely on the general experience of our staff and highly individualize our interviews and treatments. Many ERs have taught residents and medical students to utilize the CAGE sequence of questions. These are: A) "Has anyone suggested that you **c**ut down your use of alcohol?" B) "Have others been **a**nnoyed by your drinking?" C) "Do you feel **g**uilty about your intake?" D) "Do you need an "**e**ye-opener" of alcohol in the morning?"

Similarly, some ERs employ fixed withdrawal protocols, such as the Clinical Institute Withdrawal Assessment (CIWA). This excellent instrument measures ten categories of symptoms with a range of scores in each. The categories are: agitation, anxiety, auditory disturbances, clouding of sensorium, headache, nausea or vomiting, paroxysmal sweats, tactile disturbance, tremor, and visual disturbances. Such a scale is particularly useful for incipient delirium tremens, but we find it cumbersome to use routinely and here again we individualize extensively. Vital signs are the guide. Caution is advised with the standard use of chlordiazepoxide (Librium) for withdrawal in alcoholics with severe liver damage. In these patients, we substitute equivalent dosing of lorazepam (Ativan) owing to less interference with metabolism.

For the agitated intoxicated patient, haloperidol may be indicated, but all antipsychotics lower the seizure threshold and should be avoided when possible. Chlorpromazine, less often prescribed in recent years in any case, should definitely not be utilized because of its stronger seizure-inducing proclivity. If necessary, benzodiazepines may paradoxically be helpful despite prolonging the period of intoxication. Some centers prefer oxazepam as an intermediate acting tranquilizer with a record of efficacy.

General principles for assessing and treating benzodiazepine and other sedative hypnotic misuse are similar. Broad samples of benzodiazepine levels are generally screened in almost all EDs, but levels of lorazepam and clonazepam, frequently abused minor tranquilizer/anxiolytics, are often undetected. These drugs are all cross-tolerant with alcohol, so withdrawal protocols, often started (if not completed) in ERs, are similar. The public and some staff may be unaware that the more selective hypnotics, which cause subunit modulation of the GABA A-receptor complex, are also potentially addictive. Patients on these medications, such as zolpidem (Ambien) and zaleplon (Sonata), may come into the ER in withdrawal without awareness of the cause. Patients on these drugs may also present to the ER with transient confusion and other acute abnormalities, such as sleepwalking or erratic behavior. It is unclear, however, if this reaction is in any way peculiar to these newer hypnotics or truly dissimilar to that potentially caused by the standard benzodiazepines. Certainly we have seen similar responses to alprazalom and the rapidly absorbed diazepam. Withdrawal from all these drugs, especially longer acting ones like clonazepam, are often less severe than from heavy use of alcohol or barbiturates, but can also lead to seizures if the use or misuse has been long-standing and then interrupted precipitously.

Barbiturate abuse has dramatically decreased in recent years as this class of drug has declined in use. Risks in overdose and in withdrawal can be quite serious and even life-threatening, so a level of suspicion about barbiturates should continue. As with all sedative hypnotics, patients may attempt to use ERs to gain access to scripts for these medications. The substitution of other sedative hypnotics for these drugs is sound practice and very rarely should a patient be prescribed barbiturates in an ER. The most common avenue for their misuse is in compounds for pain management, such as Fioricet.

Much more frequent in today's drug culture is abuse of amphetamine-type compounds. ERs should be alert to the frequent false positives which show up as "amphetamine" abuse on screening panels. Commonly employed stimulants for attention deficit disorder and cold remedies like ephedrine can mislead. Consideration in the ER when the widely abused methamphetamine is suspected include cardiac screening as the drug is associated with QTc prolongation. Methamphetamine is more cardiotoxic than cocaine and can lead to valvular disease, cardiomyopathy, various arrhythmias, and sudden cardiac death. Medical clearance is warranted in all cases of suspected abuse. Also quite commonly presenting to ERs are those who abuse narcotics. Medical clearance is critical; sometimes these patients deteriorate quickly after being brought to the ER as their respiratory depression worsens. Skilled use of naloxone (Narcan) may be critical. Withdrawals are painful, although less dangerous than with the sedative hypnotics. In our experience patients often complain of withdrawal with clonidine, compared to use of narcotic equivalents. We remain open, however, to various approaches, including tapers with clonidine; we attempt to work with the individual, but,

again, emphasize use of the vital signs rather than the subjective experience of the patient. We make it a rule to check with methadone programs for the dosages used for their clients. We have noted a trend upward in that direction and generally cut down the total dose at least partially in the ER before full planning proceeds, with alternative options considered in consultation with outside agencies or treaters. Use of buprenorphine has changed the pattern of treatment for many patients in the last few years. At least on our service we see fewer patients with chronic narcotic abuse, but, as in all ERs, acute overdoses and new onset addictions are not unusual.

Most problematic diagnostically to ERs are those drugs new enough to be rarely suspected by, or unknown to, clinicians and/or those not picked up via our more routine lab tests. For instance, dextromethorphan (DMX), widely abused by teens because of its availability in households as a cough suppressant, is generally not screened. Yet a local survey in our county found that 5–9% of middle schoolers had tried cough syrups (what is known as "Robotripping") or cold medication to get high. DXM itself at the high doses often ingested can result in vomiting, elevated blood pressure, fainting, seizures, coma, and even death.

Similarly unavailable to labs are most of the so-called "club drugs," around for some time but not on lab panels, including Ecstasy (MDMA), GHB (gamma hydroxybutyrate), Special K (ketamine), Rohypnol (flunitrazepam) and the diverse group of hallucinogens. Although they differ in mechanism of action and subjective effects, they share a few commonalities from the ER standpoint. The club/disco/rave culture is associated with particularly high prevalence rates for these drugs, so they should be strongly suspected in those drawn to that milieu.

Some of these "club" compounds are highly adulterated; for instance, what is locally sold as "Ecstasy" may contain no MDMA at all and this variant is frequently associated with hyperthermia in initial clinical presentation. The unique activity in the central nervous system (CNS) of MDMA itself bridges the effects of both stimulants and hallucinogens. The acute intoxication state is notable for sympathomimetic effects, including tachycardia, hyperthermia, diaphoresis, and hypertension. Benzodiazepines are generally considered first-line ER treatment for sedative purposes and will often indirectly treat tachycardia and hypertension. In the treatment of MDMA-induced hypertension, pure beta-blocking antihypertensives are contraindicated as the direct catecholamine effects of MDMA lead to unopposed alpha receptor stimulation, which in turn worsens hypertension; mixed alpha/beta-blocking drugs (e.g. labetalol) are indicated instead.

GHB is an endogenously produced metabolite of GABA, though recreational doses produce concentrations thousands of times larger than those that the body produces. It is legally used for treatment of cataplexy in narcoleptics. In addition to its euphoric and sedative effects, intoxication can cause anterograde amnesia. It is widely known as a "date rape" drug; ER inquiry should include the possibility of rape or unsafe sexual practices. There is a narrow margin between euphoric doses and toxic doses, and the ER presentation is often one of CNS depression or coma, with bradycardia, hypotension, and respiratory depression. Treatment is largely supportive. Flumazenil has been shown to be ineffective in reversing effects. GHB intoxication/overdose should be suspected in cases with this presentation if standard toxicology screens are negative. It should also be suspected when a patient displays a sudden change from a comatose state to that of a normal or hyperactive psychomotor arousal.

Treatment of ketamine and of PCP, with abuse of the latter somewhat rarer in our ER in recent years, is similar. Both drugs were developed as dissociative anesthetics, but were found to have psychotomimetic effects. There is an association of ketamine with unsafe sexual behavior in gay/bisexual populations presenting to emergency services. More generally, ER management is supportive. In addition to symptoms of psychosis, intoxication is associated with cardiac and respiratory effects, hypertension, hyperthermia, and seizures. Benzodiazepines are therefore first-line treatment for sedative and antiepileptic effects. Antipsychotics may be necessary to control psychotic symptoms but also have the potential to provoke seizures with these drugs and to worsen hyperthermia. Non-pharmacologic "control procedures" (*vide infra*) may become necessary.

Rohypnol (flunitrazepam) is made in Switzerland and is illegal in the US. Essentially, it is the most potent of the benzodiazepines, estimated to be up to 10 times as potent as diazepam. It is abused recreationally for its sedative and euphoric effects. Symptoms of intoxication include respiratory and CNS depression. It has a long half-life and quick onset of action. Treatment is supportive. While intoxication may be briefly reversed by flumazenil, sedation tends to recur owing to the long half-life of the drug, and the potential to provoke seizures with repeated dosing of flumazenil is quite high.

The hallucinogens per se are a diverse group of substances with different mechanisms of action, though generally all are active at the 5-HT$_2$ receptor. Clinically, the psychosis of the intoxication/overdose state can be distinguished from symptoms of psychotic disorders on the basis of sympathomimetic effects which are common to all – mydriasis, hypertension, tachycardia, and hyperthermia – which in turn may lead to rhabdomyolysis, renal failure, hepatic necrosis, disseminated intravascular coagulation, tachypnea, and diaphoresis. In the ER, the main benefit of toxicology screening is to rule out other drugs of abuse. ER care includes a quiet, monitored environment and supportive management. Benzodiazepines are again the first choice of treatment for agitation and may indirectly treat hypertension and tachycardia. Haloperidol is a second choice for sedative purposes and treatment of psychotic symptoms. Hyperthermia requires more intensive medical management – IV hydration, muscle relaxants, cooling blankets, and lab monitoring. These are patients who should be treated in the medical ER and on the floors.

There has also been a spike in many US urban areas and college settings of the use of *Salvia divinorum*, originally native to southern Mexico. Also known as "Diviner's Sage," this psychoactive herb can induce strong dissociative effects. It is not screened and is legal in many places, but has recently become a serious concern to ERs. Inhalant abuse, from an array of products used in homes, represents another category of substance abuse increasing in use, but not tested in ERs. Some estimates suggest that up to 20% of our youth has utilized inhalants at some point, not surprising given their low expense as household products. Here, too, diagnosis must rely upon clinical suspicion and technical knowledge. Awareness on the part of ED staff may be critical since lethalities due to inhalant use are not uncommon. The peak age to suspect is the middle teens, with some cases reported as young as 5 and 6 years of age. Experimental use may start in grammar school and last through to high school, at which point this abuse tends to decline. ERs which deal with children and teenagers should be on alert. The patient may present with short-lived euphoria or become stuporous. Psychotic symptoms such as hallucinations and a degree of panic are not unusual. Multiple medical consequences can result, including respiratory depression, aspiration, asphyxiation, and cardiac irregularities. Clinicians should look for rashes around the patient's mouth and nasal passages and irritation of the eyes and lungs. Strong, unusual odors and residue on the body and clothes may also be telltale signs.

A discussion of the growing dangers involved with inhalants serves as a good example of the need for emergency services to conduct recurrent, in-service updates. It is important that ERs keep their staff up-to-date with the latest technical information about laboratory screening for drugs of abuse and the frequent limitations of such testing. Drugs are often abused in combinations, and the most easily screened drugs are not always the most salient. ED clinicians must keep abreast, as well, of recent patterns of use of the substances themselves, especially in their local area. Regional use of drugs is enormously variable and it is unrealistic for ER personnel to know intimately the characteristic presentations and dangers of all such possibilities nationwide. ERs should ensure that databases and poison control hotlines are readily available to staff dealing with diagnostic and treatment dilemmas. The need for sustained updating of expertise is another argument for staff specialization in dealing with psychiatric and substance abuse problems. Medical personnel require this advanced education, as well, for medical clearances.

As noted, patients themselves are unaware of the complexity and limitations of our toxicology tests and knowledge sets. Informing them of the substance abuse testing may be sufficient to stimulate their cooperation in acknowledging their habits, despite a frequent, initial reluctance.

Finally, a thorough psychosocial assessment should be done on all suitable patients. As important as the physical exam, lab findings, and drug screens to the proper evaluation is a good psychological one. Patients' abuse of alcohol or drugs may have precipitated a recent change in living situation or deterioration in mental functioning from an already precarious baseline. Patients often appear in EDs not because their intoxicated state or incipient withdrawal is unusual for them, but because the immediate circumstances of their lives have changed significantly. Perhaps the family is no longer tolerant of their substance use. Perhaps they have recently separated from a significant partner. Possibly they have lost their employment because of substance abuse or they are depleting their financial resources.

The discipline of psychiatry, we have argued, should take the key role at this point, if not earlier. Medical personnel are generally too preoccupied to elicit much detail about these matters. Further, most medical ED staffs openly acknowledge their lack of skill (or patience!) in this area. Mental health clinicians have been trained to attend to affective cues, resistance, and avoidance of problems. Most observers of ED settings agree that psychologically trained personnel have the most interest and expertise in conducting a thorough survey of both substance abuse and these psychological issues, once medical clearance has been addressed.

As critical as the attempt to gather a complete and detailed assessment itself is the manner in which the subject of abuse is broached. It is often a sensitive matter. Many patients are reluctant to offer a true account if family members, especially parents, are around; ensuring privacy in interviews is important. Denial or at least severe minimization is often to be expected. Mental health clinicians routinely have the training and experience to monitor their own impact upon the success of the interview and to be sensitive to their own counter-transference (*vide infra*, Psychodynamic considerations in the ED).

General treatment recommendations

Once a careful assessment has been conducted and the acute risks addressed, there remain, of course, different approaches for dealing with ED patients known or suspected of alcohol or substance abuse. A high suspicion for patient prevarication is indicated, as these patients will often attempt at this stage to deceive the clinician to obtain psychoactive medication. The paramount need is to maintain the rapport, one hopes, begun during the assessment. This dialog becomes focused now upon the ongoing recommended care and follow-up. "Motivational interviewing" and "brief interventions" have become state-of-the-art in ER settings for this purpose.

The busy staff must continue to avoid overly judgmental, simplistic, or rushed attitudes toward these patients. It is especially crucial to monitor one's tone with patients in physical distress from withdrawal states or with impaired judgment due to excitement, paranoia, agitation, or clouded consciousness. These patients require a high degree of interviewing acumen and self-monitoring from the ED clinician. Without skilled interaction they more readily become dangerous to others as well as to themselves. Their state of consciousness may fluctuate. Many may wish to bolt from the ED. Frequently staff are too willing to let the "difficult" patient leave before full treatment options have been arranged.

Simple courtesies, answering questions in a timely manner, and feeding ER patients, all go a long way toward fostering their cooperation. No attempt will be made to dictate specific treatment "techniques" to engage the patient. "Standardized" approaches tend to be a little rigid in their recommendations and may require expensive training sessions. Here, too, we prefer to conduct more informal, periodic in-service discussions and to rely on supervision. Some experts advocate more confrontational strategies with these patients. This approach is often characteristic of some twelve-step programs and of many hospital units, residential programs, and therapeutic communities. At times we bring AA colleagues or sponsors of patients into the ER and periodically a rigorous approach to the patient's resistance may work well. If time permits, we have arranged speedily assembled, more formalized "interventions" in the ED, often a wonderfully effective technique. Other experts lean toward an approach of "gentle persuasion" (Scheck, 2006).

Standardized strategies employing each of these models have been strongly advocated for EDs. Individuals bring their own styles to such a dialogue and there is no one right methodology, in our view. It is difficult to get staff to rally behind a particular approach when their own styles in relating to these patients vary so greatly. Within limits, we recommend letting staff "be themselves" in the discussion of options.

Typical treatment examples

Several particularly common case scenarios may illustrate the complexities and rewards of working with these patients.

1. A frequent visitor to our ER is the cocaine abuser, commonly the patient recently using cocaine, but now "crashing." This patient is often significantly depressed at entry and becomes suicidal for a day or two. If not too acutely disturbed, the cocaine abuser at first welcomes the respite. Arrangements to keep the patient safe are initially critical. Use of antipsychotics is invaluable in quelling the often transient paranoia. The value of a short-stay EOB bed is particularly helpful with this population.

These patients almost invariably want to leave the hospital once their acute depression and self-destructiveness have passed as they quickly develop their cravings again. These patients statistically are a high-risk group for suicide as they may undergo this cycle repeatedly. Expert, caring help in the ED may well cement an otherwise shaky treatment alliance, always a challenge with such patients. In the face of their common wish to leave and to use again, their ER stay may finally prompt them to face their need for longer term interventions and can be life-saving.

2. Severe alcoholics present with a wide variety of complaints to ERs, many initially physical in nature. Medical clearance is almost always advisable. We do not set an arbitrary alcohol level to initiate our discussion, as patients' tolerance for ethanol varies markedly. We do wait for the worst of the intoxication to pass before attempting a real dialog.

Frequently these evaluations soon involve acute "behavioral" issues, such as dyscontrol, confusion, or outright belligerence. It is a primary time for self-destructiveness to manifest itself. As with most substance abusers, frustration tolerance is generally low and the patient is soon dealing with powerful cravings for alcohol. If the patient is ready to flee, sensitive and skilled immediate interventions are often critical. Prescribing benzodiazepines in sufficient quantity may address not only the physiological withdrawal but also allay the mistrust, panic, and severe physical discomfort of the patient simultaneously.

As the withdrawal is addressed, precious time may be used to plan further interventions. We attempt to mobilize collaterals – especially family members and AA sponsors – as quickly as feasible. ERs are often the most suitable place to attend to the family tensions and despair brought on by an episode. The family or other supports are reassured that the situation is under control, but are also challenged to grab the opportunity to help implement a more decisive plan of treatment.

During this brief window of resolution of the acute emergency, when the patient feels safe and the family feels their problem is at least temporarily contained, all involved for once get the chance to think through the next, effective steps. Often family members have never been given an opportunity to consult with knowledgeable staff about their realistic options. Emergency visits, too, may provide the best opportunity for a dialog about psychological issues, such as the family's "enabling" behavior or self-defeating despair. These hindrances may have been present for years. Silently endured struggles and complex family dynamics may surface. Nowhere more evident is the power of an emergency service to make a huge difference in the trajectory of a disorder than in such a case. None of these salutary outcomes will occur if ER staff do not take the time to address the crisis in its full dimension.

3. Users of excitatory substances, such as PCP (or ketamine, many inhalants, Ecstasy, etc.), are likely to present initially with extremely impaired judgment and impulse control. Abusers of a wide variety of these illicit substances present to an ER in an agitated state. Fluctuating courses are the rule. Assuming there are no pressing medical complications, psychiatrically trained staffs are generally the most suitable clinicians to deal with the sometimes prolonged need to monitor and "talk such patients down." If the situation can be handled without restraints, a seclusion room may or may not become necessary and access to such areas should be assured.

Here, too, short-stay ER visits are generally ideal, although transfers to inpatient units are more practical in cases of ongoing dyscontrol requiring extended periods of monitoring. Access to mental health personnel is advisable from the start. Absolutes in assumptions, however, should be avoided. Certain recreational, thrill-seeking users of the various "club drugs" frequently seen in ERs may be judged ultimately to have no frank psychological problems. Nevertheless, consultation with psychiatric staff appears the safest option to employ in these cases warranting the seriousness of an ER visit. In our hospital setting, we make it the rule, if only to educate the often naïve patient about the dangerousness of his or her behavior.

Aftercare/triage issues

ERs, with access to medical expertise and inpatient beds, are the most suitable places to triage substance users in acute or confusing stages of their disorder. The most immediate triage decision is whether hospitalization is indicated. Those medically unstable or confusing in their ER presentations generally require a medically monitored environment. This population includes individuals with serious overdoses and those in withdrawal and at risk for further complications (e.g. delirium tremens). Patients whose general medical status is compromised (e.g. cardiac cases, etc.) may need an inpatient service, too. So do individuals with serious psychiatric issues or acute substance abuse leading to direct self-destructiveness. Finally, individuals who have a clear history of non-compliance or non-response to less intensive efforts and whose substance abuse is seriously jeopardizing their health or safety may also benefit from a monitored course in a medically supervised setting for a time.

If the patient is well controlled and medically stable, other aftercare options can be considered. We prefer to initiate this planning in the ER, capitalizing on the momentum and captive audience. There is little scientific consensus as to the most effective substance abuse treatment options, once hospitalization is not indicated. Recommendations should be presented to patients with confidence but openness to individual preferences and practical concerns, like insurance and finances. ER staff should acknowledge the lack of consensus as to optimal aftercare, but strongly challenge the patient to follow through on recommendations as soon as practical.

Depending on availability and preference, partial hospitalization, residential treatments, therapeutic communities, and halfway facilities should be considered for those most chronic or recalcitrant to previous efforts of assistance. For non-residential outpatient referrals, we are non-doctrinaire but advocate a multifaceted plan. We prefer to recommend a combination of modalities, along the lines advocated by those whom we regard as the most authoritative experts (Khantzian & Albanese, 2008). We encourage reliance on group support, outpatient clinics, psychiatric treatment, and medication if indicated, and abstinence reinforcers, such as mandatory urine testing, probation, and pharmacologic substitutes or antagonists. We do not eschew a recommendation for psychotherapy at the appropriate time. From the ER, however, we generally emphasize, first, a referral to an individual coordinator of the overall substance abuse care, rather than a specific psychotherapeutic practitioner at that point. Khantzian's concept of a "primary care therapist" overseeing all aspects of the plan, seems a valuable one for an ER to promote (Khantzian & Albanese, 2008).

Treatment plans and protocols

No emergency setting can deal with the volume and complexity of alcoholic and substance abusing patients without routines of care, including for treating states of withdrawal. As noted above, some EDs follow relatively fixed withdrawal regimens. A voluminous literature in monographs and textbooks addresses the technical aspects of such protocols. An excellent resource is the APA Practice Guidelines, widely available and comprehensive (American Psychiatric Association, 2006). Training staff in such methodology is important. Many ERs, such as ours, use strict protocols selectively.

We see a significant variability among patient preference and tolerability of fixed orders. A considerable assertiveness is required with substance abusing individuals in this regard. Patients are frequently informed that changes in vital signs dictate withdrawal dosages, rather than patient wishes. Conversely, acceding to patient preferences and suggestions selectively may sometimes foster an alliance.

We rarely initiate in the ED longer term pharmacotherapy for drug and alcohol abuse, such as naltrexone (now available in depot form), disulfiram or buprenorphine. We prefer to offer the next clinicians latitude regarding continuing medication strategies. The emphasis with our ED staff is the acute stabilization and initial referrals. Some EDs, however, do tend to start such medication with good results.

Psychodynamic considerations in the ED

No universal psychodynamic pattern characterizes the variety of individuals who suffer from alcoholism and substance abuse. Characteristic psychological features may be present, although it is not easy to separate cause from effect of the disorders involved. Whenever feasible, a general psychodynamic evaluation is preferable, although a more in-depth interview must wait until issues of acute intoxication have passed. Concrete issues should generally be emphasized, such as the pros and cons of the abuse, the role substance use plays in one's coping, etc. Issues of self-esteem, problematic relationships, and affect disturbances are common. Psychiatric comorbidities with attendant dependency or belligerence are also extremely frequent.

The demanding or help-rejecting nature of this population may drain staff. Caregivers in ERs accustomed to rapid turnover of patients may need to emotionally distance themselves. Rationalization of brusque treatment is common, typified, for instance, by the view that providing "too much" help, such as meals or dollops of courtesy, may result in over-utilization of ER services (Hackenschmidt, 2003).

While not all substance abusers are personality-disordered, there are similarities in the ways ER staffs react to these two groups. As typical of clinicians working with the character-disordered (paradigmatically, borderline personality disorders), moralistic and harsh cultural attitudes toward substance abuse may play an inordinate role in staff–patient interactions. Counter-transference attitudes on the part of ER staff may make it impossible for patients to discuss their concerns at all.

Two problematic counter-transference paradigms predominate. Some staff gravitate toward a "parental" style of relating. The unspoken fantasy involves the idea that these patients would comply and progress if shown maximal empathy and nurturing. Splitting, so ubiquitous a phenomenon on inpatient units, may wreak havoc in ERs, too, as certain staff feel the need to be the "good object" and denigrate subtly their more realistic colleagues. Rescue fantasies are rife. These clinicians may be naïve and can become burnt out when patients do not live up to expectations.

ED personnel are more traditionally noted for an assertive, even aggressive, style of relating. They may adapt the more confrontational model and become almost militaristic in challenging patient denial and resistance. These staff often attempt to counter strongly patients' lack of cooperation. They may be uncomfortable except in authoritarian modes of relating. These clinicians may be playing out dependency issues of their own and denying their own fears of these individuals. They may project pessimistic feelings onto the "bad" patient. The more general risk in dealing with these patients daily is burnout. As in working with chronic psychiatric patients, clinicians become discouraged when they see the "revolving door" of substance abusing patients. ER staffs need to be reminded of the "clinician's fallacy," the observation that medical staffs see the recidivists and "frequent fliers," and only more rarely the multiple success stories who "graduate" from the system. Those staffs most prone to unrealistic expectations of nurturing the patient to health are often the most easily disillusioned. They need reminders that substance abusing patients often require a few "passes" through the treatment system before the message "takes" and these individuals incorporate fully the advice and recommendations given in ER settings.

A final word

Patients with histories of alcohol and other substance abuse, who present to our ERs, are numerous, complex, and challenging. Care for these high-risk patients by a knowledgeable staff, neither hurried nor harried and organized in ways that permit full assessments and interventions, can be extremely critical to the course of these disorders. EDs often find dealing with this population taxing and sometimes relegate it to secondary consideration. The work can be quite rewarding, however, when conditions for good care in ERs permit the time and expertise for truly successful treatment.

References

American Psychiatric Association (2006). *Practice Guideline for the Treatment of Patients with Substance Use Disorder*, 2nd edn. Washington, DC: APA Press.

Lee, L. W. (2008). Bolting ER early linked to self-harm. *American Psychiatry News*, **1**, 20.

Curran, G., Sullivan, G., Williams, K. *et al.* (2008). The association of psychiatric comorbidity and use of the emergency department among persons with substance use disorders: an observation cohort study. *BMC Emergency Medicine*, **8**, 17.

Currier, G., Trenton, A. & Walsh, P. (2006). Relative accuracy of breath and serum alcohol readings in the psychiatric emergency service. *Psychiatric Services*, **57(1)**, 34–6.

Hackenschmidt, A. (2003). Should access to emergency departments be limited for "frequent fliers"? *Journal of Emergency Nursing*, **29**(5), 486–8.

Illinois Hospital Association (2005). *Emergency Utilization Survey*, p. 33. Chicago, IL.

Khantzian, E. & Albanese, M. (2008). *Understanding Addiction as Self Medication: Finding Hope Behind the Pain*. Lanham, MD: Rowman & Littlefield, passim.

Nawar, E. W., Niska, R. W. & Xu, J. (2007). National hospital ambulatory medical care survey: 2005 emergency department summary. *Advanced Data*, **386**, 1–32.

Scheck, A. (2006). Brief ED interventions lower drug and alcohol abuse. *Emergency Medicine News*, **28**(1), 36–7.

Substance Abuse and Mental Health Services Administration (2002). *Treatment Improvement Protocols 9: Assessment and Treatment of Patients with Coexisting Mental Illness and Alcohol and Other Drug Abuse*. Rockville, MD: United States Department of Health and Human Services.

Viccellio, P. (2008). Overcrowding of Emergency Rooms in the United States. American College of Emergency Physicians, Annual Meeting.

Ear acupuncture in addiction treatment

Michael Smith

Acupuncture is currently used in the treatment of addictions by approximately 2500 addiction treatment programs globally. Clinical evidence supports that it is effective in ameliorating withdrawal and craving symptoms associated with alcohol, opiate, and cocaine dependence, as well as symptoms associated with most other addictions. Acupuncture for cocaine dependence has been particularly recognized as an important innovation, since there are presently no established pharmaceutical treatments for this condition. Acupuncture is used by programs as a foundation for later psychosocial recovery. It is a non-verbal, non-threatening, "first step" intervention that has an immediate calming effect on patients regardless of the specific substance used and regardless of whether a coexisting psychiatric disorder has been diagnosed. Initial participation with acupuncture has been found to improve patients' overall treatment retention, and to facilitate their subsequent involvement. In most programs patients receive needling in three to five ear acupuncture points while seated together in a large group room so that a substantial number of patients can be treated conveniently. This safe and cost-efficient procedure has gained increasing acceptance from agencies responsible for overseeing addiction treatment. Evidence for the benefit of acupuncture in coexisting psychiatric conditions and other behavioral health settings is also presented. This article describes the practical use and research findings relating to acupuncture for addiction. Mechanisms of action that involve physiology and psychosocial process will be covered.

Acupuncture basics

History and method

Acupuncture is a major component of the ancient tradition of Chinese medicine. The principles and goals of this form of treatment have remained constant through time. The textbook that is still used today, the *Nei Jing*, was written 2000 years ago. Acupuncture was used by numerous 19th century US practitioners, including Sir William Osler, "The father of modern medicine," and the eminent physician/chemist Franklin Bache, the grandson of Benjamin Franklin. In the early 1970s, American interest was renewed when relations with China were opened. In the US, most states have acupuncture licensing laws. Acupuncture is recognized by established medical organizations in virtually every part of the world. Veterinary medical journals cite many examples of objective clinical success, including treatment of potentially lethal arthritis in horses and congenital hip dysplasia in dogs. Effective treatment of animals is usually cited as proof that acupuncture is not merely a placebo procedure.

Acupuncture consists of the stimulation of specified locations on the surface of the body that alters and improves bodily function. The Chinese term for a treatment location is *xue*, which means opening. The traditional Chinese names for these locations often refer to flow on the surface of the Earth such as valley, marsh, crevice, or stream. In the west the term *point* is used. Acupuncture points are physiologically distinct from the immediate environment; they have less electrical resistance and, therefore, greater electrical conductivity. The points are warmer than the surrounding area by 0.1–0.2 °C. The difference in warmth and electrical activity can be detected by the human hand as well as by instruments. A painful response to pressure may also be used as a point indicator. The precise location of these phenomena varies within a small area that corresponds to the acupuncture point as denoted on an acupuncture chart. Descriptions of the location and functions of these points have remained fairly constant through the centuries.

Acupuncture points can be stimulated by various means: touch, movement, heat, and electricity, as well as needling. Health-related procedures such as acupressure, shiatsu, reiki, and tai ji chuan work on the same principles as acupuncture even though no nee-dles are used. Needling is the most convenient and efficient means of stimulating acupuncture points.

Acupuncture needles are stainless steel shafts of varying length and thickness. The handle of the needle usually has an additional spiral winding made of copper. The needles may be cleaned, sterilized, and re-used as is the case with surgical equipment. Most western facilities use the needles once and discard them. Acupuncture needles are provided in conven-ient sterile packages. Needles are inserted with a brief but steady movement. Ear needles penetrate 1/8 inch, contacting the cartilage if it is present in that location. Needles are twirled by 180° for smoother insertion. The patient may feel a momentary sensation like a pinch. Occasionally there is a brief sharper sensation that may cause the patient to complain. The procedure is nearly painless and causes the rapid onset of a grati-fying sense of relaxation. On first exposure, most patients express fear of the pain of needle insertion and are confused by the idea that little needles can cope with their big problems. This fear is easily solved by letting prospective patients observe other patients undergoing the actual process of treatment. It is a mis-take to rely on leaflets and verbal explanation alone.

What the patients experience

Patients may notice local paresthesia effects such as warmth and tingling. There may be sensations of warmth, electrical movement, or heaviness in other parts of the body, although these reactions are more typical of body acupuncture rather than ear acupunc-ture. Patients may feel quite sleepy after each of the first several treatments. This reaction is part of the acute recovery process and passes readily. A few patients develop a headache at the end of a treatment session. Shortening the length of the session or redu-cing the number of needles resolves this problem. Rarely, a needling reaction occurs in which the patient feels dizzy, light-headed, and may actually faint. This reaction (postural hypotension) also occurs in many medical and dental settings. When it occurs, one should remove the needles and help the patient lie on a flat surface. The syncope will resolve within a few minutes and the patient will exhibit relaxed behavior as though the full duration treatment had been given. Needling reactions occur more often in persons with a relatively labile autonomic nervous system. Fortu-nately these reactions are quite rare in the treatment of addiction. Patients should be told to eat before com-ing for treatment to reduce the possibility of a nee-dling reaction.

The insertion of acupuncture needles never causes bleeding. Hence, there is no need for special blood contact precautions during application of treatment. Based on our experience, treatment sites in the ear bleed about 1% of the time after the needles are removed. Thus 10–20% of patients will have such a reaction. There are several methods used to cope with this problem in terms of appropriate risk management precautions. Commonly, patients are asked to remove their own needles and place them directly in a sharps container. Staff may remove needles by only touching the handle and giving the patient a cotton pad to use if bleeding is noted. A small hematoma may also occur. Staff may press each location with a Q-tip as neces-sary. Most gloves do not provide dexterity in grasping small needles. It should be noted that ear needles are inserted so shallowly that about 10% fall out during the period of treatment. Therefore many needles must be retrieved which have fallen on the patient's cloth-ing. Even wearing gloves will not protect staff who might try to search for such needles. Hence, the patients must be instructed to locate any fallen nee-dles and discard them properly. Often programs use a needle count procedure. Patients place needles in a paper cup or bowl so that staff can verify that all nee-dles are present before they are discarded in the sharps container. This procedure is particularly appropriate if acupuncture is conducted in a room that is used for other purposes.

Suggested physiological mechanisms

There have been many efforts to determine the under-lying physiological mechanisms of acupuncture. Some of these efforts were based on the misleading assump-tion that acupuncture is primarily a treatment for pain relief. Many acupuncture functions, such as autonomic and gastrointestinal effects, are independent of any aspect that relates to pain. In other cases, such as the treatment of frozen shoulder, pain is actually tempor-arily increased after successful acupuncture needling. More accurately, acupuncture is frequently an effective treatment for the circulatory, neurological, or inflam-matory causes of pain.

Acupuncture charts have a superficial resemblance to western neuroanatomical charts. The functions of the meridian channels on acupuncture charts differ substantially, however, from those of nearby peripheral nerve trunks. Ear acupuncture is a particularly clear example in this regard. The acupuncture chart of the external ear identifies more than 100 separate acupuncture points. These points relate primarily to different body locations and to various organic functions. One can easily verify some of these correlations by noting that the shoulder point on the ear shows abnormally low electrical resistance in patients with shoulder injuries, as does the ureter point on inpatients who are passing a kidney stone. The simple innervation pattern of the external ear cannot be used to explain these effects.

Researchers have noted the following variety of specific physiological effects associated with acupuncture, as cited in Brewington *et al.* (1994). It has been reported that acupuncture at traditional points produced dramatic effects in EEG, galvanic skin response (GSR), blood flow, and breathing rate. Various studies have linked acupuncture to the production of endogenous opiate peptides, such as beta-endorphin and metenkephalins, and this has been speculated as a physiological mechanism behind the treatment's effects on withdrawal discomfort.

Acupuncture has also been related to changes regarding other neurotransmitters, including ACTH and cortisol levels, serotonin, and norepinephrine. The impact of these neurotransmitters in addiction and behavioral health is well established. They are thought to be of key importance in understanding drug and medication effects in addiction and psychiatry. A review of research linking endogenous opiate peptide (EOP) production to optimal immune system functioning concluded that acupuncture appears to have beneficial effects on the immune system. A substantial literature thus exists supporting that acupuncture has a variety of neurochemical and other physiological effects.

It should be noted that certain medications – namely, methadone, corticosteroids, and benzodiazepines – seem to suppress part of the acupuncture effect. Patients taking these medications in substantial quantity have clearly less relaxation effect during treatment and may have a slower response to treatment. Nevertheless, acupuncture is an effective treatment for secondary addiction in high-dose methadone patients and in reducing benzodiazepine withdrawal symptoms. Acupuncture is also widely used to treat patients with adrenal suppression who need to be weaned off corticosteroid medication. This may suggest that part of the initial relaxation response is endorphin- and

steroid-dependent but that the more important mechanisms relate to a different type of process.

Acupuncture effects have been documented in a wide range of organisms. Needling the stem of a plant at a low resistance point will correlate with a rapid increase in the temperature of the tips of the leaves as measured by thermography. Needling a point of normal resistance will produce no such effect (Eory, 1995).

It is too restrictive to define acupuncture mechanisms in terms of highly evolved structures such as the human brain and the endocrine system. Rather it seems clear that acupuncture involves the primitive and pervasive functions that are common to all life. Such functions include circulation on a microscopic level, homeostasis, wound healing, immune function, and microneurological functioning. Acupuncture has an obvious impact on the autonomic nervous system, which is an example of a relatively primitive and homeostatic system in human beings. Acupuncture seems to enhance the integrity of these basic life functions. Pharmaceutical medicine, at best, can only suppress one or more parts of these systems. The Society for Acupuncture Research (SAR) meets yearly to discuss these issues of mechanism and research. Acupuncture research may provide a window of opportunity to enhance our understanding of basic and pervasive vital processes (Smith, 1995).

NADA protocol
Lincoln Hospital experience

Acupuncture treatment for drug and alcohol problems was primarily developed at Lincoln Hospital, a New York City-owned facility in the impoverished South Bronx. The Lincoln Recovery Center is a state-licensed treatment program that has provided more than 800 000 acupuncture treatments in the past 34 years. Dr. Yoshiaki Omura was the consultant who began the program (Omura *et al.*, 1975).

Lincoln Hospital has trained more than 7000 clinicians, usually referred to as Acu Detox Specialists (ADS), in the past 20 years. The National Acupuncture Detoxification Association (NADA) was established in 1985 to increase the use of the Lincoln model and to maintain quality and responsibility in the field. Registered trainers from NADA have trained many thousands of ADS practitioners. The Center for Substance Abuse Treatment (CSAT), part of the Substance and

Mental Services Administration (SAMHSA), publishes a series of *Treatment Improvement Protocols* (TIPs). In 2006, CSAT TIP# 45 on "Detoxification and Substance Abuse" included the use of acupuncture in its best practice guidelines for the treatment of addiction.

Initially, in 1974, Lincoln used Dr. H. L. Wen's method, applying electrical stimulation to the lung point in the ear (Wen & Cheung, 1973). Lincoln was a methadone detoxification program at that time; therefore, acupuncture was used as an adjunctive treatment for prolonged withdrawal symptoms after the 10-day detoxification cycle. Patients reported less malaise and better relaxation in symptom surveys. Subsequently, twice daily acupuncture was used concurrently with tapering methadone doses. Reduction in opiate withdrawal symptoms and prolonged program retention were noted.

It was accidentally discovered that electrical stimulation was not necessary to produce symptomatic relief. Simple manual needling produced a more prolonged effect. Patients were able to use acupuncture only once a day and still experience a suppression of their withdrawal symptoms. A reduction in craving for alcohol and heroin was described for the first time. This observation corresponds to the general rule in acupuncture that strong stimulation has primarily a symptom-suppressing or dispersing effect and that more gentle stimulation has more of a long-term, preventive or tonification effect.

Gradually the acupuncture protocol was expanded by adding the shen men (spirit gate), a point known for producing relaxation. Other ear points were tried on the basis of lower resistance, pain sensitivity, and clinical indication during a several-year developmental process. The author added the sympathetic, kidney, and liver points to create a basic five-point formula. Numerous other point formulas using body acupuncture points were tried on an individual basis without any significant improvement.

A standard acupuncture textbook (Landgren, 2008) describes the functions of each of the five points in the basic formula as follows:

1. *Sympathetic* is used for numerous diseases related to disruption in both sympathetic and parasympathetic nervous systems. It has strong analgesic and relaxant effects upon internal organs. It dilates blood vessels.

2. *Shenmen* regulates excitation and inhibition of the cerebral cortex. It produces sedative and anti-allergy effects. It is used for many neuropsychiatric disorders.

3. *Lung* is used for analgesia, sweating, and various respiratory conditions.

4. *Liver* is used for hepatitis, anemia, neuralgia, muscle spasms, and eye diseases.

5. *Kidney* is a strengthening point for the cerebrum, hematopoietic system, and kidneys. It is used for neurasthenia, lassitude, headache, and urogenital problems.

Traditional Chinese theory associates the lung with the grieving process; the liver with resolving aggression; and the kidney with willpower, coping with fear, and new growth.

Clinical value of a standard protocol

The value of using one standard group of acupuncture points became increasingly clear. The standard formula seemed to be equally effective for different drugs of abuse and at different stages of treatment. Patients responded better when acupuncture treatment was administered quickly without an intrusive, diagnostic prelude. Since acupuncture produces a homeostatic response, it was not necessary to adjust the formula for mood swings, agitation, or energy levels.

From the point of view of Chinese theory, using a single basic formula for such generally depleted patients is appropriate. In traditional Chinese medicine, the lack of a calm inner tone in a person is described as a condition of empty fire (*xu huo*), because the heat of aggressiveness burns out of control when the calm inner tone is lost. It is easy to be confused by the empty fire that many addicts exhibit and to conclude that the main goal should be the sedation of excess fire. Addicts themselves take this approach in the extreme by using sedative drugs. The empty fire condition represents the illusion of power, an illusion that leads to more desperate use of chemicals and to senseless violence. Acupuncture helps patients with this condition to restore their inner control.

A group setting enhances the acupuncture effect. A group size of less than six members seems to diminish symptom relief and retention significantly. Patients receiving acupuncture in an individual setting are often self-conscious and easily distracted. These problems are more evident in the management of new patients. General acupuncture treatment sessions need to last 20–25 minutes. Because chemical dependency patients are more resistant and dysfunctional, they should be instructed to remain in the acupuncture group setting for 40–45 minutes so that a full effect is obtained. The atmosphere of the treatment room should be adjusted to fit varying clinical circumstances. Programs with a significant number of new intakes and/or socially isolated patients should use a well lit room and allow a moderate amount of conversation to minimize alienation and encourage social bonding. On the other hand, programs with relatively consistent clientele who relate to each other frequently in other group settings should dim the lights and not allow any conversation to minimize distracting cross talk. Background music is often used in the latter circumstance.

The location of ear points and the technique of insertion can be taught effectively in a 70-hour apprenticeship-based program. Most acupuncture components can be staffed by a wide range of addiction clinicians such as counselors, social workers, nurses, medical doctors, and psychologists. Training must include a clinical apprenticeship because coping with the individual distractions and group process is more important and more difficult to learn than the technical skill of repetitive needle insertion. Each clinician can provide about 15 treatments per hour in a group setting. General supervision should be provided by licensed or certified acupuncturists or medical doctors. This arrangement allows for acupuncture to be integrated with existing services in a flexible and cost-effective manner. Numerous states have enacted specific ADS laws and/or regulations. These states include Arizona, Connecticut, Georgia, Indiana, Louisiana, Maryland, Missouri, New Mexico, New York, South Carolina, Tennessee, Texas, Vermont, and Virginia. Other states have specific arrangements that allow nurses and counselors to provide NADA acupuncture services. According to SAMHSA statistics (N-SSATS-2002), acupuncture is used in more than 900 state-licensed chemical dependency programs. Almost all of these programs are located in states with ADS laws. The limited availability of fully licensed acupuncturists (or physicians) and the expenses of hiring such providers seems to be a limiting factor.

Summary of NADA protocol

The NADA model can be summarized and defined as follows: 1) clinicians use three to five ear acupuncture points, including sympathetic, shenmen, lung, kidney, and liver. Three points (sympathetic, shenmen,

and lung) are used in developing country settings to save money without any apparent loss of effectiveness; 2) treatment is provided in a group setting for a duration of 40–45 minutes; 3) acupuncture treatment is integrated with conventional elements of psychosocial rehabilitation; 4) several components of the Lincoln program are frequently combined with acupuncture in other treatment facilities. These items include: a supportive non-confrontational approach to individual counseling; an emphasis on Narcotics Anonymous and other twelve-step activities early in the treatment process; an absence of screening for appropriate patients; the use of herbal sleep mix; the use of frequent toxicologies; a willingness to work with court-related agencies; and a tolerant, informal, family-like atmosphere (Smith & Khan, 1989).

The author developed a herbal formula known as sleep mix which is used in most acupuncture for addiction settings and many other healthcare settings as well. The formula includes chamomile, peppermint, yarrow, skullcap, hops, and catnip. These are inexpensive herbs, traditionally used in Europe, which are reputed to calm and soothe the nervous system and tend to stimulate circulation and the elimination of waste products. The herb formula is taken as a tea on a nightly basis or frequently during the day as symptoms indicate. Sleep mix can be used for the treatment of conventional stress and insomnia as well as providing an adjunctive support in addiction treatment settings. Sleep mix is particularly appropriate for the management of alcohol withdrawal symptoms. Patients receiving conventional benzodiazepine treatment will often voluntarily refuse this medication if sleep mix is available. Lincoln has used a reiki circle for the past 10 years. Reiki is a type of therapeutic touch which is related to acupuncture. A reiki circle can involve 20 people if several practitioners are involved. Reiki provides similar benefits to NADA acupuncture. In addition, reiki is more socially interactive and helps patients learn more about their own process of change. Lincoln and many programs use magnetic beads for weekend treatments. The beads are attached to a square of adhesive. They are usually placed on the lung point, the shenmen point, or on the back of the ear on a "reverse shenmen" position. Only one point should be used bilaterally. Beads remain in place for 1–2 weeks if necessary. In addition to addiction-related treatment, beads have been used for general stress relief and for ADHD and other childhood problems. A pilot study at Reed Academy in

Framingham, MA shows potentially promising results for autism spectrum disorders (Smith & Lee, 2003).

Controlled studies

Randomized placebo trials

H. L. Wen, MD, of Hong Kong was the first physician to report successful use of acupuncture treatment of addiction withdrawal symptoms (Wen & Cheung, 1973). He observed that opium addicts receiving electroacupuncture (EA) as post-surgical analgesia experienced relief of withdrawal symptoms. The lung ear point was used. Subsequently, Wen conducted several basic clinical pilot studies that formed the basis of subsequent research.

Results from available placebo-design studies support the conclusion that acupuncture's effectiveness in facilitating abstinence with alcohol, opiate, and cocaine abusers is not due to a simple placebo effect (Brewington et al., 1994). Seven published studies involving animal subjects (i.e. mice or rats) indicate that EA reduces opiate withdrawal symptoms with morphine-addicted subjects. In these studies, experimental and control animals show behavioral differences regarding rodent opiate withdrawal symptoms, such as hyperactivity, wet dog shakes, and teeth chattering. Each of these studies notes significantly less withdrawal symptoms with subjects receiving EA relative to controls. Significantly different hormonal and beta-endorphin levels post-EA are noted between experimental and control subjects in several of these studies.

A number of controlled studies have been conducted on human subjects using various modified versions of the Lincoln Hospital ear point formula. Washburn reported that opiate-addicted individuals receiving correct site acupuncture showed significantly better program attendance relative to subjects receiving acupuncture on placebo sites (Washburn et al., 1993). Two placebo-design studies provide strong support regarding acupuncture's use as a treatment for alcoholics. Bullock studied 54 chronic alcoholics randomly assigned

to receive acupuncture either at points related to addiction or at nearby point locations not specifically related to addiction (Bullock et al., 1987). Subjects were treated in an inpatient setting but were free to leave the program each day. The setting also provided frequent twelve-step meetings and a supportive atmosphere typical of an aftercare facility.

Throughout the study, experimental subjects showed significantly better outcomes regarding attendance and their self-reported need for alcohol. Significant differences favoring the experimental group were also found regarding: 1) the number of self-reported drinking episodes; 2) self-reports concerning the effectiveness of acupuncture in affecting the desire to drink; and 3) the number of subjects admitted to a local detoxification unit for alcohol-related treatment. Bullock et al. (1989) replicated earlier work (Bullock et al., 1987) using a larger ($n = 80$) sample over a longer (6 months) follow-up period. Of 40 patients in the treatment group, 21 completed the 8-week treatment period as compared with 1 of 40 controls. Significant differences favoring the experimental group were again noted. Placebo subjects self-reported over twice the number of drinking episodes reported by experimental subjects. Placebo subjects were also re-admitted to the local hospital alcohol detoxification unit at over twice the rate as experimental subjects during the follow-up period (Table 23.1).

Research problems

There are several potential distortions of research data that are particular to acudetox studies. Controlled studies must often rely on "soft outcomes," including interim measurements from questionnaires or short-term attendance or toxicology. Acupuncture is not "valium in a needle." Conventional researchers usually assume that acupuncture has an exclusively sedating effect. They assume that treatment success can be measured by responses on a one-time, one-dimensional questionnaire which equates more relaxation with a greater treatment effect. The reality of NADA

Table 23.1 Completion rates in HENNEPIN study. Reproduced with permission from Bullock et al., 1989

	Treatment group	Control	P
Phase I (daily acupuncture for 2 weeks)	37 (92%)	21 (52%)	0.001
Phase II (three times a week for 4 weeks)	26 (65%)	3 (7%)	0.001
Phase III (twice a week for 2 weeks)	21 (52%)	1 (2.1%)	0.001

acupuncture is quite different. It has a balancing effect, which includes arousal and increased energy in some treatments. Some other acupuncture treatments lead to a moderate sense of wellbeing; the significant effects primarily occur hours or days after treatment. The most important effects of acudetox have little to do with immediate sedation effects. Meditation and rejuvenation are very different to sedation.

Addiction treatment is not merely the suppression of the indications of illness. Most people in the field agree that the best outcome of addiction treatment is the development of self-responsibility. We focus our effort so that the patient takes charge of his or her own recovery. This situation is very different to the conventional model in which there is an active pharmacologic agent and a passive patient. From the point of view of research design, patients' own efforts become an unwanted variable. How do we know if the medicine did it or the patient did it?

Note the results of the pilot study from Reed Academy cited in this article (Smith & Lee, 2003). Halfway through the study, four boys decided they wanted to "take control of their lives" and have the magnetic beads removed. Statistically, they were removed from the study database. But, clinically, they continued to do well and gained a level of success that had not seemed possible before. This effect is widely accepted in the outcome evaluation of long-term treatment. Patients who drop out of therapeutic communities after 6 months are seen to have a comparable success rate to those who complete the whole program. Self-actualization, not simple obedience, is the more significant trait. Many forms of treatment do not fit easily with the process of self-actualization. Other forms of treatment – acupuncture, twelve-step, Drug Court, for example – fit easily with a patient's growing independence.

The social context for a research study is often a critical variable that is overlooked. The pilot study for the Cocaine Alternative Treatment Study (CATS) at Yale (Avants *et al.*, 2000) showed promising results. In this case acupuncture was embedded in a well functioning methadone program and the link between the patients, program, and the study was constructive. When the large CATS study was done, the Yale site data showed no significant effect. The intervention and controls were identical; the variable was a less functional social bond between the program and patients which led to the need-to-pay patients to get enough research participants (Margolin *et al.*, 2002b).

It is often difficult to design or identify a social context which will be appropriate to test a claim that acupuncture is an effective supportive context-dependent treatment. The CATS study tested an inappropriately optimistic claim that acupuncture can reduce cocaine use as a virtual stand-alone treatment (Margolin *et al.*, 2002a). The Fairview study by Bullock sought to measure a treatment enhancement where little enhancement was possible owing to the already comprehensive schedule in that rehab program (Bullock *et al.*, 2002).

Placebo points may be active

The five NADA points are not the only acupuncture points for acudetox. Several points can give about the same effect. This causes problems when researchers look for placebo points. Konefal examined the efficacy of different acupuncture point protocols with patients with various alcohol and other drug problems. Subjects ($n = 321$) were randomly assigned to one of three groups: a one-needle auricular treatment protocol using the shenmen point; the five-needle Lincoln protocol; or the five-needle Lincoln protocol plus selected body points for self-reported symptoms. All groups showed an increase in the proportion of drug-free urine tests over the course of treatment. Subjects with the single-needle protocol, however, showed significantly less improvement compared to the other two groups (Konefal *et al.*, 1995).

During the trial and error search conducted at Lincoln Hospital for a more effective ear acupuncture formula for addiction treatment, it was clear that a large number of points had some effect on acute withdrawal symptoms. Ear acupuncture charts indicate that all areas on the anterior surface of the ear are identified as active treatment locations. Using a placebo or sham acupuncture technique is actually an effort to use relatively ineffective points in contrast to the conventional use of totally ineffective sugar pills in pharmaceutical trials. Sham points are usually located on the external helix or rim of the ear, although there is no consensus about the level of effectiveness of this procedure. Bullock's alcoholism studies used highly failure-prone subjects and hence may have revealed the difference between active and sham points more effectively.

Landmark Schwartz study

While focusing on the complexities of randomized controlled double-blind studies, it is easy to forget that a controlled study is never more than an approximation of reality. Real life surveys tend to have explicit "hard" outcomes that represent prolonged significant change. Consequently, the large Boston Target Cities study conveys more potentially valid information than any of the randomized controlled studies that have been done on acudetox (Schwartz et al., 1999).

Schwartz surveyed 8011 complete treatment episodes that were totally blinded because no "study" was being conducted. Low volume studies must be carefully monitored (controlled) because relatively small variations can create significant distortions in the results. Surveying a high volume of treatments tends to minimize this problem.

The Schwartz study uses data from the federally funded Target Cities program which provided assessment and referral of all detoxification patients in Boston during 1993–4. Consequently, Target Cities provided a uniquely convenient database for referral and subsequent referral comparison. At the time of the study, Boston had three outpatient detoxification programs that used acupuncture instead of pharmaceutical medication. These were long-standing programs so the study measured outcomes from existing established programs rather than a new or experimental design. Schwartz compared the recidivism rates of the three outpatient detoxification programs to the recidivism of four residential detoxification programs. Recidivism is defined as re-admission for detoxification within 6 months of discharge from the prior admission for detoxification.

Of 8011 patients discharged during the study period, 6907 (86%) had their first detox discharge from an inpatient program and 1104 (14%) from an outpatient acupuncture program. As might be expected, the acupuncture group tended to be more educated, employed, and well-housed. The modality of outpatient acupuncture treatment was selected by the clinical referral staff. Patients had to be educated about acupuncture before they agreed to this modality.

Schwartz et al. took the necessary step of matching 740 of the acupuncture patients with a similar group of residential patients with similar baseline characteristics. So 67% of the acupuncture patients with a similar group of residential patients were able to be included in the matched sample.

The outcomes of the study were fairly clearcut. The odds that an acupuncture patient was re-admitted within 6 months were 0.71 of the odds that a residential patient was re-admitted ($P = 0.02$, 95% CI 0.53–0.95). Acupuncture appeared particularly beneficial for those patients with a primary alcohol diagnosis (odds 0.53) (Table 23.2) and those patients with two or more detox admissions in the past year (Table 23.3). Looking at the overall database, repeat recent detox admissions are the primary predictor of recidivism.

The characteristics of the two modalities being compared in the Schwartz study need to be examined. Residential detoxification lasts about 1 week and was billed at $850–900 in Boston in 1993. Most patients are referred to other treatment after detoxification. Outpatient detoxification has an initial intensive period of daily treatment and then a stabilization period up to a total average duration of 4 months.

Outpatient detoxification involves a lot of individual and group counseling as well as acupuncture. Acupuncture is valuable in the initial retention of patients and helping the patient to be calm and receptive to benefit from counseling and social support. Target cities processed a mixed group of addicts (alcohol 42%, cocaine and crack 33%, heroin 24%). Outpatient use of pharmaceutics is not a useful method of detoxification for most of this population, especially the cocaine subgroup.

Residential detoxification is more expensive than outpatient detoxification. The greater cost is usually

Table 23.2 Percentage of clients readmitted to residential detox or acupuncture within 6 months and the multivariate model odds ratio associated with acupuncture readmission as a function of primary drug. Reproduced with permission from Schwartz et al., 1999

		Residential detox		Acupuncture	Multivariate model
Primary drug	n	Readmitted (%)	n	Readmitted (%)	Odds ratio[a]
Alcohol	2 919	37.3	358	10.9	0.53 (0.29–0.98)
Cocaine	1122	31.0	183	19.7	1.03 (0.52–2.04)
Crack	1099	28.8	223	21.5	0.97 (0.54–1.74)
Heroin	1699	40.6	210	31.4	1.11 (0.63–1.96)

[a]Odds ratio associated with acupuncture admission (95% confidence interval).

Table 23.3 Percentage of clients readmitted to residential detox or acupuncture within 6 months and odds ratio associated with acupuncture as a function of number of detox admissions in the year preceding the index admission. Reproduced with permission from Schwartz *et al.*, 1999

		Residential detox		Acupuncture detox	Multivariate model
Admissions in year preceding the index admission	*n*	Readmitted (%)	*n*	Readmitted (%)[a]	Odds ratio
No acupuncture admissions	3781	0.0	821	0.0 (0.64)	–[b]
One residential detox admission	1326	65.6	113	72.6 (0.13)	1.37 (0.89–2.12)[c]
Two or more residential detox admissions	1518	89.4	61	78.7 (0.01)	0.47 (0.25–0.88)[c]
One acupuncture and no residential detox admissions	124	78.2	69	40.6 (<0.01)	–

[a]Numbers in parentheses under readmitted are the *P* values for a test of the null hypothesis that readmission rates of residential detox and acupuncture clients are similar; [b]too few readmission cases to develop a model; [c]odds ratio (acupuncture clients compared to the reference group of residential detox clients) and 95% confidence interval for the odds ratio.

justified by greater retention. Residential treatment is thought to have more impact on the patient so that further treatment will be sought. This study does not reveal how many successful referrals were made by the residential programs. However, the net effect of those referrals has been measured by the recidivism rate. Outpatient acupuncture treatment is less expensive and more flexible than residential detoxification. Showing that outpatient detoxification is even equally effective on a large scale review has clear policy implications. This finding is especially pertinent because the outcomes are better with the most common drug of abuse (alcohol) and for the most problematic subgroup (multiple prior admissions.)

Tweed study

An article from the Centre for Addiction and Mental Health in Toronto shows that acupuncture is an effective supportive treatment in a comprehensive treatment program for women with concurrent mental health and substance use problems. The Jean Tweed Centre (JTC) in Toronto provides a 21-day residential/day treatment program for women experiencing problems with alcohol and/or drugs. Women are either self-referred to the program or referred by others, such as physicians and self-help groups. The structured program offers daily therapeutic activities that address diverse aspects of women's psychological and physical health. These aspects include group and individual therapy, addiction education, self-esteem, anger management, family and relationships, recreation and leisure in recovery, women's health, life skills and relapse prevention, relaxation and stress management,

sexuality, assertiveness training, journal writing, nature walks, reading, and self-reflection (Courbasson *et al.*, 2007).

A NADA acupuncture component was added to the basic program for eight 21-day cycles. As a control five cycles were monitored without the acupuncture enhancement. Randomizing patients within each cycle was not possible because almost all of the patients wanted the acupuncture experience once they saw it. By alternating cycles the control patients were not aware of acupuncture in any manner. The control patients were given a time for meditation and reflection comparable to the time the other patients spent on acupuncture.

The most commonly abused substance was alcohol (44%). Demographics showed 40% employed, 10% university graduates, and 64% single or separated. Anxiety and depression were the primary mental health findings. Women with psychotic symptoms are excluded from the unit. Results showed that women receiving acupuncture (*n* = 185) reported having reduced physiological cravings for substances, felt significantly less depressed, less anxious, and were better able to reflect on and resolve difficulties than women in the control (*n* = 101).

Possible broader range of effectiveness

NADA acupuncture can have an effect on symptoms not related to addiction. A British researcher, Beverley de Valois, used NADA acupuncture as a treatment for hot flashes and night sweats in women using adjuvant hormonal treatment for breast cancer. Women who had had the treatment were invited to retrospective focus groups. Most of the 16 attendees found that acupuncture was helpful and relaxing. Many reported a reduction in hot flash frequency as well as improvements in overall emotional and physical wellbeing (Walker *et al.*, 2007).

Impact on different abuse patterns

Acupuncture is being used in numerous diverse treatment settings. Outcome reports have been published only to a limited degree because of the journals' emphasis on placebo-controlled studies. Unless otherwise noted, these outcomes are based on clinical experiences at Lincoln Hospital or personal observation of other programs made by the author.

Opiates

Opiate addiction was first treated by Dr. Wen in Hong Kong and has been treated at Lincoln Hospital since 1974. Acupuncture provides nearly complete relief of acute observable opiate withdrawal symptoms in 5–30 minutes. This effect lasts for 8–24 hours. The duration of this effect increases with the number of serial treatments provided. Patients often sleep during the first session and may feel hungry afterward. Patients who are acutely intoxicated at the time acupuncture is administered will behave in a much less intoxicated manner after the session. Surprisingly these patients are gratified by this result, in contrast to patient reports of discomfort after Narcan administration.

Acupuncture for opiate addiction is typically administered two to three times daily in acute inpatient settings. Alternatively, it may be administered only once a day with clonidine or methadone on an outpatient basis. Many patients do well on once-daily acupuncture because they taper their illicit opiate usage over a 3–4-day period. Heroin addicts usually seek detox to reduce the size of their habit, so this arrangement fits their immediate goals. The addition of an acupuncture component to an opiate detoxification program typically leads to a 50% increase in retention for completion of the recommended length of stay.

Alcohol

Directors of the acupuncture social setting detox program conducted by the Tulalip Tribe at Marysville, Washington, have estimated a yearly saving of $148 000 owing to less frequent referrals to hospital programs. Inpatient alcohol detoxification units typically combine acupuncture and herbal "sleep mix" with a tapering benzodiazepine protocol. Patients report fewer symptoms and better sleep. Their vital signs indicate stability; hence, there is much less use of benzodiazepines. One residential program in Connecticut noted a 90% decrease in Valium use when only herbal "sleep mix" was added to their protocol.

Retention of alcohol detox patients generally increases by 50% when an acupuncture component is added to conventional settings. Some alcoholics who receive acupuncture actually report an aversion to alcohol. Woodhull Hospital in Brooklyn reported that 94% of the patients in the acupuncture supplement group remained abstinent as compared to 43% of the control group who only received conventional outpatient services (Lao, 1995). The widely quoted controlled study by Bullock *et al.* (1989) showed 52% retention of alcoholism patients as compared to a 2% sham acupuncture retention rate.

Cocaine

Cocaine addiction has provided the most important challenge for conventional treatment because there are no significant pharmaceutical agents for this condition. Acupuncture patients report more calmness and reduced craving for cocaine even after the first treatment. The acute psychological indications of cocaine toxicity are visibly reduced during the treatment session. This improvement is sustained for a variable length of time after the first acupuncture treatment. After three to seven sequential treatments, the anti-craving effect is more-or-less continuous as long as acupuncture is received on a regular basis.

Urinalysis outcomes were examined for Lincoln Hospital patients using cocaine or crack who had more than 20 treatment visits and were active during the 1-week study period in March 1991. At Lincoln, patients typically provide urine samples for testing during each visit. Of the entire study group of 226 patients, 149 had more than 80% negative tests during their entire treatment involvement. Of the remaining patients, 39 had at least 80% negative tests during the 2 weeks prior to data collection.

Methamphetamine

Methamphetamine-using patients experience similar dramatic increases in treatment retention. The Hooper Foundation, the public detoxification center

239

in Portland, Oregon, reported 5% retention of meth-amphetamine users prior to the use of acupuncture and 90% retention after adding acupuncture to their protocol. Increased psychological stability and decreased craving were cited.

Methadone

Methadone maintenance patients receive acupuncture in a number of different settings. Patients report a decrease in secondary symptoms of methadone use such as constipation, sweating, and sleep problems. Typically there is a substantial drop in requests for symptomatic medication. Treatment staffs usually notice decreased hostility and increased compliance in methadone–acupuncture patients. The most important impact of acupuncture in maintenance programs is reduction of secondary substance abuse – primarily involving cocaine, even in patients with minimal motivation (Margolin et al., 1993). Reductions in secondary alcohol use are also frequently described. Acupuncture is effective with patients in any dosage level of methadone.

Lincoln Hospital used methadone and acupuncture together from 1974 to 1978. Several hundred methadone maintenance patients were detoxified during that period using tapered doses of methadone and acupuncture. Based on our previous non-acupuncture experience, we observed that patients were much more comfortable and confident when they received acupuncture. Even though patients regularly complained about withdrawal symptoms, there were very few requests for dosage increase. The large majority of patients completed the entire detoxification process and provided at least one negative toxicology after the cessation of methadone.

Methadone dosages were decreased 5–10 mg per week, with a slower schedule during the final 10 mg. Starting levels of methadone ranged from 20 mg to 90 mg with a median of 60 mg. Acupuncture was provided 6 days per week and continued up to 2 months after the last methadone dose. Although many of these patients had been referred for administrative or mandatory detoxification owing to secondary drug use, toxicologies were usually drug-free after the first 2–3 weeks of treatment.

Methadone withdrawal is notable for unpredictable variations in symptoms and significant post-withdrawal malaise. Symptoms such as depression, low energy, and atypical insomnia are quite difficult to manage without acupuncture. Patients are usually fearful and have considerable difficulty participating in psychosocial therapy during the detoxification period. Acupuncture is particularly valuable in the methadone-to-abstinence (MTA) setting, because the patient's future wellbeing depends on their ability to utilize psychosocial support during the detoxification period.

Marijuana

At Lincoln, we have had a significant number of primary marijuana users seeking care. These patients usually report a rapid reduction in craving and improved mental wellbeing. Secondary marijuana use is usually eliminated along with the detoxification of the primary drug (e.g. cocaine).

Tobacco

The use of the NADA protocol can be helpful in residential treatment where the patients are not able to continue tobacco use. Its use in a 90-day inpatient, tobacco-free, dual diagnosis treatment program demonstrated improved retention in treatment with longer length of stay and improved participation in those patients who received the needles. The use of the acupuncture appeared to help both those planning to re-start smoking after discharge as well as those wanting to continue abstinence after discharge. For those planning to smoke as soon as possible after discharge, significantly more successfully completed the program if they had eight or more acudetox sessions, 57% versus 24% with fewer than eight sessions ($P < 0.0001$). For those planning to remain abstinent, significantly more successfully completed if they had eight or more sessions, 90% versus 69% with fewer than eight sessions ($P < 0.05$). The patients receiving needles reported significant improvement in sleep, anger, pain, concentration, and energy compared to those not receiving needles. Combined with education, the acudetox allows patients to move forward in their stage of change regarding tobacco use after discharge (Stuyt & Meeker, 2006).

For patients in outpatient treatment who are motivated to quit smoking, the NADA protocol can be very helpful. Bier et al. demonstrated that the combination of acupuncture with education resulted in an effectiveness rate of 40% cessation and 53% post-treatment reduction in total cigarettes smoked. This result is comparable to that produced by pharmacological treatment of nicotine addiction combined with behavioral support (Bier et al., 2002).

Clinical effectiveness

Retention and recidivism

The beneficial effects of acupuncture in cocaine treatment often lead to dramatic increases in retention of cocaine-using patients. Women in Need, a program located near Times Square in New York, reported the following outcome figures in their treatment for pregnant crack-using women.

1. Patients with conventional outpatient treatment averaged three visits/year.
2. Patients who took acupuncture in addition to conventional treatment averaged 27 visits/year.
3. Patients who participated in an educational component in addition to acupuncture and conventional treatment averaged 67 visits/year. Patients averaging three visits per year would be unlikely to participate in an educational component.

Therefore, it seems likely that the increased retention correlated with acupuncture set a foundation for successful participation in the educational component.

Acupuncture detoxification programs report substantial reduction in their recidivism rates. The Hooper Foundation cited a decrease from 25% to 6% in comparison to the previous non-acupuncture year. Kent-Sussex Detoxification Center (in Delaware) reported a decrease in recidivism from 87% to 18%.

Substance Abuse Recovery (Flint, MI) noted that 83% of a group of 100 General Motors employees were drug- and alcohol-free productive workers a year after entering acupuncture-based treatment. Most of these patients had repeated prior attempts at treatment and frequent relapse. The entire 17% failure group had less than five program visits. Of the success group, 74% continued to attend AA and NA meetings after completing the treatment program. Programs specifically designed for adolescents, such as the Alcohol Treatment Center in Chicago and a Job Corps-related program in Brooklyn, have shown retention rates comparable to adult programs.

Frequency and duration of treatment

Acupuncture treatment is generally made available to patients 5–6 days per week. Lincoln offers treatment during an 8-hour period, but many smaller programs offer acupuncture during 1–2-hour time periods each day. Morning treatment hours seem to be more bene-ficial. Active patients will receive treatment 3–6 times per week. Initially, acupuncture should be defined as an expected part of the program. If one describes acupuncture as a voluntary or optional part of the program, this description is easily misunderstood by a crisis-ridden addicted person. Such a person cannot handle choice and ambivalence effectively. Initially, patients need direction and clarity. They should be asked to sit in the treatment room without needles if they are unsure about receiving acupuncture. New patients will learn about acupuncture from other more experienced patients and they will observe the process of treatment on a first hand basis. Sometimes a patient will be willing to try just one or two needles at first. Eventually a high percentage of patients will be active participants.

The duration of acupuncture treatment depends on many factors. Inpatient programs will want to stress acupuncture in the beginning for detoxification and stabilization and prior to discharge for separation anxiety. Outpatients in a drug-free setting typically receive acupuncture for 1–3 months on an active basis. About 10% of these outpatients will choose to take acupuncture for more than 1 year if possible. Such patients usually have significant difficulties bonding on a psychosocial basis.

Lincoln Hospital used to provide acupuncture 7 days a week for the benefit of patients in crisis. Eventually it became clear that full weekend coverage did not appreciably improve clinical results. Patients who began the treatment program on Friday have essentially the same outcomes as patients who begin the program on Monday. Acupuncture is not primarily a dose-related phenomenon as is pharmaceutical treatment. Acupuncture more appropriately represents a qualitative service comparable to a school room class or psychotherapy session.

Patients who are using acupuncture appropriately should be allowed to choose how often they receive acupuncture treatment. Duration of the effect of each individual treatment increases as the patient becomes more stable. Since this treatment is a private personal process, it should come under the patient's control as soon as possible. Some patients will discontinue acupuncture too quickly, but they should be able to learn from the resultant loss of wellbeing to make better decisions in the future. Participation in acupuncture is a different kind of decision than participation in group or individual psychotherapy.

Effect on the whole treatment process

Relapsing patients are often able to continue to be involved in acupuncture even though they are no longer constructive participants in psychotherapy. Acupuncture patients do not tend to burn their bridges as quickly; hence, retention and eventual success are increased in an acupuncture-based program. A wide range of patients can be accepted for the initial stage of treatment because there is no verbal motivational requirement. Also, acupuncture is effective for most drugs and a wide range of psychological states. A low threshold, easily staffed, program can be established for new patients.

Ambivalent street-wise patients find the acupuncture setting almost impossible to manipulate. The setting is so soothing and self-protective that even extremely antisocial people are able to fit in. Problems relating to language and cultural differences are diminished. For new patients, frequent acupuncture treatment permits the gradual completion of assessment on a more accurate basis. Patients can be evaluated and triaged according to their daily response to treatment and testing rather than merely on the basis of the initial interview.

The tolerant, non-verbal aspect of acupuncture facilitates retention during periods when the patient would otherwise be ambivalent, fearful, or resentful within a more intense verbal interpersonal setting. Ear acupuncture makes it easy to provide outpatient treatment on demand, without appointments, while the patients are being acclimated to the interpersonal treatment setting. Patients are often willing to be tested even when they know that their toxicology result is positive, thereby showing respect for the value system of the overall treatment process. Those same patients may be unable or unwilling to share their crisis and failure verbally until they have time to reach more solid ground. In the acupuncture setting, time is on our side.

Acupuncture has many characteristics in common with twelve-step programs such as AA and NA. It uses a group process in a tolerant, supportive, and present time-oriented manner. Participation is independent of diagnosis and level of recovery. Both approaches are simple, reinforcing, nurturing, and conveniently available. The emphasis on self-responsibility is common to both systems. In practice, acupuncture provides an excellent foundation for twelve-step recovery. Patients seem less fearful and more receptive when they first enter the meetings. The traditional advice "listen to learn and learn to listen" fits this model well.

Acupuncture reduces white knuckle sobriety considerably. There is less guarding and greater ability to support each other warmly. The increased ability to use twelve-step meetings provides more stable support for continuing treatment on an outpatient basis.

AIDS-related treatment

Easy access and better retention encourage the outpatient management of difficult patients with less need for additional drugs or services. One can select times for hospitalization more appropriately. An outpatient continuum also facilitates primary healthcare management for AIDS, tuberculosis, and STDs. Acupuncture is used in a large proportion of AIDS prevention and outreach programs in New York and London, as well as other cities. These facilities include needle exchange and harm reduction programs; recovery readiness and pre-treatment programs, as well as health service providers for HIV-positive and AIDS patients. In relationship to addiction treatment, each of these programs faces similar dilemmas. Their clients are likely to have ever-increasing addiction-related problems; however, these clients minimize their need for help. Furthermore, the clients are often overwhelmed by problems relating to immune deficiency. Acupuncture is uniquely appropriate entry-level treatment because it is convenient, relaxing, and not dependent on any mutually agreed upon diagnosis or treatment plan. Acupuncture also provides treatment for emotions such as fear and depression. Many of these clients may be ashamed and confused, not knowing how to describe their ever-changing feelings in a conventional therapeutic context.

Maternal treatment

The use of acupuncture has led to a considerable expansion of treatment services for cocaine- and crack-using women. The Lincoln program was cited as a model innovative program for prenatal care in a monograph, *Hospital and Community Partnership*, issued by the American Hospital Association in 1991.

The average birth weight for babies at Lincoln with more than ten maternal visits is 6 pounds, 10 ounces. The average birth weight for less than ten visits is 4 pounds, 8 ounces, which is typical of high-risk cocaine mothers. There is a high correlation between clean toxicologies, retention in the clinic program, and higher birth weights. Of our pregnant intakes, 76% are retained in long-term treatment and give birth to nontoxic infants.

Premature birth is a serious health risk. The Hospital of St. Raphael in New Haven used the Lincoln acupuncture model for 8 years. The director of obstetrics, Dr. Wilfredo Requero, reported a drop in perinatal death rate from 18.5 to 7.1 from 1990 to 1992, following the use of acupuncture and other innovative outreach techniques. Special acupuncture-based components have also been developed for women with children in long-term foster care in the Drug Strategies Institute program in Baltimore. Acupuncture is used during high-risk prenatal home visits conducted by public health nurses in Washington State.

Female patients are often trapped in destructive and exploitative relationships and therefore have special difficulty with any therapeutic relationship. A consistently tolerant and non-confrontational approach prepares the way to establish a trauma survivor support service for patients at an early sobriety stage of recovery. The supportive atmosphere makes it relatively easy for patients to keep children with them during treatment activities. The acupuncture point formula used for addictions is also specific for the kind of emotional and muscular guarding associated with early sexual trauma. These patients will suffer intermittent crises and experience profound challenges to their physical and spiritual identity. All of their relationships will be strained and transformed. Acupuncture is a very appropriate adjunct to trauma survivors' support work.

Criminal justice-related treatment

Patients referred by court-related agencies often enter treatment in total denial or with a basic conflict with the referring agency. The non-verbal aspect of acupuncture allows the intake staff to get beyond these protests and offer acupuncture for stress relief instead of forcing the issue. By using acupuncture one is able to wait until the patients feel more comfortable and less threatened so they can admit their addiction and ask for help.

Addicts have trouble with discipline. They need order in their lives but cannot develop internal structure. Addicts have trouble liking themselves. They are depressed and depersonalized, and cannot accept good things. The end result is self-destruction and adherence to a masochistic lifestyle. The ability to like oneself builds the foundation for internal discipline. Acupuncture provides a significant advantage in meeting the paradoxical requirement of tough love. Verbal interpersonal intensity is reduced. Patients feel that

their immediate needs and their urges toward independence have been satisfied. A tolerant, flexible atmosphere exists. Acupuncture delivered in a consistent and caring manner provides the basis for the love side of the equation. The foundation for the development of more effective discipline has been set.

Frequent urine testing provides an objective non-personalized measure of success that can be accepted equally by all parties. In this system, the counselor is the good cop and the urine machine is the bad cop. The counseling process can be totally separated from the process of judgment and evaluation. Discipline is separated from the difficulties of interpersonal relationships. Within this context, discipline or leniency by the judicial authority leads to constructive, not escapist, behavior. Positive toxicology results are primarily used to require a more prolonged or intense commitment to treatment.

The well-known Drug Court program in Miami uses the acupuncture-based model we have described. This program diverts thousands of felony drug possession arrestees into treatment each year. More than 50% of these patients eventually graduate the program on the basis of providing 90 consecutive negative toxicologies over the period of a year or more. Drug Court diversion and treatment programs have been established in thousands of settings nationwide. This expansion represents a valuable increased commitment to addiction treatment throughout the US. The majority of the largest and oldest Drug Court programs (Miami, Broward, Las Vegas, and Portland) used acupuncture as a primary component of their protocol. Acupuncture is also being used in many jails and prisons in the US and abroad. A follow-up study in Santa Barbara, CA, for example, showed that women who received acupuncture were 50% less likely to be re-arrested after being released from the county jail (Brumbaugh, 1993). Sex offenders in a maximum security prison in Oak Park Heights, Minnesota, received acupuncture on a regular basis. There was a significant reduction in anger and violent intrusive sexual fantasies as compared to a control population (Culliton & Leaf, 1996, personal communication).

Coexisting mental health problems
Serious and persistent mental illness
There is little substantive published literature on the use of acupuncture in the treatment of primary psychiatric problems. During the past 20 years at Lincoln

Hospital we have noted numerous effects of acupuncture on patients with coexisting addiction and psychiatric conditions. Agitated patients routinely fall asleep while receiving acupuncture. Chronic paranoid patients have a higher than average retention rate. We have seen many examples in which grossly paranoid addicted persons have made special efforts to access acupuncture treatment. Our patients do not express paranoid ideas about acupuncture although they may remain otherwise quite paranoid. These patients experience a gradual reduction in psychiatric symptoms as well as a typical response in terms of craving and withdrawal symptoms. Psychotropic medication does not interact with acupuncture. Patients should remain on psychotropic medicines while using acupuncture, since the improved level of compliance that correlates with acupuncture often makes the process of medication more reliable and effective.

A pilot program used acupuncture according to the Lincoln model in the public mental health system in Waco, Texas, with a goal of the reduction in the rate of re-hospitalization. Highly disturbed, non-compliant, drug-addicted, severely and persistent mentally ill (SPMI) patients were deliberately selected for this trial. Rates of hospitalization dropped from 50% to 6% in the group of 15 patients. Harbor House, a residential program for mentally ill chemical abusers (MICA) in the Bronx, reported a 50% reduction in psychiatric hospitalization in the first year of acupuncture utilization. Their dropout rate during the first month of treatment decreased by 85%. The patients in Waco, Texas, participated more enthusiastically. They listened better and were more cooperative. The context of treatment became even more important to these patients.

Acupuncture has an obvious advantage in the treatment of MICA patients, especially those with SPMI. MICA patients have particular difficulty with bonding and verbal relationships. Acupuncture facilitates the required lenient supportive process; however, at the same time it provides an acute anti-craving treatment that is also necessary. The use of acupuncture can resolve the contradictory needs of MICA patients.

In the past decade the NADA acupuncture protocol has been widely used in large general psychiatric hospitals in Germany and Scandinavia. In Sweden, some hospitals have requested training for 50–150 nurses. Training is conducted for 24 nurses at a time. One Swedish nurse summarized the changes: "Acupuncture reduces anxiety even for patients who are waiting for hours in the emergency unit. With quite aggressive people we use acupuncture. It seems to reduce hallucinations and make them less frightening. The more paranoid the patient is, the greater the effect from acupuncture. Depressed patients often get more active. Their antidepressant medications seem to work better. Prescriptions for benzodiazepines are often reduced."

Dr. Elizabeth Stuyt of Pueblo State Hospital in Colorado reports similarly that "the worse patients seem to do better with acupuncture."

Trauma and violence

The World Trade Center in New York City was attacked on September 11, 2001. St. Vincent's Hospital became the receiving hospital where volunteer medical personnel gathered. As the stress intensified, a nurse from the hospital's alcoholism program offered their acupuncture protocol for stress relief for staff and visitors. More than 1000 people received the ear acupuncture protocol during the next 2 weeks. This response led to a realization that this protocol has a much wider applicability than just addiction-related treatment. A full-time acupuncture service is still used by the New York City Fire Department for 9/11-related stress. Acupuncturists were invited to New Orleans after hurricane Katrina, specifically to treat the homeless, and police and fire personnel. These treatments have been so successful that the medical board and the State of Louisiana are planning to have all first responders and community members have access to ear acupuncture training.

In recent years the ear acupuncture protocol has been used in a wide variety of settings: parenting classes (Washington), suicide prevention in a security force (India), schools for violent youth (England), recovery programs for commercial sex workers (San Francisco and Ethiopia), street children (Mexico, Peru, and Philippines), victims of sexual abuse (US), and menopause-like side effects of tamoxifen (UK).

Ear acupuncture was used for stress relief for the inmates of Dartmoor Prison (UK) in the 1990s. Correction officials discovered a dramatic reduction of inmate violence and a greater interest in drug-free dormitories. Support for acupuncture spread quickly through the prison system. By 2006, 130 prisons in England were using ear acupuncture. More than 500 correctional officers have been trained to provide ear acupuncture in the prisons. The atmosphere between the officers and inmates has changed very positively as a result of this systemic transformation.

Psychosocial mechanisms of action

Personal behavior

It is essential to understand acupuncture's psychological and social mechanisms of action to use this modality effectively. Acupuncture has an impact on the patients' thoughts and feelings that is different from conventional pharmaceutical treatments. Subsequently, one can discuss how the use of acupuncture has a valuable and profound impact on the dynamics of the treatment processes as a whole. We should emphasize that acupuncture for addictions is provided in a group setting. The new acupuncture patient is immediately introduced to a calm and supportive group process. Patients describe acupuncture as a unique kind of balancing experience. "I was relaxed but alert. I was able to relax without losing control." Patients who are depressed or tired say that they feel more energetic. This encouraging and balancing group experience becomes a critically important basis for the entire treatment process.

The perception that a person can be both relaxed and alert is rather unusual in western culture. We are used to associating relaxation with somewhat lazy or spacey behavior and alertness with a certain degree of anxiety. The relaxed and alert state is basic to the concept of health in all Asian culture. Acupuncture encourages a centering, focusing process that is typical of meditation and yoga. Therapists report that patients are able to listen and remember what we tell them. Restless impulsive behavior is greatly reduced. On the other hand, discouragement and apathy are reduced as well. It is a balancing, centering process.

One of the striking characteristics of the NADA acupuncture treatment setting is that each patient seems comfortable in their own space and in their own thinking process. One patient explained, "I sat and thought about things in a slow way like I did when I was 10 years old." Acupuncture treatment causes the perception of various relaxing bodily processes. Patients gradually gain confidence that their minds and bodies can function in a more balanced and autonomous manner. A hopeful process is developed on a private and personal basis, laying a foundation for the development of increasing self-awareness and self-responsibility.

Addiction is about trading present experience for past and future realities. Patients hang onto the present, because the past and future seem to offer nothing but pain. Unfortunately conventional treatment efforts tend to focus on assessment of past activities and planning for the future. Patients are obsessed by present sensations and problems. They often feel alienated and resentful that we cannot focus on their immediate needs. Acupuncture is one of the only ways that treatment staff can respond to a patient's immediate needs without using addictive drugs. We can meet the patient in the present time reality – validating their needs and providing substantial relief. Once a comfortable day-to-day reality support is established, we can approach past and future issues with a better alliance with the patient.

The nature of recovery from addiction is that patients often have quickly changing needs for crisis relief and wellness treatment. Many persons in recovery have relatively high levels of wellness functioning. Even so, a crisis of craving or past association may reappear at any time. Conventional treatment settings have trouble coping with such intense and confusing behavioral swings. Often merely the fear of a possible crisis can sabotage clinical progress. Acupuncture provides either crisis or wellness treatment using the same ear point formula. The non-verbal, present-time aspects of the treatment make it easy to respond to a patient in whatever stage of crisis or denial that may exist.

Internal change

Patients readily accept that it is possible to improve their acute addictive status. They seek external help to provide hospitalization and medication for withdrawal symptoms. The challenge develops when they encounter the necessity for internal change. Addicts and others perceive themselves as being unable to change from within. Their whole life revolves around powerful external change agents. Each addict remembers countless examples of weakness, poor choices, and overwhelming circumstance that lead to the conclusion that they cannot help themselves become drug-free. Indeed, many influential members of society agree that once an addict, always an addict.

Many of the complicating factors in our patients' lives echo this challenge of past internal failure. Persons leaving prison are confronted with a bleak uncaring world. Their own feelings of inadequacy frequently become so overwhelming that a return to prior drug and alcohol use may occur within hours of release. When a person learns they are HIV-positive, their self-esteem drops precipitously. A drug-abusing seropositive person typically feels punished for past weaknesses by their HIV status. How can such a person have the confidence to seek out internal personal strength in the future?

Victims of incest and childhood abuse are well known to have been robbed of an internal sense of value. Their innermost physical and emotional responses have become sources of betrayal. It is not surprising, therefore, that a large majority of female addicts have been injured in this way.

All of us pass through a period of fearful internal inadequacy during the process of adolescence. Powerful trends of self-doubt and internal vulnerability are manifested at that time. No amount of external support will eliminate the need to confront internal fears on a private, personal basis. Hopefully, adolescents gradually learn to accept and appreciate themselves. They may also learn to rely on internal resources in their efforts to improve their circumstances. This archetypal challenge of adolescence is echoed in the struggle to become drug-free, as well as countless other efforts to become more internally resourceful and resilient in daily life. The question "does treatment work?" is comparable to asking whether internal self-discovery and re-definition are possible.

Acupuncture provides uniquely valuable assistance in coping with this challenge of internal re-definition. Patients often begin acupuncture treatment seeking external escape and sedation as they do when they use drugs. When there is a rapid calming effect, they often assume there was some sort of chemical agent in the acupuncture needle. After a few treatments they come to the astonishing conclusion that acupuncture works by revealing and employing their internal capability rather than by inserting an external chemical. Patients begin to realize that their mind is capable of calm, focused thoughts on a regular basis. There seems to be no indication of permanent damage to their thinking and consciousness. On the contrary, their ability to listen, think, and learn seems to be growing steadily each day.

Inevitably, a critical point will be reached. The newly drug-free patient will enter treatment one day with the feeling that "I don't deserve to be relaxed today because of all the bad things that I have done in the past." Such feelings frequently sabotage early

treatment achievements. In an acupuncture program, however, the patient realizes that their mind can become calm and clear even in the face of such overwhelming feelings of inadequacy. This lesson demonstrates that change based on internal resources is possible. In other words, successful treatment is possible. Regular participation in acupuncture helps a patient take advantage of their internal resources much faster than conventional treatment processes. This effect contributes to the calm cooperative atmosphere in most acupuncture settings. It reduces dropouts based on fears of failure and low self-esteem that typify the early stage of treatment.

Foundation for autonomy

The use of acupuncture sets a foundation so that patients can have more autonomy in developing their own plan of treatment. A calmer, less resentful atmosphere is created. The tolerant, self-validating process helps patients find their level and type of involvement in a productive manner. Patients must choose to talk sincerely with their counselor just as they must choose to avoid temptation and return to the program each day. These choices may fluctuate widely and be mistaken at times, but such independence is the only path toward growing up. When a program properly encourages structure but ignores the patient's own independence efforts, these actions undermine future success. Acupuncture creates a better atmosphere so that treatment staff can spend their energies helping patients make choices rather than being fatigued by trying to impose authority on a resistant clientele.

One can describe acupuncture as a foundation for psychosocial rehabilitation. In the beginning of treatment, building a proper foundation is very important. If we are building on a weak "sandy" personality, work on the foundation may take many months or years before it is strong enough to support any significant psychosocial treatment efforts. However, once a foundation is established, the focus of treatment should shift away from acupuncture toward building a house of psychosocial recovery on that foundation. When one of our patients testified at city council hearings, she described how important it was to attend daily NA meetings and barely mentioned acupuncture. For a patient with 3 months' sobriety this emphasis was appropriate. Of course, during her first 2 weeks in our program, she was quite angry and ambivalent and was only able to relate to the acupuncture component of the program.

Non-verbal therapy

Acupuncture is a non-verbal type of therapy. Words and verbal relationships are not necessary components of this treatment. We do not mean that the therapist should not talk with the patient. Verbal interaction can be quite flexible so that a patient who does not feel like talking can be accommodated easily and naturally. Acupuncture will be just as effective even when the patient lies to us.

The most difficult paradox in this field is the common reality that addicted persons usually deny their need for help. Such patients do not say anything helpful to the treatment process. Nevertheless, resistant patients often find themselves in a treatment setting due to referral or other pressures. Using acupuncture can bypass much of the verbal denial and resistance that otherwise limit retention of new and relapsed patients. Addicts are frequently ambivalent. Acupuncture helps us reach the needy part of their psyche that wants help. Acupuncture can reduce stress and craving so that patients gradually become more ready to participate in the treatment process.

Addiction patients often cannot tolerate intense interpersonal relationships. Using a conventional one-to-one approach often creates a brittle therapeutic connection. It is easily broken by events or any stress. Patients have difficulty trusting a counselor's words when they can hardly trust themselves. Even after confiding to a counselor during an intake session, a patient may feel frightened and confused about expanding that relationship. Many of their concerns are so complex and troublesome that talking honestly about their lives could be difficult in the best of circumstances. The ambivalence typical of addicts makes it easy to develop misunderstandings. All of these factors support the usefulness of non-verbal technique during early and critical relapse phases of treatment and critical periods of relapse.

A woman who was 6 months' pregnant entered our clinic several years ago. She said, "I can't tell you much about myself because my husband is out in the street with a baseball bat; he'll hit me in my knees if I say too much." We provided an emergency acupuncture treatment and conducted a simplified intake interview. Two weeks later this patient told us, "This is my husband, he doesn't have a drug problem, but he is nervous, can you help him?" Both of them received acupuncture that day. The woman needed non-verbal access to treatment because of real physical danger. Overprotective spouses often forcefully oppose all social contacts outside the marriage. This patient was protected because there was no premature verbal bonding that would have threatened the husband. The whole process was so supportive that the husband was able to trust his wife and seek help himself. Like many fearful people, he was literally unable to make any verbal approach on his own.

A certain mistake in treatment interaction should be highlighted. One should avoid re-verbalizing the acupuncture interaction. Anxiety and depression are common indications for acupuncture. However, it is a mistake to require that the patient admit to anxiety or depression to qualify for acupuncture. Addicts who have significant anxiety or depression will usually not admit these feelings. They will avoid anyone who asks such questions. At a later stage of sobriety and recovery, talking about these feelings will be important, but at an early stage of treatment verbalizing these feelings can lead to dropout. Likewise, it is not productive to ask patients why they have missed a previous acupuncture session. Use the advantage that acupuncture will be effective even if we don't know the issues involved.

Improving treatment program function

Treatment programs without acupuncture are compelled to screen for patients who are able to talk readily with authority figures. Many verbally needy patients become quite dependent on the program and quite involved with numerous staff members. Such patients may be the focus of many conferences, but they are often too needy to remain drug-free outside the hospital. In contrast, acupuncture-assisted intake can retain patients who are relatively more paranoid, independent, assertive, and hostile. Noisy, troublesome patients who are frustrated with the world and with themselves actually may be more likely to sustain a drug-free lifestyle than patients with verbal dependency needs.

Acupuncture helps a program develop an underlying environment of acceptance, tolerance, and patience. There is ample space for the ambivalence and temporary setbacks that are a necessary part of any transformation. Patients can have a quiet day by attending the program and receiving acupuncture without having to discuss their status with a therapeutic authority figure. Since acupuncture reduces the agitated defensive tone in the whole clinical environment, patients are able to interact with each other on a much more comfortable level. Their increased ability to listen to others and accept internal changes has a profound effect on the quality and depth of communication in group therapy sessions and twelve-step meetings. Being a sympathetic witness to a description of past tragedies can be easier to achieve in a setting that is not charged with defensive self-centered associations. The primary community agenda can focus on the acceptance of each person and a tolerant encouragement of change rather than coping with defensive and antagonistic interactions.

Clinical examples

Using acupuncture can be a catalyst for unique personal developmental as the following two examples show.

In the first case, the author was demonstrating ear acupuncture at a dual-diagnosis program in a university medical center. The patients were able to see sample acupuncture treatments, but they were not specifically introduced to me. After sitting for a few minutes, one woman asked me in a strong voice, "Does this treatment help incest survivors?" I answered "sometimes." The patient volunteered for the treatment and soon after she fell asleep. Later on, she asked me if she could talk to the local professional acupuncturists who were sitting nearby. She said "This treatment helps me; I want to make an appointment in your office… I can pay for the treatment." I was impressed and shared this experience with the rest of the staff.

The staff replied that they could have made the appointment and could have paid for the treatment. The process of observing and requesting acupuncture was part of this patient's survival process. She was able to express herself and make decisions on her own. A potentially cumbersome therapeutic and case management issue was resolved by the patient's healthy initiative.

In the second case, the author was visiting an outpatient treatment program run for the Cook County Jail in Chicago. In an effort to reduce overcrowding, jail officials would release 50 pre-trial inmates per month to a brief intervention program. Part of the program was a large acupuncture group. One of the patients came to me and said, "Do you see the blue ribbon on my belt. That means I belong to XXX gang. I have to kill anyone with a red ribbon on his belt, like this guy in YYY gang walking toward us." I didn't know what to do. "Why are you telling me these things?" I said. The two men met in the middle of the room. They gave each other a big hug. "This is a peace zone," they said. "Who made it a peace zone?" I said. "We did," they replied. Gang members are separated in jail lock-up, but referral to the program had not taken that simple measure. The acupuncture led to self-affirming, gentle communication, and a simple special outcome that no amount of counseling could have achieved.

Conclusion: patients' own stories

To really know the power of acupuncture in the treatment of addiction, listen to clients who have experienced it as part of their recovery transformation.

Client 1

Acupuncture has gotten me where I don't have a really manic life and I'm not depressed. I'm able to deal with everything that comes my direction because I have a lot of support also. I am energized, not miserable. I feel great about myself. I can smile today and the smile has feelings behind it. Acupuncture has hooked me up spiritually. I found my higher power – God – and he leads me each and every day.

Client 2

I was into prostitution and pornography – a violent woman… I behave differently today. I live with principles that I believe were ignited, sparked in me with acupuncture. As cumulative as acupuncture is, it has reached me in this level that I am able to change my beliefs more comfortably. I am given courage to take a look at my beliefs and empower myself, and now empower other women. I stand under reality strong truth that women can recover, and I know that acupuncture is the most valuable tool I know for recovery.

Client 3

Talking to [counselors], getting acupuncture treatment – hate, anger, jealousy, vengefulness, vindictiveness, all that changed into compassion and love. The acupuncture treatment just helped the process change in the detoxin (sic) and everything.

Client 4

Someone helped me find a simple way to just be with myself long enough to see what I need to work on – where I was wounded and how I could heal. And it is like a quiet way for one person to help to give treatment to another person. Acupuncture is a way to help sand the rough edges of what is going to be changed. It will give you a place to take all your other things into, and help create the change

Source: Voyles, 2000.

References

Avants, S. K., Margolin, A., Hofford, T. R. & Kosten, T. R. (2000). A randomized controlled trial of auricular acupuncture for cocaine dependence. *Archives of Internal Medicine*, **160**(115), 14–28.

Bier, I. D., Wilson, J., Studt, P. & Shakleton, M. (2002). Auricular acupuncture, education, and smoking cessation: a randomized, sham-controlled trial. *American Journal of Public Health*, **92**, 1642–7.

Brewington, V., Smith, M. & Lipton, D. (1994). Acupuncture as a detoxification treatment: an analysis of controlled research. *Journal of Substance Abuse Treatment*, **11**(4), 298–307.

Brumbaugh, A. (1993). *Transformation and Recovery: A Guide for the Design and Development of Acupuncture Based Chemical Dependency Treatment Programs.* Santa Barbara, CA: Still Point Press.

Bullock, M. L., Umen, A. J., Culliton, P. D. & Olander, R. T. (1987). Acupuncture treatment of alcoholism recidivism: a pilot study. *Alcoholism: Clinical and Experimental Research*, **11**(3), 292–5.

Bullock, M. L., Cullington, P. D. & Olander, R. T. (1989). Controlled trial of acupuncture for severe recidivist alcoholism. *Lancet*, **24**, 1435–9.

Bullock, M. L., Kiresuk, T. J., Sherman, R. E. *et al.* (2002). A large randomized placebo controlled study of auricular acupuncture for alcohol dependence. *Journal of Substance Abuse Treatment*, **22**(2), 71–7.

Courbasson, C., Araulo de Sorkin, A., Dullerud, B. & ssVan Wyk, L. (2007). Acupuncture treatment with concurrent substance use and anxiety/depression: an effective alternative therapy? *Evidence-based Practices in Family and Community Health*, **30**(2), 112–20.

Eory, A. (1995). *Society for Acupuncture Research*, discussion.

Konefal, J., Duncan, R. & Clemence, C. (1995). Comparison of three levels of auricular acupuncture in an outpatient substance abuse treatment program. *Alternative Medicine Journal*, **2**, 5.

Landgren, K. (2008). *Ear Acupuncture: A Practical Guide.* Edinburgh: Churchill Livingstone.

Lao, H. (1995). A retrospective study on the use of acupuncture for the prevention of alcoholic recidivism. *American Journal of Acupuncture*, **23**(1), 29–33.

Margolin, A., Avants, K. S., Chang, P. & Kosten, T. R. (1993). Acupuncture for the treatment of cocaine dependence in methadone-maintained patients. *The American Journal on Addictions*, **2**(3), 194–201.

Margolin, A., Avants, S. K. & Holford, T. R. (2002a). Interpreting conflicting findings from clinical trials of auricular acupuncture for cocaine addiction: does treatment context influence outcome? *Journal of Alternative and Complementary Medicine*, **8**(2), 111–21.

Margolin, A., Kleber, H. D., Avants, S. K. *et al.* (2002b). Acupuncture for the treatment of cocaine addiction. A randomized controlled trial. *Journal of the American Medical Association*, **287**, 55–63.

Omura, Y., Smith, M., Wong, F. *et al.* (1975). Electro acupuncture for drug addiction withdrawal. *Acupuncture and Electrotherapeutics Research International Journal*, **1**, 231–3.

Schwartz, M., Saitz, R., Mulvey, K. & Brannigan, P. (1999). The value of acupuncture detoxification programs in a substance abuse treatment system. *Journal of Substance Abuse Treatment*, **17**(4), 305–12.

Smith, M. & Lee, C. (2003). *The Reed Academy Experience.* Columbia, MO: NADA Clearinghouse.

Smith, M. O. (1995). *Nature of Qi.* Society for Acupuncture Research, proceedings. Vancouver: J & M Reports.

Smith, M. O. & Khan, I. (1989). Acupuncture program for treatment of drug addicted persons. *Bulletin on Narcotics*, XL, **1**.

Stuyt, E. B. & Meeker, J. L. (2006). Benefits of auricular acupuncture in tobacco-free inpatient dual-diagnosis treatment. *Journal of Dual Diagnosis*, **2**, 41–52.

Voyles, C. (2000). *Some Lessons Learned.* Vancouver: J & M Reports.

Walker, G., de Valois, B., Davies, R., Young, T. & Maher, J. (2007). Ear acupuncture for hot flushes – the perceptions of women with breast cancer. *Complementary Therapies in Clinical Practice*, **13**, 250–7.

Washburn, A. M., Fullilove, M. T., Keenan, P. A. *et al.* (1993). Acupuncture heroin detoxification: a single-blind clinical trial. *Journal of Substance Abuse Treatment*, **10**, 345–51.

Wen, H. L. & Cheung, S. Y. C. (1973). Treatment of drug addiction by acupuncture and electrical stimulation. *Asian Journal of Medicine*, **9**, 139–41.

Index

abstinence
  as a therapeutic concept, 48
  meanings and connotations, 45
abstinence as a goal
  Alcoholics Anonymous (AA), 46
  defining abstinence, 45
  harm reduction model, 47
  historical concepts of abstinence,
    45–46
  moderation management (MM),
    46–47
  Overeaters Anonymous, 47
  Sexual Compulsives Anonymous,
    47–48
  therapeutic approaches to
    abstinence, 48
acamprosate, 188
  alcohol dependence
    meta-analyses, 199
  clinical predictors of efficacy, 193
  compliance with acamprosate
    therapy, 193
  differences from naltrexone,
    188–189
  efficacy in treating alcohol
    dependence, 189–193
  safety and tolerability, 193
  similarities to naltrexone, 188
  use in combination with naltrexone,
    199–201
  use in patients with comorbid
    psychiatric disorders, 193
  usefulness in alcohol dependence,
    201–202
acupressure, 230
acupuncture
  history, 230
  Lincoln model, 232–235
  method, 230–231
  NADA protocol, 232–235
  possible broader range of
    effectiveness, 238–239
  role in addiction treatment
    programs, 230
  safety issues, 231
  suggested physiological mechanisms,
    231–232
  what patients experience, 231
acupuncture and abuse patterns,
    239–241
  alcohol, 239
  cocaine, 239

marijuana, 133–134
methadone treatment, 240
methamphetamine, 239–240
opiates, 239
tobacco, 240
acupuncture effectiveness
  addiction patients' own stories,
    248–249
  AIDS-related treatment, 242
  criminal justice related treatment,
    243
  effect on the whole treatment
    process, 242
  effects of trauma and violence,
    244–245
  frequency and duration of
    treatment, 241–242
  maternal treatment, 242–243
  range of applications, 244–245
  retention and recidivism, 241
  serious and persistent mental illness,
    243–244
acupuncture psychosocial mechanisms
  clinical examples, 248
  foundation for autonomy, 246–247
  improving treatment program
    functions, 247–248
  internal change, 245–246
  non-verbal therapy, 247
  personal behavior, 245
acupuncture studies
  activity in placebo points, 236
  randomized placebo trials, 235
  research problems, 235–236
  Schwartz study, 236–238
  Tweed study, 238
Adderall, 28
  nonmedical use, 137
addiction treatment success, 92–94
  addressing trauma and negative life
    events, 94
  perspective on success, 94
  readiness for treatment, 92–93
  rebuilding relationships, 93–94
  reconnecting with strengths, 93
  treatment-resistant patients, 93
  treatment-resistant treatment, 93
ADHD medications
  non-medical use, 157
aerosol propellants
  abuse as inhalants, 32
AIDS-related acupuncture treatment, 242

alcohol dependence
  pharmacotherapies, 188
  acamprosate and naltrexone in
    combination, 199–201
  acamprosate compliance, 193
  acamprosate safety and tolerability,
    193
  acamprosate studies, 189–193
  clinical predictors of acamprosate
    efficacy, 193
  clinical predictors of naltrexone
    efficacy, 197–198
  differences between acamprosate
    and naltrexone, 188–189
  meta-analyses of acamprosate and
    naltrexone, 199
  naltrexone compliance, 198
  naltrexone efficacy studies, 194
  naltrexone safety and tolerability,
    194–197
  patients with comorbid psychiatric
    disorders, 193
  similarities between acamprosate
    and naltrexone, 188
  usefulness of new
    pharmacotherapies, 201–202
alcohol use
  acute complications, 24
  and creativity, 83
  delirium tremens (DTs) 25
  extent of use, 24
  fetal alcohol syndrome, 25–26
  long-term consequences, 25
  with cocaine, 139
  with stimulants, 138, 139
  withdrawal syndrome, 24–25
Alcoholics Anonymous (AA) 143
  and the Oxford Group, 45
  attributing meaning to experiences,
    99–100
  complexity of the AA phenomenon,
    100
  defining recovery on the basis of
    spirituality, 100
  experience of spiritual redemption,
    97–98
  goal of abstinence, 46
  outcome evaluations, 97
  place in American society, 98
  positive psychology, 99
  psychological perspective on the
    disease, 98–99

251

religious tradition, 98
role in a treatment plan, 119
spiritual recovery movements, 100
spiritual fellowship, 98
worldwide membership, 97
alcoholism
  addressing mortality, 119
  adoption studies, 104
  alcoholic rage, 108–109
  animal studies, 104–105
  biological factors, 103–106
  biopsychosocial nature of the
      disease, 103–109
  diagnosis, 112
  difficulties in evaluating
      prevalence, 102
  ear acupuncture, 239
  emotional–psychological factors,
      107–109
  empirical research findings, 114–115
  existential factors, 118–119
  family history studies, 105
  genetic risk factors, 103–106
  learning theory models, 112–114
  life's loss of meaning, 118–119
  personality factors, 107–109
  prevalence data, 102–103
  psychodynamic theories, 115–118
  psychological theories, 112–115
  role of culture and environment,
      106–107
  role of heredity, 103–106
  social cultural factors, 106–107
  twin studies, 104
alcoholism in primary care
  assessment of the patient, 129–130
  definitions of alcohol-related
      disorders, 126
  equivocal attitudes of doctors, 125
  intervention, 130–131
  laboratory tests, 129
  medical complications of
      alcoholism, 126
  negotiating a plan, 130
  patient history, 129
  physical examination, 129
  physicians' responses to alcoholics,
      126–127
  presenting the diagnosis, 130
  prevalence of alcoholism, 125–126
  referral strategies, 131
  screening for alcoholism, 127
  where to refer, 131
alcoholism treatment, 119–121
  case example, 120–121
  multimodal approach, 119
  planning treatment, 119–121
  role of Alcoholics
      Anonymous (AA) 119
  stages of change theory, 119–120

therapeutic model, 120
alcoholism typographies, 109–111
  Cloninger, 111
  Jellinek, 109–110
  Knight, 110–111
  Winokur, Rimmer and Reich, 111
alcohol-related birth defects, 26
alert-state training, 182
alpha training, 173–174
alpha-theta training, 182
alprazolam, 156
Ambien, 24
American Academy of Pain Medicine
    (AAPM)
  purpose and mission statement, 163
American Pain Society (APS)
  purpose and mission statement, 163
American Society of Addiction
    Medicine (ASAM)
  mission statement, 163–164
amotivational syndrome, 28
amphetamines, 28
  non-medical use, 137
  prescription drug abuse, 157–158
amyl nitrite, 32
anabolic androgenic steriods (AAS)
  and sports performance, 78–79
Angel dust. See phencyclidine
Antabuse, 142
anxiolytics
  prescription drug abuse, 155–156
arts
  preoccupation with notions of
      death, 3–4
  the price of peak experience, 3–4
ayahuasca, 81

barbiturates, 24, 72
  withdrawal syndrome, 156
Becker, Ernst 19, 3
behavioral marital therapy, 89
benzodiazepines
  and stimulants, 138
  prescription drug abuse, 156
  withdrawal syndrome, 156
  See also sedatives
biofeedback. See EEG neurofeedback
bipolar disorder
  and creative states, 4–4
blood doping in sports, 80
blues musicians
  destructive lifestyles of the greatest, 4–5
  selling your soul to the devil, 5–5
body sculpting with drugs, 76
borderline personality disorder
  co-occurrence with substance use
      disorders (SUDs), 207
borderline personality disorder
    and SUDs
  case example, 207–208

commitment to DBT-S
    treatment, 212
DBT-S attachment strategies, 212
DBT-S case management, 213–214
DBT-S skills training, 212–213
DBT-S treatment and session
    structure, 210–211
DBT-S treatment concept,
    209–210
DBT-S treatment overview, 209
empirical support for DBT-S,
    214–215
establishing DBT-S treatment goals,
    211–212
orientation to DBT-S treatment,
    211–212
overlap between, 208–209
pharmacotherapy, 214
Budzynski, Tom, 174
buprenorphine, 151–152
bupropion
  use in smoking cessation, 134
butalbital, 24
butyl nitrite, 32

caffeine
  performance enhancement, 73–74
Campral. See acamprosate
Chantix, 51–53
chlordiazepoxide, 24, 156
chronic cannabis syndrome, 28
chronic obstructive pulmonary disease
    (COPD), 26
Clapton, Eric
  price of being the greatest, 5–8
client–therapist relationship
  building the relationship, 10–11
  how the therapist feels, 10
  the client's viewpoint, 10
cocaethylene, 139
cocaine, 28, 157
  effects of fetal exposure, 141
  medical uses, 138
Cocaine Anonymous (CA), 143
cocaine dependence
  acute psychoactive effects, 138
  ear acupuncture, 239
  history of cocaine use in the
      US, 137
  hypersexual behavior, 141–142
  medical consequences, 140–141
  patterns of use, 139–140
  pharmacotherapy, 142
  phases of treatment, 143–144
  post-stimulant "crash", 138–139
  preparation of the drug, 137–138
  psychiatric complications, 140
  psychosocial treatment, 142–144
  routes of administration, 137–138
  tolerance, 139

treatment approach, 137
withdrawal, 139
codeine, 139, 155
community reinforcement, 142
Concerta, 137
contingency management, 142
contractual therapies, 88
cosmetic psychopharmacology
    amphetamine use in sport, 80
    anabolic androgenic steroids (ASS)
        in sport, 78–79
    athletic performance enhancement,
        76–80
    blood doping in sports, 80
    body sculpting with drugs, 76
    caffeine, 73–74
    creative inspiration and expression,
        82–83
    drug-assisted psychotherapy, 81
    energy drinks, 74
    ethical issues, 72–76
    ethical issues in sport, 76–77
    genetic manipulation, 80
    hallucinogenic drugs, 80–82
    history of, 72
    human desire for
        self-improvement, 72
    improving everyday function, 72–76
    methylphenidate use in sports, 80
    nicotine, 80
    non-medical use of ADHD
        medications, 74–76
    non-medical use of
        methylphenidate, 74–76
    non-medical use of modafinil,
        74–76
    prescribed medications in sport,
        77–78
    prescription stimulants, 74–76
    psychotherapeutic exploration using
        drugs, 80–82
    search for transcendent experiences,
        80–82
    sports performance enhancement,
        76–80
    stimulant use by athletes, 80
    supplements in sport, 78
    therapy versus enhancement debate,
        72–76
crack cocaine, 137, 138
CRAFT family intervention, 89
crank. See methamphetamine
creative states
    and psychiatric illness, 4
creativity
    enhancement through drugs,
        82–83
criminal justice-related acupuncture
    treatment, 243
crystal meth. See methamphetamine

Crystal Meth
    Anonymous (CMA), 143
Cylert, 137

DBT-S (dialectical behavior therapy
    adaptation), 207
    attachment strategies, 212
    biosocial theory of DBT, 208–209
    BPT and substance abuse case
        example, 207–208
    case management, 213–214
    commitment to treatment, 212
    comparison with other addiction
        treatment models, 209–210
    empirical support for use in BPD
        and SUDs, 214–215
    establishing treatment goals,
        211–212
    orientation to treatment, 211–212
    overlap between BPD and SUDs,
        208–209
    pharmacotherapy, 214
    skills training, 212–213
    training in DBT-S, 215
    treatment and session structure,
        210–211
    treatment overview, 209
death
    romantic allure of, 4–4
    spiritual release from, 3–4
deep-state training, 173, 182
delirium tremens ("DTs"), 25
designer drugs, 28, 31
dexedrine, 137
dextroamphetamine/levoamphetamine.
    See Adderall
diazepam, 24, 156
DiFranza, Joseph, 134–135
Dilaudid, 30
disulfiram, 142
Dole, Vincent, 147
Dolophine, 148
dopamine hypothesis of drug
    dependence, 133
Drug Enforcement Administration
    (DEA), 163
drug treatments for addiction, 88–90
    Antabuse, 88
    contractual therapies, 88
    experiential therapies, 89–90
    theurgic approach to therapy, 88
dry cleaning fluids
    (carbon tetrachloride)
    abuse as inhalant, 32
Duragesic, 30

ear acupuncture
    history of acupuncture, 230
    Lincoln model, 232–235
    method, 230–231

NADA protocol, 232–235
    possible broader range of
        effectiveness, 238–239
    range of applications, 244–245
    role in addiction treatment
        programs, 230
    safety issues, 231
    suggested physiological
        mechanisms, 231–232
    what patients experience, 231
ear acupuncture and abuse patterns,
    239–241
    alcohol, 239
    cocaine, 239
    marijuana, 133–134
    methadone treatment, 240
    methamphetamine, 239–240
    opiates, 239
    tobacco, 240
ear acupuncture effectiveness
    addiction patients' own stories,
        248–249
    AIDS-related treatment, 242
    criminal justice-related
        treatment, 243
    effect on the whole treatment
        process, 242
    effects of trauma and violence,
        244–245
    frequency and duration of
        treatment, 241–242
    maternal treatment, 242–243
    retention and recidivism, 241
    serious and persistent mental
        illness, 243–244
ear acupuncture psychosocial
    mechanisms
    clinical examples, 248
    foundation for autonomy, 246–247
    improving treatment program
        functions, 247–248
    internal change, 245–246
    non-verbal therapy, 247
    personal behavior, 245
ear acupuncture studies
    activity in placebo points, 236
    randomized placebo
        trials, 235
    research problems, 235–236
    Schwartz study, 236–238
    Tweed study, 238
Ecstasy (MDMA), 28
EEG neurofeedback mechanism, 170–172
    architecture of neuronal networks,
        170–171
    brain plasticity in the adult, 170
    dynamic management of
        states, 688, 172
    neuronal growth in the adult
        brain, 170

organization of network functions, 171
"small-world" model of networks, 170–171
EEG neurofeedback therapy
alert-state training, 182
alpha-theta training, 182
alpha training, 173–174
current status of the approach, 181–182
deep-state training, 173, 182
definition, 169
historical development of neurofeedback, 173–174
influencing addiction comorbidities, 170
interconnection and normalization, 182–183
minor traumatic brain injury (MTBI), 183
neuronal network functions, 169
origins of use in addiction, 169–170
psychological trauma, 182–183
research on addictions treatment, 174–181
restoration of brain regulatory function, 185
role and treatment of trauma, 173
satiety, behavior, and the brain, 172–173
self-regulation aspect, 170
supporting model of brain function, 170–172
transformative event, 183–185
emergency care of substance abusers
acute treatment, 221–225
aftercare/triage issues, 227–228
assessment of the patient, 221–225
challenges for ER staff, 228–229
general treatment recommendations, 225–226
organization of emergency services, 219–221
pressures on emergency departments, 218
psychiatric patients, 219–221
psychodynamic considerations in the ED, 228–229
range of substances of abuse, 221–225
steps of emergency treatment, 221–226
substance abuse rates in EDs, 218–219
treatment plans and protocols, 228
typical treatment examples, 226–227
energy drinks
performance enhancement, 74
erythropoietin (EPO)
blood doping in sports, 80

eszopiclone, 24
ethelchlorvynal, 156
ether
abuse as inhalant, 32
experiential therapies, 89–90

Farmer, Simon, 171
Faust motif in the arts, 3–4
Fehmi, Lester, 174
Fenichel, Otto, 116–116
Fen-Phen weight loss drug, 76
fentanyl, 30
Fentora, 30
fetal alcohol effects, 26
fetal alcohol spectrum disorder, 26
fetal alcohol syndrome, 25–26
Fiorinal, 24
flumazenil, 24
flurazepam, 156
Freeman, Walter, 172
Freud, Sigmund, 115–116

gasoline
abuse as inhalant, 32
Glover, Edward, 116
glue
abuse as inhalant, 32
glutethemide, 156
Green, Elmer, 174
Green, Peter, 8–9

hallucinogens, 31–32
acute complications, 113, 32
and creativity, 82–83
experimentation with, 80–82
flashbacks, 115, 32
long-term consequences of use, 115, 32
ranges of drugs used, 31
haloperidol, 32
Hardt, Jim, 174
Harm Reduction model of abstinence, 47
hepatitis B risk in drug abusers, 30
hepatitis C risk in drug abusers, 30
heroin and cocaine ("speedball") 139
heroin use
extent of use in the US, 30
long-term consequences, 30–31
signs of opioid intoxication, 30
withdrawal syndrome, 30
HIV risk in intravenous drug users, 30
HIV transmission
stimulant users, 137, 140
Hooked on Nicotine Checklist (HONC), 134
hydrocodone, 30, 139, 154, 155
hydromorphone, 30

hyperalgesia in opioid drug abusers, 31
hypersexual behavior
and stimulant drugs, 141–142

ibogaine
cytochrome P450 metabolism, 55–56
effects of noribogaine, 56–57
effects on opiate withdrawal symptoms, 53–54
experiences of drug-dependent patients, 52–53
historical overview, 50–51
history of use in addiction, 50–51
identification of a primary metabolite, 54
influence of genetic polymorphisms on metabolism, 55–56
mechanisms underlying beneficial effects, 56–57
noribogaine activity, 57–58
noribogaine as pharmacological therapy, 57–58
noribogaine effects, 56–57
noribogaine metabolite, 55–56
pharmacokinetics, 55–56
potential therapy for substance abuse, 50–58
prodrug, 57–58
source of, 50
traditional uses, 50
use in Bwiti religious rituals, 51–52
use in opiate detoxification, 53
use in treating drug dependence, 50
varieties of human experiences with, 51–53
inhalant abuse
acute complications, 32
extent of abuse, 32
long-term consequences, 32
range of substances used, 32
intensive outpatient programs (IOPs), 142
interpersonal psychotherapy, 143
intranasal insufflation of drugs, 30

James, William, 4, 97
Jarvik, Murray E., 133–134
Johnson, Robert, 8
pact with the devil, 5
Jones, Brian, 5
Jung, Carl, 118

Kamiya, Joe, 173
ketamine, 31
acute complications, 31
Khantzian, Edward, 116–117

Kierkegaard, Soren, 3
Kohut, Hans, 117–118
Kreek, Mary Jeanne, 147
Krystal, H., 117–117

LAAM (*levo*-alpha-acetylmethadol), 152
Lambarene, 50
Linehan, Marsha, 207
lorazepam, 156
Lortab, 30
LSD (lysergic acid
    diethylamide), 81
Lunesta, 24
lung cancer and smoking, 26

maintenance therapy, 151–152
    See also methadone, 152
Mann, Thomas, 5
marijuana use, 27–28
    acute complications, 27
    and creativity, 82
    chronic cannabis syndrome, 28
    ear acupuncture, 133–134
    effects during pregnancy, 28
    long-term consequences, 27–28
    prevalence, 27
    with stimulants, 138
    withdrawal syndrome, 27
Marlowe, Christopher, 5
Matrix Model, 142
Mayall, John, 7
MDMA, 28
MDMA-assisted psychotherapy, 81
medical sequelae of addiction
    alcohol, 24–26
    hallucinogens, 31–32
    inhalants, 32
    marijuana, 27–28
    opioids, 30–31
    sedatives, 24–26
    stimulants, 28–30
    tobacco, 26–27
    variations between classes of
        substances, 32–33
Menninger, Karl, 174
mental illness
    acupuncture treatment,
        243–244
meperidine, 30
meprobamates, 155
mescaline, 81
methadone, 30, 159
    history of development and use,
        147–148
    pharmacological properties,
        147–148
methadone treatment
    approach to opiate/opioid
        dependency, 147
    future of, 151–152

practical pharmacology of
    methadone, 147–148
use of ear acupuncture, 240
methadone treatment program
    funding, 149–150
    governance, 149
    other drugs used by patients, 151
    patient demographics, 150–151
    regulations and rules, 148
    staffing, 148–149
    what patients want, 150–151
methamphetamine, 28
    effects of fetal exposure, 141
methamphetamine dependence
    acute psychoactive effects, 138
    ear acupuncture, 239–240
    emergence of methamphetamine
        use, 137
    hypersexual behavior, 141–142
    medical consequences, 140–141
    patterns of use, 139–140
    pharmacotherapy, 142
    phases of treatment, 143–144
    post-stimulant "crash", 138–139
    preparation of the drug, 138
    psychiatric complications, 140
    psychosocial treatment, 142–144
    routes of administration, 138
    tolerance, 139
    treatment approach, 137
    withdrawal, 139
methylenedioxymethamphetamine.
    See Ecstasy; MDMA
methylphenidate, 28
    non-medical use, 137, 157
    use for performance enhancement,
        74–76
minor traumatic brain injury
    (MTBI), 183
modafinil, 137
    use for performance enhancement,
        74–76
moderation management (MM),
    46–47
modified dynamic group
    psychotherapy, 143
morphine, 155
Motivational Interviewing (MI)
    techniques, 143
Murray, Thomas, 76–77

NADA (National Acupuncture
    Detoxification Association)
    protocol, 232–235
naloxone, 151–152
naltrexone
    alcohol dependence
        meta-analyses, 199
    clinical predictors of efficacy,
        197–198

compliance with naltrexone
    therapy, 198
differences from acamprosate,
    188–189
efficacy in alcohol dependence,
    194
safety and tolerability, 194–197
similarities to acamprosate, 188
use in combination with
    acamprosate, 199–201
use in patients with comorbid
    psychiatric disorders, 198–199
usefulness in alcohol dependence,
    201–202
Narcotics Anonymous (NA), 143
nicotine
    use in sports, 80
nicotine addiction in smokers, 133
    smoking cessation research,
        133–135
    See also smoking; tobacco
nicotine patch development, 134
nicotine research
    therapeutic applications for
        smokeless nicotine, 135
nitrous oxide
    abuse as inhalant, 32
noribogaine, 50
    active metabolite of ibogaine,
        57–58
    beneficial effects of, 56–57
    pharmacological therapy for drug
        dependence, 57–58
Nyswander, Marie, 147

oceanic bliss
    and psychiatric illness, 4
    destructive pursuit of, 4
opiate abuse
    ear acupuncture, 239
opiate detoxification
    use of ibogaine, 53–54
opiate maintenance therapy, 151–152
    See also methadone, 152
opioid abuse
    acute complications, 30
    and stimulants, 138
    long-term consequences, 30–31
    prescription drug abuse, 155
    prescription opioid analgesic
        drugs, 30
    range of drugs used, 30
    signs of opioid intoxication, 30
    withdrawal syndrome, 30
opioid addiction
    prescription drugs, 159–160
Overeaters Anonymous (OA), 47
Oxford Group, 45, 98
oxycodone, 30, 139, 154, 155
OxyContin, 30, 154, 155

pain management
    professional societies, 163–164
pain management and addiction
    treatment
    case scenarios, 166
    treatment and management issues,
        166–168
pain relief medications
    prescription drug abuse, 155
PCP. *See* phencyclidine
peak experience,
    the price of, 3–4
pemoline, 137
Peniston, Eugene, 169, 174–181
Percocet, 30
performance enhancement. *See*
    cosmetic psychopharmacology
phencyclidine, 31
    acute complications of intoxication,
        13, 32
polamidon, 148
Pope, Harrison, 76
post-traumatic stress
    disorder (PTSD), 169
pregnancy and substance abuse
    ear acupuncture treatment, 242–243
prescription opioid analgesics
    acute complications of abuse, 30
    long-term consequences of abuse,
        30–31
    range of drugs of abuse, 30
    withdrawal syndrome, 30
prescription psychoactive drug abuse
    adolescents, 158
    anxiolytics, 155–156
    commonly abused classes of drugs, 154
    contributory factors, 154
    definition, 154
    elderly people, 158
    opioid addiction treatment, 159–160
    opioids, 155
    pain relief medications, 155
    prevention, 159
    rates of misuse, 154
    rates of prescribing, 154
    sedative hypnotic addiction
        treatment, 160
    sedative hypnotics, 156–157
    stimulant addiction treatment, 160
    stimulants, 157–158
    treatment of prescription drug
        addiction, 159–160
    types of people who abuse drugs,
        154–155
    vulnerable populations, 158–159
propoxyphene, 30
Provigil, 137
psilocybin, 81–82

Rado, Sandor, 116

Raskin, H., 117
Redfield Jamison, Kay, 4
reiki, 230
ReVia. *See* naltrexone
Ritalin, 28, 137
rock & roll
    destructive lifestyles of the
        greatest, 4–5
Romazicon, 24
Rose, Jed, 133–134

Sbutex, 159
sedative-hypnotics
    prescription drug abuse, 156–157
sedatives
    acute complications, 24
    delirium tremens ("DTs"), 25
    effects on the fetus, 25–26
    long-term consequences, 25
    neonatal abstinence syndrome, 26
    range of substances used, 24
    withdrawal syndrome, 24–25
Sexual Compulsives Anonymous, 47–48
shiatsu, 230
"small-world" model of networks, 170
SMART Recovery, 143
smoking
    development of the nicotine
        patch, 134
    dopamine hypothesis of drug
        dependence, 133
    history of tobacco use, 133
    morbidity and mortality rates, 133
    neurochemical determinants, 133
    nicotine addiction, 133
    smoking cessation research, 133–135
    See also nicotine; tobacco
speed. *See* methamphetamine
sport
    blood doping, 80
    ethics of performance
        enhancement, 76–77
    use of anabolic androgenic steroids
        (AAS), 78–79
    use of prescribed medications, 77–78
    use of stimulants, 308, 80
    use of supplements, 78
stages of change theory, 119–120
Sterman, M. Barry, 174
stimulant use, 28–30
    acute complications, 102, 29
    for performance enhancement,
        74–76
    hypersexual behavior, 141–142
    long-term consequences, 105, 30
    prescription drug abuse, 137,
        157–158
    range of drugs used, 28–28
    treatment of addiction, 160
    withdrawal syndrome, 29

Suboxone, 151–152, 159
suicide, 37–42
    assessment of risk, 40–42
    conditioned behavior model of
        addictive behavior, 39–40
    disorders co-occurring with
        substance abuse, 38–39
    epidemiology, 37–38
    high-risk population, 39
    mood disorders and substance
        abuse, 38–39
    phenomenology of addictive
        behavior, 39–40
    prevention initiatives, 40–42
    raising awareness of risk factors,
        40–42
    rates among different groups, 37–38
    risk factors, 39
    role of substance abuse, 38
    substance abuse prevention and
        treatment programs, 40–42

Tabernanthe iboga, 51–52
tai ji chuan, 230
tattooing, 30
Taylor, Michael (Mick), 9–10
tetrahydrocannabinol (THC), 27
therapeutic communities
    approach, 61
    method and model, 63
    mutual self-help, 63–64
    peer confrontation and
        affirmation, 63–64
    peers as role models, 64
    social structure, 63
    staff members as rational
        authorities, 64
    work as education and therapy, 63
therapeutic communities model
    challenges and developments, 69
    evolution, 68–69
    modifications and applications, 68–69
    staff issues, 69
therapeutic communities
    perspective, 61–63
    motivation for recovery, 62
    recovery as developmental learning, 62
    self-help and mutual self-help, 62
    social learning, 62
    view of recovery, 62
    view of right living, 62
    view of the disorder, 61
    view of the person, 61–62
therapeutic communities research
    effectiveness, 67
    enhancing retention in TCs, 68
    predictors of dropout, 67–68
    retention, 67
    retention rates, 67–68
    treatment process research, 68

therapeutic communities, 61
therapeutic communities treatment
    process
    aftercare, 67
    community and clinical
        management elements, 65
    community enhancement activities, 65
    disciplinary sanctions, 65–66
    elements of the treatment process, 64
    privileges, 65
    program stages and phases, 66–67
    surveillance (house runs), 66
    therapeutic-educative activities,
        64–65
    urine testing, 66
theurgic approach to therapy, 88
thiazolam, 156
tobacco, 26–27
    acute complications of smoking, 26
    ear acupuncture to help stop
        smoking, 240

effects of secondhand smoke,
    26–27
effects of smoking during
    pregnancy, 27
extent of use, 26–26
long-term consequences of
    smoking, 26
types of tobacco products, 26
withdrawal syndrome, 26
See also nicotine; smoking
tramadol, 30
trauma
    acupuncture treatment, 244–245
treatment success in addiction,
    92–94
    addressing trauma and negative life
        events, 94
    perspective on success, 94
    readiness for treatment, 92–94
    reconnecting with strengths, 93
    treatment-resistant patients, 93

treatment-resistant treatment,
    92–93
rebuilding relationships, 93–94
Twelve Step Approach. See Alcoholics
    Anonymous (AA)

Vaillant, George, 108–108
Valium, 24
varenicline, 51–53
Vicodin, 30, 154
violence
    acupuncture treatment, 244–245
Vivitrol See naltrexone

Wilson, Bill, 116, 97–98

Xanax, 24

zapelon, 156
zolpidem, 24, 156
Zyban, 134